SO-EJV-194

# INORGANIC AND NUTRITIONAL ASPECTS OF CANCER

# ADVANCES IN EXPERIMENTAL MEDICINE AND BIOLOGY

Editorial Board:

Nathan Back          *State University of New York at Buffalo*

N. R. Di Luzio       *Tulane University School of Medicine*

Bernard Halpern      *Collège de France and Institute of Immuno-Biology*

Ephraim Katchalski   *The Weizmann Institute of Science*

David Kritchevsky    *Wistar Institute*

Abel Lajtha          *New York State Research Institute for Neurochemistry and Drug Addiction*

Rodolfo Paoletti     *University of Milan*

## Recent Volumes in this Series

*Conference on*

# INORGANIC AND NUTRITIONAL ASPECTS OF CANCER

Proceedings of the First Conference of the International Association of
Bioinorganic Scientists, Inc. held in La Jolla, California, January 3–5, 1977

Edited by

## G. N. Schrauzer

University of California at San Diego
La Jolla, California

RC 262
C 545
1978

PLENUM PRESS • NEW YORK AND LONDON

335184

Library of Congress Cataloging in Publication Data

Conference on Inorganic and Nutritional Aspects of Cancer, La Jolla, Calif., 1977.
   Inorganic and nutritional aspects of cancer.

   (Advances in experimental medicine and biology; 91)
   Includes indexes.
   1. Cancer—Nutritional aspects—Congresses. 2. Trace elements—Physiological effect—
Congresses. 3. Carcinogenesis—Congresses. 4. Cancer—Chemotherapy—Congresses.
I. Schrauzer, G. N., 1932-       II. International Association of Bioinorganic Scien-
tists. III. Title. IV. Series. [DNLM: 1. Neoplasms—Congresses. 2. Minerals—Con-
gresses. 3. Metals—Congresses. 4. Drug therapy—Congresses. 5. Nutrition—Con-
gresses. 6. Trace elements—Congresses. W1 AD559 v. 91 1977/QZ200 C746i 1977]
RC262.C545  1977                       616.9'94                       77-13974
ISBN 0-306-32691-4

The Conference on Inorganic and Nutritional Aspects of Cancer was sponsored by
Grant 1 R13 CA21031-01A1 of the National Cancer Institute, Department of Health,
Education and Welfare and the International Association of Bioinorganic Scientists, Inc.

© 1978 Plenum Press, New York
A Division of Plenum Publishing Corporation
227 West 17th Street, New York, N.Y. 10011

All rights reserved

No part of this book may be reproduced, stored in a retrieval system, or transmitted,
in any form or by any means, electronic, mechanical, photocopying, microfilming,
recording, or otherwise, without written permission from the Publisher

Printed in the United States of America

*INVITED SPEAKERS AND DISCUSSION LEADERS*

Brada, Zbynek
Papanicolaou Institute for
  Cancer Research
Miami, Florida 33136

Eskin, Bernard A.
The Medical College of
  Pennsylvania
Philadelphia, Pennsylvania 19129

*Flessel, Peter
Department of Biology
University of San Francisco
San Francisco, California 94117

French, Frederic A.
Department of Medicine
Mount Zion Hospital and Medical
  Center
San Francisco, California 94115

Frost, Douglas V.
17 Rosa Street
Schenectady, New York 12308

*Furst, Arthur
Institute of Chemical Biology
University of San Francisco
San Francisco, California 94117

*Groth, David
National Institute of Occupa-
  tional Safety and Health
Cincinnati, Ohio 45226

Houten, Lorne
Roswell Park Memorial Institute
Buffalo, New York 14221

Jacobs, Maryce
University of Texas System Cancer
  Center
M. D. Anderson Hospital and Tumor
  Institute
Texas Medical Center
Houston, Texas 77030

Jansson, Birger
University of Texas System Cancer
  Center
M. D. Anderson Hospital and Tumor
  Institute
Texas Medical Center
Houston, Texas 77030

Jasmin, Gaëtan
Université de Montréal
Faculté de Médicine
Montréal 101, Canada

Kirschner, Stanley
Department of Chemistry
Wayne State University
Detroit, Michigan 48202

Langer, Arthur M.
Mount Sinai School of Medicine
The City University of New York
New York, New York 10029

*Discussion Leaders

*Levinson, Warren
Department of Microbiology
University of California
San Francisco School of
  Medicine
San Francisco, California 94143

*Loeb, Lawrence
Institute for Cancer Research
Fox Chase Center for Cancer
  and Medical Sciences
Philadelphia, Pennsylvania 19111

*Petering, David H.
Department of Chemistry
The University of Wisconsin
  at Milwaukee
Milwaukee, Wisconsin 53201

Petering, Harold G.
University of Cincinnati
  and
Department of Environmental
  Health
Kettering Laboratory
Cincinnati, Ohio 45219

Pories, Walter
Case Western Reserve University
  School of Medicine
Cleveland, Ohio 44109

Reeves, Andrew L.
Wayne State University
Detroit, Michigan 48226

Rosenberg, Barnett
Department of Biophysics
Michigan State University
East Lansing, Michigan 48824

*Schrauzer, Gerhard N.
Department of Chemistry
University of California, San Diego
Revelle College
La Jolla, California 92093

*Schwarz, Klaus
UCLA and Veterans Administration
  Hospital
Long Beach, California 90801

*Shimkin, Michael B.
Department of Community Medicine
University of California, San Diego
Medical School
La Jolla, California 92093

Stoner, Gary D.
Department of Health, Education,
  and Welfare
National Cancer Institute
Bethesda, Maryland 20014

*Sunderman, F. William, Jr.
Department of Laboratory Science
University of Connecticut School
  of Medicine
Farmington, Connecticut 06032

Vitale, Joseph J.
Department of Pathology
Boston University School of
  Medicine
Boston, Massachusetts 02118

*PREFACE*

For many decades, cancer research concentrated heavily on "organic" aspects of the disease and ignored the role of trace elements and minerals in carcinogenesis and tumor growth. However, in recent years, spectacular progress has been made in "inorganic" cancer research: numerous inorganic substances were shown to possess carcinogenic properties. Quite unexpectedly, certain coordination compounds of platinum were found to have powerful antineoplastic properties, and a number of essential trace elements were demonstrated to have profound effects on the genesis and growth of spontaneous, induced, or transplanted tumors. It therefore appeared desirable to call upon leading authorities in the field of inorganic cancer research to present their views in a conference dedicated specifically to their discipline. But since trace elements are normal constituents of foods, it seemed advantageous to include nutritional aspects into the program. The fact that diet and nutrition influence tumor growth and development has been known or suspected for a long time. However, too little research has been done in this important field, resulting in a serious retardation of knowledge. Hence, this opportunity to cover nutritional aspects of cancer was taken, even though it was clear from the beginning that this broad field could not really be treated in the available time. It was necessary, for example, to exclude entirely the vast area of nutrition as an adjuvant in cancer therapy, and even then, further limitation of the scope of topics to be covered had to be made. The importance of the emerging *Conference on Inorganic and Nutritional Aspects of Cancer* was recognized by the National Cancer Institute, DHEW, who provided generous financial support. The conference was further supported by the *International Association of Bioinorganic Scientists* (I.A.B.S.), an independent interdisciplinary scientific organization founded in 1975.

I would like to acknowledge the invaluable assistance of my friends, colleagues, and fellow I.A.B.S. members, Drs. Michael B. Shimkin (Department of Community Medicine, School of Medicine) and Elvin Harper (Department of Chemistry), both at UCSD, in the plan-

ning and execution of the conference.  In addition, I received
numerous suggestions from Drs. Arthur Furst (San Francisco),
F. William Sunderman, Jr. (Farmington, Conn.), Harold G. and David
H. Petering (Cincinnati and Milwaukee), as well as from Dr. Klaus
Schwarz (Long Beach), which contributed to the success of the
conference.

*G. N. Schrauzer*

*Department of Chemistry*
*University of California*
   *at San Diego*
*La Jolla, California*

# CONTENTS

## PART I

### CARCINOGENESIS BY INORGANIC COMPOUNDS AND MINERALS

PART IV

TRACE ELEMENTS AND NUTRITION IN CANCER PREVENTION

# Part I

## Carcinogenesis by
## Inorganic Compounds and Minerals

## CHAPTER 1

# AN OVERVIEW OF METAL CARCINOGENESIS

Arthur Furst

Institute of Chemical Biology
University of San Francisco
San Francisco, California
and
Department of Pharmacology
Stanford University School of Medicine
Stanford, California
(By Courtesy)

Metal or inorganic carcinogenesis has come of age. Originally considered an obscure phase of the cancer problem, it was neglected for many years. Reviews on the topic carcinogenesis either failed to mention metals as causative agents or simply included a few ions as examples of an unusual class. Another area of neglect has been the association of occupational exposure to dusts, fumes, and even vapors of inorganic chemicals with an increase in various types of cancer among certain industrial workers. This phenomenon was first noted in the 1880s but did not result in laboratory investigations. Virchow, one of the early pioneering pathologists, suggested that this cancer rise could be linked to a "chronic irritation theory", but this explanation stirred no imaginative research.

In an early study of an inorganic compound, BAGG(1) injected zinc chloride into the testes of roosters and reported the formation of teratomas. SCHINZ and UELINGER(2), also among the first to study metal carcinogenesis, implanted the metals intramuscularly and found sarcomas at the injection site. However, the systematic study of metals and their compounds as primary carcinogens in animals was carried out by HUEPER and his associates. HUEPER summarized much of his work in the book co-authored by CONWAY(3). He also wrote a number of compendia and gave impetus to much of what we know today about the relationship of exposure to inorganic agents and occupational cancer.(4)

For those new to this more obscure field of carcinogenesis, overviews of metal carcinogenesis are now available. Several have been published in the past few years; among them are reviews by FURST(5,6,7), FURST and HARO(8), SUNDERMAN(9), and ROE and LANCASTER(10), as well as two sections in the World Health Organization/ARC monographs, Vol. 2(11) and Vol. 11(12). An excellent review on the subject has also been published in Japanese by KANISAWA(13), but unfortunately, a translation is not available. Also recently published is a detailed overview of environmental exposure to carcinogenic and potentially carcinogenic metals. The origin of these metals, both natural and manmade, is listed, as are the exposure levels.(14) Three more reviews on metal carcinogenesis are in press; one of these is by LUCKEY (noted in a letter in Chemical Engineering News, May 12, 1976), one by SUNDERMAN, and one by FURST. The latter two independent reviews will appear in separate volumes of Advances in Modern Toxicology.

Parenthetically, any conference on carcinogenesis must come to grips with the following problem: How do we relate to and define terms? For example, are tumorigenic and carcinogenic synonymous? A recent editorial(15), suggesting terms to be used, failed to include tumorigenic as acceptable. There must also be strict criteria for malignancy. In the review mentioned above, FURST and HARO(8) included the criteria they believed must be met before a metal could be called carcinogenic. These criteria are:

> Tumors must appear at a site distant from the point of application; more than one route must be effective; more than one species must respond; the growth should be transplantable; and, if malignant, invasion and/or metastasis must be noted. Most important, all histological slides must be evaluated by a pathologist knowledgeable in animal tumors.

Few if any researchers have ever agreed with, or even paid attention to these criteria. The significant question is still: Can a tumor be called malignant without the attendant phenomenon of invasion and/or metastasis? This to me is the crux of a definition of malignancy and must be applied to all chemicals considered carcinogenic.

All evaluations of metals, or their insoluble compounds or complexes, as potential carcinogens by any injection route, especially intramuscular or subcutaneous, must include consideration of the phenomenon of nonspecific, solid-state, or foreign-body carcinogenesis. Often, the physical state or the viscosity of a particular solution of the injected substance may be a factor in determining whether that substance will play a role in the development of

any growth.(16)   Preneoplastic changes resulting from a variety of
sheets and foils have been studied.(17)   Recent attention has been
focused on the so-called Oppenheimer effect; i.e., a local sarcoma
can easily appear at the site of subcutaneous implantation of almost any solid metal disc or foil(18), or for that matter, of a
variety of films.(19)   It is simply impossible to conclude that any
solid, implanted subcutaneously or intramuscularly, is ipso facto
a carcinogen.

Asbestos will be discussed.(20,21)   Where does asbestos fit
into the framework of metal carcinogenesis?  Is it mainly a repository for the carcinogenic nickel or chromium compounds?(22,23,24,25)
Is the carcinogenic property of asbestos a function of the nature
of the fiber only?  Or is the carcinogenic property of asbestos
possibly a matter of the ratio of diameter-to-length of special
fibers?(26)

Perhaps this conference will stimulate granting agencies to
fund more research in this area.  Answers need to be found for a
host of questions:

- What is the relationship of the carcinogenic activity
  of any pure metal to its compounds; both inorganic
  and organic (Table 1)?

TABLE 1

ELEMENTS POSITIVE IN MANY ANIMAL EXPERIMENTS

| ELEMENT | COMPOUNDS |
|---------|-----------|
| Ni | $Ni_2S_3$  $Ni(CO)_4$  $NiO$ |
|  | $NiAc_2$  $NiCO_3$  $Ni_3(PO_4)_2$ |
|  | $Ni(C_5H_5)_2$ |
| Cd | $CdSO_4$  $CdO$  $CdS$  $CdCl_2$ |

- How many pure metallic elements are active while
  their compounds are not (Table 2)?

TABLE 2

| ELEMENT ONLY | NO COMPOUNDS |
|--------------|--------------|
| Co | |

• Does the situation hold true in reverse (Table 3)?

TABLE 3

COMPOUNDS TESTED IN ANIMALS AND FOUND POSITIVE
ELEMENTS NEGATIVE (OR NOT TESTED)

| | |
|---|---|
| Pb | $PbCrO_4$   $PbAc_2$ and Basic $Ac_2$ |
| Cr | $CrO_4^=$ |
| Fe | Dextran   Dextrin |
| Be | $BeSO_4$   BeO |
| Pd | Pd   ? |
| Ti | Titanocene   ?? |
| Zn | $ZnSO_4$   ??   $ZnCl_2$ |
| Mn | $MnCl_2$   ?? |

?? = Doubtful experiments

Nickel will be discussed in detail.  Powdered nickel seems to be active, as are many nickel compounds of diverse structure[27] including the gaseous nickel carbonyl.[28]  A number of strains of rats may respond, although with differing degrees of susceptibility.[29]  Powdered nickel is active when injected by different routes;[30] the subsulfide can induce renal tumors[31] (Table 1). This will also be covered in the Conference.

Cadmium, not to be reviewed at this conference, also may be an example of the carcinogenicity of both the element and its compounds (see Table 1).[12,32,33]  For a time, cadmium seemed carcinogenic only for rodents; however, human exposure has recently also been associated with carcinogenic risk.[34]

The element lead may be an example of inverse possibility.  In its acetate form, lead has been reported to induce renal tumors;[35,36] as the free element, lead does not appear to be active.[37]

Lead chromate did induce fibrosarcomas at the site of injection,(37) but there is some question as to whether this action was due to the lead.  Chromates were among the first inorganic compounds implicated as carcinogens; they also may be examples of compounds that are active, although the free element (chromium) is not (Table 3).  Chromate compounds are the agents responsible for perforation of the nasal septum (38) and have been associated with cancers in humans since the 1930s.  Over a period of years, there have been reports that implicate chromates as the causative agents for human tumors.(39,40,41)  A question to be considered at this conference is whether Cr(VI) is the only chromium compound active as a carcinogen in experimental animals.(42)

Why, at this late date, has the arsenic question not been laid to rest?  Are the extensive epidemiological studies, especially those of LEE and FRAUMINI(43) and OTT(44) adequate?  Will the absence of activity of arsenic in animals be convincing?(11,45)  Is man uniquely sensitive to this agent?  Perhaps these questions will be answered at this conference.

Is zinc a real carcinogen?  The answer seems to depend upon which publication is read.  Interestingly enough, zinc figured in the first references on metal carcinogenesis, when BAGG(1) injected zinc chloride into the testes of roosters and reported teratomas. Zinc itself does not appear to be carcinogenic;(46) its compounds have been reported to be inhibitors to tumor growth.(47,48)  This conference should provide more information on this subject.

Where does cobalt fit in?(49)  Should manganese be studied in detail?  Both these elements are assuming greater industrial importance.

Also among the elements about which more information should be acquired is selenium.  Is it an inducer of hepatomas,(50,51) or is it not?(52)  Is it antitumorigenic (Table 4 )?(53,54)  How valid are the experiments that purport to demonstrate the carcinogenicity of selenium?  How important is the manipulation of protein in the diet in feeding experiments?  These pressing questions should be considered here.


TABLE   4

MORE ANIMAL WORK NEEDED:

| | |
|---|---|
| Group A | As  Se  Zr  V  Mo  Mn  Zn |
| Group B | Rare Earths |

Not enough importance is placed on those metals tested and found to be noncarcinogenic, at least by specific experimental design (Table 5). Are there better methods for testing the carcinogenicity of metals than intramuscular injection or inhalation? What are some novel procedures?(55) Are we paying enough attention to the health of our animals?(56) Does species or strain in some way determine the extent of susceptibility to carcinogenic action?

To repeat, if we do not know enough about metals as carcinogens (free element versus inorganic compound versus salt versus organometallic compound versus chelate, or oxidation state A versus oxidation state B) do we have any hint as to how a cell recognizes a metal carcinogen as opposed to the noncarcinogenic element? Body tissues can dissolve many metals,(57) and the ions are readily excreted.(58) Is there a difference in action between carcinogenic and noncarcinogenic metals? What is the role of trace elements in cancer?(59) It appears that simple analysis of trace metals in tumors gives us no basic information;(60) but what information is needed?

TABLE 5

METALS TESTED IN ANIMALS AND FOUND NEGATIVE
IN ONE OR MORE LABORATORIES

Al  Cu  Ag  Au  Sn  Ge  W

How do we approach a theory of mechanism? Do metals fit a scheme that has been developed for organic dyes or polynuclear hydrocarbons or nitroso compounds? Metals do not seem to follow a two-stage hypothesis. To what extent, then, will Berenblum's(61) ideas fit this class? Mechanisms proposed for the action of hydrocarbons and amines, which might explain metabolic activation to "true" carcinogens, are not applicable to metals.(62,63) If metal ions are just other examples of electrophiles,(64) then how does one account for the activity of Cr(VI) and not Cr(III); or must we question the data derived from the experiments?

The study of metal coordination and enzyme activity(65) has been disappointing as it relates to metal carcinogenesis, even though we now have a plethora of information on the function and role of transition metal ions in metalloenzymes(66) and in enzyme activation.(67,68)

Carcinogenic metals, nickel in particular, can inhibit a number of enzymes, especially P-450 cytochromes(69) and polymerases of nucleic acids.(70,71) Are these general properties of carcinogenic ions? Will there be differences between a carcinogenic and a noncarcinogenic element, relative to these inhibitory properties?

Based on the information now available on nucleic acid-metal interactions,(72,73,74) an understanding of metal carcinogenesis seems probable. In addition, model systems using synthetic polynucleotides are shedding light on this subject.(75) There should be more information about the effect of metal ions on nucleic acids at this conference.(76) It is indeed logical that the ultimate mechanism of metal carcinogenesis action will involve the binding of a particular carcinogenic metal ion with a base from a nucleic acid, presumably DNA.(77) This combination should result in a chelate which may not readily dissociate. In order for replication to continue, one hypothesis that can be used is that the deletion of a base or a sequence of bases(78) will result in a "new" nucleic acid which gives a cell "new" information. The "new" cell may not obey normal regulatory mechanisms; this would then result in an unchecked proliferation of cells.

Any theory that involves metal ions with bases of nucleic acids must explain how carcinogenic ions can bypass the fence of magnesium ions which, acting as an outer shield, can protect the backbone of the nucleic acids. Why does a noncarcinogenic ion fail to get past the magnesium ions? If these former ions do get past, will they not also chelate with the bases, especially adenine?

Omitted in this overview are the effect of one metal on another such as the somewhat inhibitory action of manganese on nickel carcinogenesis,(79) and the carcinogenic effects of beryllium.(80)

In the long run, many more basic facts must still be obtained to determine which elements and compounds are of risk to man. Ultimately, until much more is known about the causes of cancer, our efforts must be focused on prevention.(81)

Gathered here today is a virtual "Who's Who" in Metal Carcinogenesis. With few exceptions from overseas, every important scientist who has participated in this phase of cancer research is here. I only regret that Dr. Hueper is not present. The International Association of Bioinorganic Scientists must be congratulated for organizing this conference. In these few days, not only the art of the science, but the science itself will be advanced. We shall learn about a number of aspects of metal carcinogenesis; hopefully, what is real, and above all, what is not.

*ACKNOWLEDGEMENT*

I would like to thank the co-trustees of the Carrie *Baum *Browning fund for their aid to my research endeavors.

*REFERENCES*

1.   Bagg, H. J., Am. J. Cancer 26, Page 69, 1936.

2.   Schinz, H. R. U., and Uehlinger, E., Krebsforsch, A., 52, Page 425, 1942.

3.   Hueper, W. C., and Conway, W. D., Chemical Carcinogenesis and Cancers, C. C Thomas, Springfield, Illinois, 1964.

4.   Hueper, W. C., "Recent Results Cancer Research," 3, Page 85, 1966.

5.   Furst, A., Metal-Binding in Medicine, M. J. Seven and L. A. Johnson, Editors, J. P. Lippincott Co., Philadelphia, pp 336-343, 1960.

6.   Furst, A., The Chemistry of Chelation in Cancer, C. C Thomas, Springfield, Illinois, 1963.

7.   Furst, A., "Environmental Geochemistry in Health and Disease," Memoir 123, Geological Society of America, Boulder, Colorado, pp 109-130, 1971.

8.   Furst, A., and Haro, R. T., Prog. Exp. Tumor Res. 12, Page 102, 1969.

9.   Sunderman, F. W., Jr., Fd. and Cosmet. Toxicology, 9, Page 105, 1971.

10.  Roe, F. J. C., and Lancaster, M. C., British Medical Bulletin, 20, Page 127, 1964.

11.  International Agency for Research on Cancer, Monogr. 2, 1973.

12.  International Agency for Research on Cancer, Monogr. 11, 1976.

13.  Kanisawa, M., Annual Report Institute Food and Microbiology, Chiba University, 24, Page 1, 1971.

14.  Fishbein, L., J. Toxicology Environmental Health, 2, Page 77, 1976.

15. Hecker, E., Int. J. Cancer 18, Page 22, 1976.

16. Brand, K. G., Scientific Foundations of Oncology, T. Symington and R. L. Carter, Editors, Wm. Heinemann Medical Boods, Ltd, London, pp 490-495.

17. Brand, K. G., Buoen, L. C., and Brand, I., J. National Cancer Institute 55, Page 319, 1975.

18. Oppenheimer, B. S., Oppenheimer, E. T., Danishefsky, I. I., and Stout, A. P., Cancer Res. 16, Page 439, 1956.

19. Danishefsky, I., Oppenheimer, E. T., Heritier-Watkins, O., Bella, A., Jr., and Willhite, M., Cancer Research 27, Page 833, 1967.

20. Reeves, A. L., Puro, H. E., Smith, R. G., and Vorwald, A. J., Environmental Research 4, Page 496, 1971.

21. Selikoff, I. J., and Churg, J., Editors, Annals N. Y. Academy Science 132(1), Page 1, 1965.

22. Harrington, J. S., Biological Effects of Asbestos, P. Bogovski, V. Trimbrels, J. L. Gilson and J. C. Wagner, Editors, Lyon, IARC WHO, pp 304-311, 1973.

23. Roy-Chowdhury, A. K., Muoney, J. I., and Reeves, A. L., Arch. Environ. Health 26, Page 253, 1972.

24. Dixon, J. R., Lowe, D. B., Richards, D. E., Cralley, L. J., and Stokinger, H. E., Cancer Res. 30, Page 1068, 1970.

25. Cralley, L. J., J. Am. Med. Hyg. Assoc. 32, Page 653, 1971.

26. Stanton, M. F., and Wrench, C., J. National Cancer Institute 48, Page 787, 1972.

27. Sunderman, F. W., Jr., Annals Clin. Lab. Sci. 3, Page 156, 1973.

28. Lau, T. J., Hackett, R. L., and Sunderman, W. F., Jr., Cancer Res. 32, Page 2253, 1972.

29. Sunderman, F. W., Jr., and Maenza, R. M., Res. Communs. Chem. Pathol. Pharmacol. 14, Page 319, 1976.

30. Furst, A., and Cassetta, D., Proceedings American Assoc. Cancer Research, 14, Page 31, 1973.

31. Jasmin, G., and Riopelle, J. L., Lab. Invest., in press.

31.  Jasmin, G., and Riopelle, J. L., Lab. Invest., in press.

32.  Nordberg, G. F., Ambio., 3, Page 55, 1974.

33.  Kazantzis, G., Nature 198, Page 1213, 1963.

34.  Kolonel, L. N., Cancer 37, Page 1782, 1976.

35.  Boyland, E., Dukes, C. E., Grover, P. L. and Mitchley, B. C.,
     British J. Cancer, 16, Page 283, 1962.

36.  Coogan, P., Stein, L., Hsu, G., and Hass, G., Lab. Invest., 26,
     Page 273, 1972.

37.  Furst, A., Schlauder, M. and Sasmore, D. P., Cancer Research,
     36, Page 1779, 1976.

38.  Pye, W., Ann. Surg. 1, Page 303, 1885.

39.  Baetjer, A. M., Arch. Ind. Hyg. Occup. Med., 2, Page 487, 1950.

40.  Bidstrup, D. L. and Case, R. A. M., British J. Ind. Med., 13,
     Page 260, 1956.

41.  Langard, S. and Norseth, T., British Ind. Med., 32, Page 62,
     1975.

42.  Roe, F. J. C., and Carter, R. L., British J. Cancer, 23, Page
     172, 1969.

43.  Lee, A. M., and Fraumeni, J. E., Jr., J. National Cancer Inst.,
     42, Page 1045, 1969.

44.  Ott, M. G., Holder, B. B. and Gordon, H. L., Arch. Environ.
     Health, 29, Page 250, 1974.

45.  Neubauer, O., British J. Cancer, 1, Page 192, 1947.

46.  Heath, J. C., Daniel, M. R., Dingle, J. T. and Webb, M.,
     Nature, 193, Page 592, 1962.

47.  Poswillo, D. E. and Cohen, B., Nature, 231, Page 447, 1971.

48.  De Wys, W. D. and Poires, W., J. National Cancer Inst., 48,
     Page 375, 1972.

49.  Gilman, J. P. W., Cancer Res. 22, Page 158, 1962.

50.  Nelson, A. A., Fitzhugh, O. G. and Calvan, O., Cancer Res., 3,
     Page 230, 1943.

51.  Tscherkes, L. A., Volgarev, M. N. and Aptekar, S. G., Acta
     Unio Intern. Contra Cancrum, 19, Page 632, 1963.

52.  Harr, J. R., Bone, J. F., Tinsely, J. J., Weisig, P. H. and
     Yamamoto, R. S.:  1966 Symposium, Selenium in Biomedicine,
     AVI Publishing Company, Westport, Connecticut, pp. 163-178,
     1973.

53.  Shamberger, R. J., J. National Cancer Institute, 44, Page 931,
     1970.

54.  Shamberger, R. J., Tytko, S. A. and Willis, C. E., Arch.
     Environ. Health, 31, Page 231, 1976.

55.  Stoner, G. D., Shimkin, M. B., Troxell, M. C., Thompson, T. L.,
     and Terry, L. S., Cancer Research, 36, Page 1744, 1976.

56.  Keller, R., Ogilvie, B. M. and Simpson, E., Lancet 1, Page 678,
     1971.

57.  Weinzierl, S. M. and Webb, M., British J. Cancer, 26, Page 279,
     1972.

58.  Chen, J. K. M., Haro, R. and Furst, A., Wasmann J. Biol., 29,
     Page 1, 1971.

59.  Schwartz, M. K., Cancer Research, 35, Page 3481, 1975.

60.  Addink, N. W. H. and Frank, L. J. P., Cancer, 12, Page 544, 1959.

61.  Berenblum, I., Frontiers of Biology, Vol. 34, A. Neuberger and
     E. L. Tatum, Editors, American Elsevier Publishers, New York,
     1974.

62.  Frei, J. V., Chem. Biol. Interact., 13, Page 1, 1976.

63.  Weinstein, I. B., Adv. Patholbiol. 4, Page 106, 1976.

64.  Miller, J. A. and Miller, E. C., J. National Cancer Institute,
     47(3), V, 1971.

65.  Vallee, B. L. and Colman, J. E., Comprehensive Biochemistry,
     Vol. 12, M. Florkin, Editor, American Elsevier Publishers,
     pp. 165-235, 1964.

66.  Riordan, J. F. and Vallee, B. L., Adv. Exp. Med. Biol., 48,
     Page 33, 1974.

67.  Lehninger, A. L., Physiol. Rev., 30, Page 393, 1950.

68.  Malmstrom, B. G. and Rosenberg, A., Adv. Enzymol., 21, Page
     131, 1959.

69.  Sunderman, F. W., Jr., Cancer Research, 28, Page 465, 1968.

70.  Beach, D. J. and Sunderman, F. W., Jr., Cancer Res., 30,
     Page 48, 1970.

71.  Sunderman, F. W., Jr. and Esfahani, M., Cancer Research, 28,
     Page 2565, 1968.

72.  Fuwa, K., Wacker, W. E. C., Druyan, R., Bartholomay, A. F.
     and Vallee, B. L., Proceedings National Academy Science,
     U. S. A., 46, Page 1298, 1960.

73.  Butzow, J. J. and Eichhorn, G. L., Biopolymers, 3, Page 95,
     1965.

74.  Eichhorn, G. L., Clark, P. and Tarien, E., J. Biol. Chem.,
     244, Page 937, 1969.

75.  Murray, M. J. and Flessel, C. P., Biochem. Biophys. Acta, 425,
     Page 256, 1976.

76.  Groth, D. H., Stettler, L. and Mackay, G., Effects and Dose
     Response Relationships of Toxic Metals, G. F. Nordberg, Ed.,
     Elsevier Sci. Publishing Co., Amsterdam, pp. 527-543, 1976.

77.  Furst, A. and Haro, R. T., Proceedings of the International
     Symposium, Israel Academy of Sciences and Humanities,
     "Fundamental Mechanisms of Carcinogenesis," E. D. Bergmann
     and P. Pullman, Editors, pp. 310-320, 1970.

78.  Sirover, M. A. and Loeb, L. A., Proceedings National Academy
     Science, U. S. A., 73, Page 2331, 1976.

79.  Sunderman, F. W., Jr., Kasprzak, K. S., Lau, T. J., Minghetti,
     P. P., Maenza, R. M., Becker, N., Onkelinx, C. and Goldblatt,
     P. J., Cancer Research, 36(5), Page 1790, 1976.

80.  Stokinger, H. E., Beryllium: Its Industrial Hygiene Aspects,
     Academic Press, New York, 1966.

81.  Gori, G. B. and Peters, J. A., Preventive Medicine, 4, Page
     239, 1975.

*CHAPTER 2*

BERYLLIUM CARCINOGENESIS

Andrew L. Reeves

School of Medicine
Wayne State University
Detroit, Michigan

## I.  INTRODUCTION

With an atomic number of 4, beryllium is the lightest of all solid and chemically stable substances.  Its present industrial uses are numerous, including fatigue-resistant alloys, heat-resistant ceramics, electronic and nuclear reactor parts, rocketry and classified weaponry.  All of these applications originated during the last 25 to 50 years, and the ubiquitousness of beryllium in our civilization is a relatively recent phenomenon.

Urban air contained 0.3-3.0 ng $Be/m^3$ as early as 1951,[1] and there is reason to believe that general atmospheric concentrations have increased since then.  In 1974, food crops and tobacco in West Germany were found to contain 0.08-0.8 $\alpha$ Be/g dry substance[2] and the average daily intake of the population by all routes in industrialized countries can be estimated at about 20 $\alpha$ Be/day at present.

## II.  BONE SARCOMA IN RABBITS AND MICE

Beryllium was the first inorganic substance to be found carcinogenic by experiment, and the discovery was then a great surprise.  The experiments were performed because of health problems of workers in the beryllium industry.  These included dermatitis, pneumonitis and pulmonary granulomatosis, but no known incidence of neoplasia; yet when GARDNER and HESLINGTON, in 1946[3] administered intravenous zinc beryllium silicate to rabbits, the results were osteosarcoma of the long bones, and a similar lesion was also obtained with beryllium oxide but not with zinc oxide, zinc silicate, or silicic acid.

Beryllium bone sarcoma of the rabbit was reproduced by numerous workers by way of intravenous injection (4-10) and in one experiment by inhalation.(11)   In the latter study, one of six rabbits exposed to BeO developed sarcoma of the pubic bone with extension into the contiguous musculature and with pulmonary metastasis.   There is also one report of malignant bone tumors in mice who received intravenous injections of zinc beryllium silicate.(12)   Some details of these experiments are collated in Table 1.

## III.   PULMONARY ADENOCARCINOMA IN RATS AND MONKEYS

Primary pulmonary tumors were produced in rats by inhalation exposure to beryllium sulfate (13-18) and in one case by intratracheal injection of beryllium oxide or sulfate.(19)   These tumors were alveolar adenocarcinomas of various histopathologic types, although the neoplasm after intratracheal $BeSO_4$ (observed in one of five rats who survived dosing for six months or more) was a sarcoma. Pulmonary tumor was also found in several rats and a rhesus monkey exposed to the inhalation of beryllium phosphate,(20,21) and in eight of eleven rhesus monkeys exposed to the inhalation of beryllium sulfate.(22)   The latter tumors were described as very anaplastic, with adenomatoid patterns predominating among areas of epidermoid characteristics.   These experiments are summarized in Tables 2 and 3.

## IV.   ANIMAL SPECIES
## WITH NO KNOWN NEOPLASTIC RESPONSE TO BERYLLIUM

Other animal species employed in beryllium toxicity research included guinea pigs, hamsters, chickens, dogs, cats, and goats. (16,23,24,25,26)   No neoplasms of any kind were found in these other species after contact with beryllium.   In many instances, the work was not designed for the production of neoplasia, but at least in the case of the guinea pig, the studies did include several experiments of the type and duration that should have produced tumors if there were susceptibility in that species.(3,20,25,26)

TABLE 2

OSTEOSARCOMA FROM BERYLLIUM

| Author | Year | Species | Compound | Mode of Administration | Total Dose (mg Be) | Incidence of Osteosarcoma |
|---|---|---|---|---|---|---|
| GARDNER | 1946 | rabbits | Zn Be silicate | i.v. in 20 doses | 60 | 7 in 7 |
| | | | BeO | | 360 | 1 in ? |
| | | guinea pigs | Zn Be silicate | | 60 | 0 |
| | | | BeO | | 360 | 0 |
| | | rats | Zn Be silicate | | 60 | 0 |
| | | | BeO | | 360 | 0 |
| | | rabbits | Zn Be silicate | | 17 | 4 in 5 |
| | | | BeO | | 140 | 0 |
| CLOUDMAN | 1949 | mice | Zn Be silicate | i.v. in 20-22 doses | 0.26 | "some" |
| | | | BeO | | 0.55 | 0 |
| BARNES | 1950 | rabbits | Zn Be silicate | i.v. in 6-10 doses | 7.2 | 4 in 4 |
| | | | BeO | | 15 | 2 in 3 |
| | | | BeO | | 180 | 1 in 1 |
| HOAGLAND | 1950 | rabbits | Zn Be silicate (BeO = 2.3%) | i.v. in 1-30 doses | 3-7 | 3 in 6 |
| | | | Zn Be silicate (BeO = 14%) | | 10-12 | 3 in 4 |
| | | | Be phosphate | | 130? | 0 in 5 |
| | | | BeO | | 360 | 1 in 8 |
| NASH | 1950 | rabbits | Zn Be silicate | i.v. "repeated" | 12+ | 5 in 28 |
| | 1950 | rabbits | | i.v. in 17-25 doses | 64-90 | 2 in 3 |
| | | | | i.v. in 20-26 doses | 360-700 | 6 in 6 |
| DUTRA | 1951 | rabbits | BeO | inhalation 25 hrs/wk 9-13 months | 1* | 0 in 5 |
| | | | | | 6* | 1 in 6 |
| | | | | | 30* | 0 in 8 |
| JANES | 1954 | rabbits | Zn Be silicate | i.v. in 20 doses | 12 | 5 in 10 |
| | 1956 | splenectomized rabbits | | | 12 | 7 in 7 |
| KELLY | 1961 | rabbits | | | 12 | 10 in 14 |
| HIGGINS | 1964 | rabbits | | | 3300 | "many" |

*atmospheric concentration in mg $Be/m^3$.

TABLE 2

PULMONARY CARCINOMA FROM BERYLLIUM PART 1

| Author | Year | Species | Compound | Mode of Administration or Duration of Exposure | Dose or Atm. Concn. (Be) | Incidence of Pulmonary Carcinoma |
|---|---|---|---|---|---|---|
| | | rabbits | Zn Be Mn silicate | intratracheal injection | 2.3-6.9 mg | 0 |
| | | rats | silicate | | 0.46 mg | 0 |
| | 1950 | guinea pigs | Be stearate | | 3.4 mg | 0 |
| | | | Be(OH)₂ | | 5 mg | 0 |
| | | | Be metal | | 31 mg | 0 |
| | | | | | 54 mg | 0 |
| | | | | | 75 mg | 0 |
| | 1953 | | BeO | intratracheal inj. in 3 doses | 338 γ | 1 in 4 |
| | | | | | 33 γ | 1 in 5 |
| VORWALD | 1955 | rats | | 12-14 mo. | 33-35 γ/m³ | 4 in 8 |
| | | | | 13-18 mo. | | 17 in 17 |
| | | | BeSO₄ | 3-18 mo. | 55 γ/m³ | 55 in 74 |
| | | | | 12 mo. | 180 γ/m³ | 11 in 27 |
| | 1962* | | BeSO₄ | 3-22 mo. | 18 γ/m³ | 72 in 103 |
| | | | | 8-21 mo. | | 31 in 63 |
| | | | | 9-24 mo. | | 47 in 90 |
| | | | | 11-16 mo. | | 9 in 21 |
| | | | | 8-21 mo. | 1.8-2.0 γ/m³ | 25 in 50 |
| | | | | 9-24 mo. | | 43 in 95 |
| | | | | 13-16 mo. | | 3 in 15 |
| | 1966 | | BeO | 3-12 mo. | 9 mg/m³ | 22 in 36 |
| | | | | 18 mo. | 21-42 γ/m³ | "almost all" |
| | | | BeSO₄ | 18 mo. | 2.8 γ/m³ | 13 in 21 |
| | 1968 | monkeys | BeO | inhal. av.15 hrs/wk 3 + yrs. | 38.8 γ/m³ | 8 in 11 |
| | | | BeO | bronchomural implant + intra-bronchial inj. | 18-90+ mg | 3 in 20 |

inhalation exposure on 35-38 hrs/wk. schedule

*unpublished

TABLE 3

PULMONARY CARCINOMA FROM BERYLLIUM PART 2

| Author | Year | Species | Compound | Duration of Exposure | Atmospheric Concentration Be | Incidence of Pulmonary Carcinoma |
|---|---|---|---|---|---|---|
| SCHEPERS | 1957 | rats | BeSO$_4$ | 6-9 mo. | 32-35 $\gamma/m^3$ | 58? in 136 |
| | | | Be phosphate | 1-12 mo. | 227 $\gamma/m^3$ | ca. 35-60 in 170 |
| | | | BeF$_2$ | 6-15 mo. | 9 $\gamma/m^3$ | ca. 7 in 40 |
| | 1961 | | Zn Be Mn silicate | 1-9 mo. | 0.85-1.25 $mg/m^3$ | ca. 10-12 in 200 |
| | | rabbits | | 24 mo. | 1 $mg/m^3$ | ca. 4-20 in 220 |
| | | guinea pigs | | 22 mo. | | 0 |
| | | | | | | 0 |
| | | | | | | 0 |
| | 1964 | monkeys | BeSO$_4$ | 8 mo. | 35 $\gamma/m^3$ | 0 in 4 |
| | | | BeF$_2$ | | 35-200 $\gamma/m^3$ | 0 in 4 |
| | | | | | 180 $\gamma/m^3$ | 0 in 4 |
| | | | Be phosphate | | 0.2 $mg/m^3$ | 1 in 4 |
| | | | | | 1.1 $mg/m^3$ | 0 in 4 |
| | | | | | 8.3 $mg/m^3$ | |
| REEVES | 1967 | rats | | 13 mo. | 34.25±23.66 $\gamma/m^3$ | 43 in 43 |
| | 1969 | | BeSO$_4$ | 3 mo. | 35.66+13.77 $\gamma/m^3$ | 19 in 22 |
| | | | | 6 mo. | | 33 in 33 |
| | | | | 9 mo. | | 15 in 15 |
| | | | | 12 mo. | | 21 in 21 |
| | | | | 18 mo. | | 13 in 15 |
| | 1972 | guinea pigs | | 18-24 mo. | 3.7-30.4 $\gamma/m^3$ | 0 in 58 |
| | 1976* | | | | ~15 $\gamma/m^3$ | 0 in 110 |
| WAGNER | 1969 | rats | beryl | 17+ mo. | 620 $\gamma/m^3$ | 18 in 19 |
| | | | bertrandite | | 210 $\gamma/m^3$ | 0 in 30-60 |
| | | hamsters | beryl | | 620 $\gamma/m^3$ | 0 in 48 |
| | | | bertrandite | | 210 $\gamma/m^3$ | 0 in 12 |
| | | monkeys | beryl | | 620 $\gamma/m^3$ | 0 in 12 |
| | | | hertrandite | | 210 $\gamma/m^3$ | 0 in 12 |

*unpublished

## V.  THE EVIDENCE IN MAN

The results on experimental animals summarized herein naturally led to increased watchfulness regarding the human experience.  In 1952, a "Beryllium Case Registry" was established at the Massachusetts General Hospital, which accumulated the records of all reported clinical cases with the diagnosis of beryllium disease.(27) MANCUSO et al.(28,29) have recently attempted to examine this material and other epidemiological sources, a total of more than 800 cases.  It appears from these studies that the prevalence of cancer among beryllium-exposed persons, in comparison to a control cohort, was not elevated.  However, the prevalence of lung cancer did show positive correlation with the prevalence of other pulmonary disorders, including berylliosis.  On the other hand, incidence of pulmonary cancer among beryllium workers was inversely related to length of occupational exposure.  Sporadic clinical reports on the occurrence of malignancy in beryllium-exposed persons include two cases of pulmonary carcinoma(30) and one case of osteosarcoma(31) originating from the years 1945 to 1954.  One of the pulmonary carcinomas regressed after radiation therapy.

The presently available evidence is incomplete and allows contradictory interpretations regarding the carcinogenicity of beryllium in man.  The Occupational Safety and Health authorities of the United States, Western Germany, and Sweden view beryllium as a potential human carcinogen, based essentially on the experimental animal evidence.  There are as yet no convincing human data to support that view.

## VI.   DOSE-RESPONSE RELATIONSHIPS

The experiments on rabbits resulting in bone sarcomas employed beryllium oxide and zinc beryllium silicate in total amounts of 3-3300 mg Be per animal, usually administered in divided doses. Since these studies were conducted in various laboratories, the establishment of a dose-response curve must be done with considerable reservation.  Figure 1 represents the best regression line that can be drawn across the various data points.  The slope of this line allows the as yet untested assumption that the threshold of significant induction of osteosarcoma by intravenous zinc beryllium silicate in the rabbit is in the range of 2-3 mg Be per animal.

The experiments on rats resulting in pulmonary carcinomas were conducted, for the most part, by inhalation in chambers.  The establishment of a dose-response curve in this case is even more difficult because the doses cannot be computed even approximately.  Most cancers were observed about one year after commencement of exposure, but exposures of a few months' duration, followed by transfer of

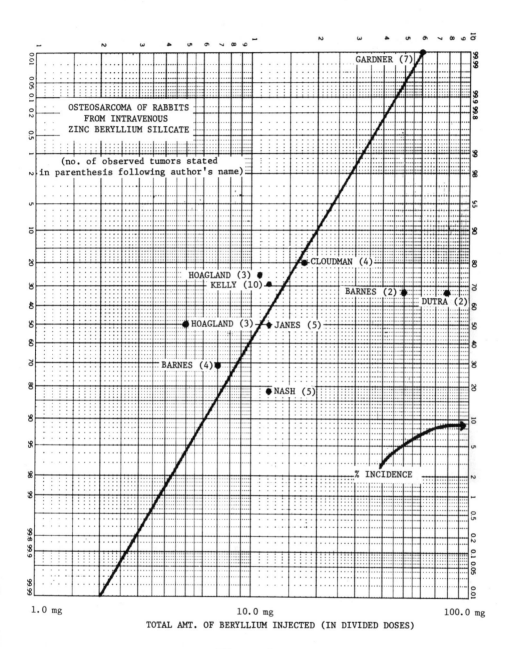

OSTEOSARCOMA OF RABBITS
FROM INTRAVENOUS
ZINC BERYLLIUM SILICATE

(no. of observed tumors stated
in parenthesis following author's name)

GARDNER (7)

CLOUDMAN (4)

HOAGLAND (3)
KELLY (10)

BARNES (2)
DUTRA (2)

HOAGLAND (3) — JANES (5)

BARNES (4)

NASH (5)

% INCIDENCE

1.0 mg                    10.0 mg                    100.0 mg

TOTAL AMT. OF BERYLLIUM INJECTED (IN DIVIDED DOSES)

Figure 1

the animals to clean air , frequently had the same effect as continuous exposures through the entire time period.  Figure 2 attempts
to plot atmospheric exposure levels versus pulmonary cancer incidence percentages.  The data points in this chart are derived from
both published and unpublished(15) sources.  Although the latter
data may be subject to more uncertainty than finished or confirmed
work, they were nonetheless quoted in a review(16) including a claim
for considerable incidence of cancer in rats from the surprisingly
low atmospheric level of 1.8-2.8 $\alpha/m^3$(in the range of the present
TLV for beryllium).  These data points on Figure 2 are at considerable distance to the left from the best regression line that can
be drawn; except for these points, the threshold of significant
induction of pulmonary carcinoma by inhaled beryllium sulfate in
the rat, with exposure lasting several months, would be in the range
of 10 $\alpha$ Be/$m^3$.

## VII.  SPECIES SPECIFICITY

Table 4 summarizes all beryllium cancer research data, with
indication of their degree of certainty.  It can be seen that much
of the evidence is fragmentary, uncontrolled, or otherwise not beyond some degree of doubt.  Only three facts can be regarded as
reasonably confirmed.  These are:

1.  Rabbits develop osteosarcoma from intravenous beryllium.

2.  Rats develop pulmonary carcinoma from inhaled beryllium.

3.  Guinea pigs do not suffer neoplastic effects from
    inhaled beryllium.

Since facts 2 and 3, above, refer to the same mode of administration, same compound, at same concentration, they must be regarded
as evidence for a genuine species specificity.  The reasons for this
specificity are not known, but it is noteworthy that guinea pigs
develop delayed cutaneous hypersensitivity to beryllium, whereas,
rats do not.(25)  Obviously, more research is needed to ascertain
that these two phenomena are not merely coincidental.  However, it
is interesting that in rabbits, the spleen appears to be involved
in the neoplastic response to intravenous beryllium, and the first
report on beryllium bone sarcomas(3) included the observation of
prompt concurrent splenic atrophy.  JANES et al.(32) had the impression that splenectomy increased the incidence of bone sarcomas
from beryllium in rabbits.  These studies allow the working hypothesis that some form of cellular immunity, with immunocompetent cells
arising from the spleen , may be a factor in determining whether the
response to beryllium will be neoplastic or not, and that various
species have partial or total resistance to beryllium cancer according to their immunocompetence.

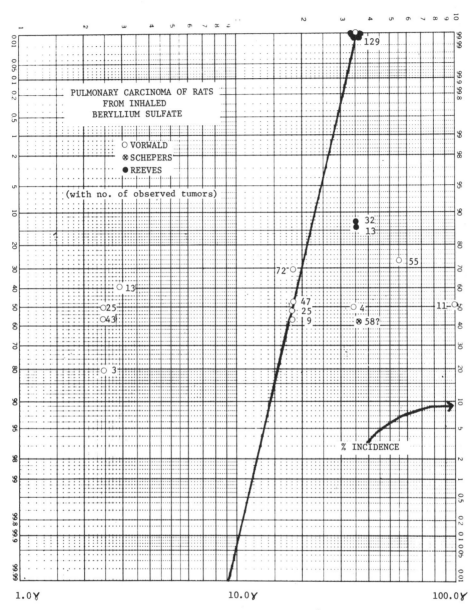

ATMOSPHERIC CONCENTRATION (PER m³ AIR)

Figure 2

TABLE 4

SUMMARY OF RESEARCH DATA ON THE CARCINOGENIC RESPONSE TO BERYLLIUM

| Species | Mode of Administration | | |
| | Intravenous Injection | Intratracheal Injection | Inhalation |
|---------|------------------------|-------------------------|------------|
| rabbits | osteosarcoma (3,4,5,6,7,8,9, 10,12) | no effect? (23) | no effect? (20) osteosarcoma? (11) |
| rats | no effect? (3) | no effect? (23) pul.carcinoma? (19) | pul.carcinoma (13,14,15,16, 17,18,19,20,24) |
| guinea pigs | no effect? (3) | no effect? (23) | no effect (20,25,26) |
| mice | osteosarcoma? (12) | 0 | 0 |
| hamsters | 0 | 0 | no effect? (24) |
| monkeys | 0 | pul.carcinoma? (16) | no effect? (24) pul.carcinoma? (16,21,22) |

Confirmed results are underlined.
Unconfirmed or contradictory results are question marked.
Figures in parenthesis are literature references.
0 = Not Done.

## VIII.   THE IMMUNE RESPONSE TO BERYLLIUM IN GUINEA PIGS

ALEKSEEVA(33) discovered that hypersensitivity to beryllium in
guinea pigs was cell mediated and passively transferable with
lymphoid cells, while the transfer of serum was ineffective.  Anti-
lymphocyte serum from rabbits(34) could inhibit all cutaneous reactions to beryllium in guinea pigs, and inhalation of beryllium
could also suppress skin reactivity.(25,35)  Furthermore, guinea
pigs in a state of beryllium hypersensitivity reacted differently
than untreated guinea pigs to beryllium inhalation and developed
less pulmonary pathology.(36,37)  It was thus apparent that immune
phenomena govern the susceptibility or resistance of the guinea pig
at least to berylliosis.

IX.  THE IMMUNE RESPONSE TO BERYLLIUM IN MAN

The human response to beryllium also contains a distinct immunological component.  CURTIS(38,39) developed a patch test to beryllium both in cases of beryllium dermatitis and pulmonary berylliosis, and other diagnostic measures involving immune reactions including lymphocyte blast transformation(40) and macrophage migration inhibition(41) appeared applicable to human disease.  It is interesting that STERNER and EISENBUD(1) had suggested an immunologic etiology to human berylliosis as early as 1951.  They noted in an epidemiologic study of chronic pulmonary berylliosis cases that dose-response relation between exposure and incidence was nonexistent, with workers from the cleanest plants and "neighborhood cases" sometimes showing the worst clinical forms.  Furthermore, the morphology of pulmonary granulomata caused by beryllium, with considerable similarity to those observed in sarcoidosis, also allowed the assumption of an immunological etiology.  The lesions typically consisted of a cluster of monocytes surrounded by a zone of lumphocytes and plasma cells.(42)  These findings, coupled with the lack of known excess incidence of neoplastic disease in beryllium-exposed humans, also create the impression that the ability of beryllium to induce various types of tissue damage , or the ability of the host to resist them, involves immune phenomena.

X.  POSSIBLE MECHANISMS OF THE NEOPLASTIC RESPONSE

Beryllium is the strongest known inhibitor of alkaline phosphatase(43) but the relevance of this finding to neoplastic bone formation is unknown.  Also unknown is the significance, if any, of the observation that beryllium inhibited the activity of aryl hydrocarbon hydroxylase, an enzyme that perhaps is instrumental in the detoxification of carcinogenic polynuclear hydrocarbons that may be present in the environment.(44)  At higher concentrations, beryllium inhibits numerous other enzymes.  Remarkable is the action of beryllium on lactate dehydrogenase because it has been found that among the molecular forms of this enzyme, the "heart-type" isozyme was more sensitive to the inhibition than the "muscle-type" isozyme, and only the former was depressed in beryllium-induced pulmonary tumors.(45)  However, the relevance of this finding to the mechanism of pulmonary carcinogenesis is also unknown.

Recent findings show that beryllium is a garbler of DNA-polymerase-induced nucleic acid replication.  It has been known since 1951(46) that beryllium inhibited cell division in the metaphase, with marked decrease in the intensity of the Feulgen reaction for DNA.  The effect was specific to DNA, with RNA biosynthesis remaining unaffected.  Preferential accumulation of radioberyllium in the nuclei of regenerating livers was noted, with increase of the sedimentation constant of DNA after contact with beryllium,(47)

but it was also shown that, while beryllium did inhibit the
replication of DNA in regenerating rat livers, it did not become
attached to DNA.(48)   There is increasing evidence that beryllium
can present interference with nucleic acid function at the transcriptional level.   Misincorporation of polydeoxyadenosylthymidine
by micrococcal DNA polymerase in the presence of beryllium, with
strong inhibition of the 3'-5' exonuclease ("editing") activity
of the enzyme, was recently noted,(49) and beryllium alone among
several divalent cations substantially affected the fidelity of
in vitro DNA transcription by single-base substitutions.(50)   The
significance of these findings with respect to the ultimate mechanism of beryllium carcinogenesis, and their relation to the immune phenomena discussed above, remains to be established.

## XI.  SUMMARY

    Beryllium is a proven bone carcinogen in rabbits, and a proven
pulmonary carcinogen in rats.   Median effective doses or concentrations can be computed only with considerable uncertainty; they
appear to be in the 10 mg area (as total dose, in divided intravenous injections, expressed as Be for zinc beryllium silicate)
for rabbits, and in the  20 $\alpha/m^3$ area (as atmospheric concentration
for inhalation exposures lasting for at least three months, expressed as Be for beryllium sulfate) for rats.   It is also proven
that, at least from inhalation, guinea pigs do not develop beryllium
cancers.   Epidemiologic studies in humans are thus far unconfirmed
but do not show increased cancer morbidity among beryllium workers.

    Current research is aimed at explaining the mechanism of car-
cinogenic action in the susceptible species, which seems to involve
nucleic acid transcriptional interference, or the species specificity, which seems to involve immune mechanisms.   No experiments
were reported thus far besides the carcinogenesis studies to show
that beryllium is a chemical mutagen.   In the species thus far tested, there appeared to be mutual exclusion of development of a delayed (cell-mediated) hypersensitivity to beryllium and development
of neoplasia from beryllium.   Further research on this subject might
lead to new possibilities in the understanding of cancer susceptibility.

*REFERENCES*

1.   Sterner, J. H., and Eisenbud, M., Arch. Indust. Hyg. 4,
     Page 123, 1951.

2.   Petzow, G., and Zorn, P., Chemiker Ztg. 98, Page 236, 1974.

3.  Gardner, L. U. and Heslington, H. F., Fed. Proceedings 5,
    Page 221, 1946.

4.  Barnes, J. M., Denz, F. A. and Sissons, H. A., British J.
    Cancer 4, Page 212, 1950.

5.  Dutra, F. R. and Largent, E. J., American J. Pathology 26,
    Page 197, 1950.

6.  Hoagland, M. B., Grier, R. S. and Hood, M. B., Cancer Res. 10,
    Page 629, 1950.

7.  Nash, P., Lancet i, Page 519, 1950.

8.  Janes, J. M., Higgins, G. M. and Herrick, J. F., J. Bone and
    Joint Surgery 36(B), Page 543, 1954.

9.  Kelly, P. J., Janes, J. M. and Peterson, L. F. A., J. Bone and
    Joint Surgery 43(A), Page 829, 1961.

10. Higgins, G. M., Levy, B. M. and Yollick, B. L., J. Bone and
    Joint Surgery 46(A), Page 289, 1964.

11. Dutra, F. R., Largent, E. J. and Roth, J. L., Arch. Path. 51,
    Page 473, 1951.

12. Cloudman, A. M., Vining, D., Barkulis, S. and Nickson, J. J.,
    American J. Pathology 25, Page 810, 1949.

13. Vorwald, A. J., Pratt, P. C. and Urban, E. J., Acta Unio
    International Contra Cancrum 11, Page 735, 1955.

14. Schepers, G. W. H., Durkan, T. M., Delahant, A. B. and
    Creedon, F. T., Arch. Indust. Health 15, Page 32, 1957.

15. Vorwald, A. J., Prog. Rep. American Cancer Society, Grant No.
    E-253-G, 1962.

16. Vorwald, A. J., Reeves, A. L. and Urban, E. J., Beryllium--
    Its Industrial Hygiene Aspects, Academic Press, New York,
    pp. 201-234, 1966.

17. Reeves, A. L., Deitch, D. and Vorwald, A. J., Cancer Res. 27(1),
    Page 439, 1967.

18. Reeves, A. L. and Deitch, D., Proceedings International Con-
    gress Occupational Health 16, Page 651, 1969.

19.  Vorwald, A. J., Cancer of the Lung--An Evaluation of the Prob-
     lem, American Cancer Society, Detroit, Michigan, pp. 103-109,
     1953.

20.  Schepers, G. W. H., Prog. Exptl. Tumor Res. 2, Page 203, 1961.

21.  Schepers, G. W. H., Indust. Med. Surg. 33, Page 1, 1964.

22.  Vorwald, A. J., Use of Nonhuman Primates in Drug Evaluation,
     University of Texas, Austin, pp. 222-228, 1968.

23.  Vorwald, A. J., Pneumoconiosis--L. U. Gardner Memorial Volume,
     P. B. Hoeber, New York, pp. 393-425, 1950.

24.  Wagner, W. D., Groth, D. H., Holtz, J. L., Madden, G. E. and
     Stokinger, H. E., Toxicol. Appl. Pharmacol. 15, Page 10, 1969.

25.  Reeves, A. L., Krivanek, N. D., Busby, E. K. and Swanborg, R. H.,
     Int. Arch. Arbeitsmed. 29, Page 209, 1972.

26.  Reeves, A. L., Prog. Rep. USPHS Grant No. ES-EC-353, 1976.

27.  Hardy, H. L., Rabe, E. W. and Lorch, S., J. Occup. Medicine 9,
     Page 271, 1967.

28.  Mancuso, T. F. and El-Attar, A. A., J. Occup. Med. 11, Page
     422, 1969.

29.  Mancuso, T. F., Environmental Research 3, Page 251, 1970.

30.  Niemöller, H. K., Int. Arch. Gew. Path. Gew. Hyg. 20,
     Page 180, 1963.

31.  Hardy, H. L., New England J. Medicine 295, Page 624, 1976.

32.  Janes, J. M., Higgins, G. M. and Herrick, J. F., J. Bone
     and Joint Surgery 38(A), Page 809, 1956.

33.  Alekseeva, O. G., Gig. Tr. Prof. Zabol. 11, Page 20, 1965.

34.  Chiappino, G., Cirla, A. and Vigliani, E. C., Arch. Path. 87,
     Page 131, 1969.

35.  Reeves, A. L., Ann. Clin. Lab. Sci. 6, Page 256, 1976.

36.  Reeves, A. L. Swanborg, R. H., Busby, E. K. and Krivanek, N. D,
     Inhaled Particles III, Unwin Bros., London, pp. 599-608, 1971.

37.  Reeves, A. L. and Krivanek, N. D., Trans. New York Academy
     Science 36, Page 78, 1974.

38.  Curtis, G. H., Arch. Dermatol. Syphilol. 64, Page 470, 1951.

39.  Curtis, G. H., Arch. Indust. Health 19, Page 150, 1959.

40.  Deodhar, S. D., Barna, B. and Van Ordstrand, H. S., Chest 63,
     Page 309, 1973.

41.  Marx, J. J. and Burrell, R., J. Immunology 111, Page 590, 1973.

42.  Vorwald, A. J., J. Occup. Med. 5, Page 684, 1948.

43.  Dubois, K. P., Cochran, K. W. and Mazur, M. Science 110,
     Page 420, 1949.

44.  Jacques, A. and Witschi, H. R., Arch. Environ. Health 27,
     Page 243, 1973.

45.  Reeves, A. L., Cancer Research 27(1), Page 1895, 1967.

46.  Chèvremont, M. and Firket, H., Nature 167, Page 772, 1951.

47.  Truhaut, R., Festy, B. and Le Talaer, J. Y., Compt. Rend.
     Acad. Science Ser. D. 266, Page 1192, 1968.

48.  Witschi, H. R., Biochem. J. 120, Page 623, 1970.

49.  Luke, M. Z., Hamilton, L. and Hollocher, T. C., Biochem.
     Biophys. Res. Commun. 62, Page 497, 1975.

50.  Sirover, M. A. and Loeb, L. A., Proceedings National Academy
     Science 73, Page 233, 1976.

*CHAPTER 3*

ASBESTOS CARCINOGENESIS*

Arthur M. Langer and Mary S. Wolff

Environmental Sciences Laboratory
Mount Sinai School of Medicine of
The City University of New York
New York, New York 10029

I.   INTRODUCTION

A.   Cancer in Western Man

In countries where vital statistics concerning causes of death have been kept and mortality and morbidity data are validated by clinical and autopsy information, cancer deaths have increased dramatically (e.g., the United States, Silverberg and Holleb, 1972.(1) Some forms of malignant tumors have increased at alarming rates; such is the case for lung cancer, colon cancer, and bladder cancer. As an example, lung cancer now accounts for one of every six male deaths in Glasgow, Scotland (Haddow, 1970).(2). Some investigators have attributed the increasing cancer incidence to the inadvertent introduction of carcinogenic agents into the environment as pollutants (Boyland, 1969).(3) These agents, which represent low-level, long-term insult to the host, may represent one of the most important factors in the etiology of malignant neoplasms in the general population (Saffioti, 1970).(4)

The suggested correlation between exposure to an agent in the environment and occurrence of excess neoplasms in the general population has come about from the study of occupational cancers.  The first such cancer was described over 200 years ago, and focused on the occurrence of scrotal cancers among chimney sweeps in London

---

*  This work was supported in part by the following grants from the NIEHS; Center Grant ES 00928; Career Award, ES 44812(AML), and Post-doctoral Fellowship, ES 02565(MSW).

(Pott, 1976).(5)   Since this time, many occupations have been scrut-
inized and studied, and agents found that have been correlated with
the etiology of specific malignant neoplasms (Hunter, 1969).(6)
Some of these tumors also have been observed in populations which
are only indirectly exposed to the agent, or which simply lived in
the local area where the agent was used.   This has been defined in
some detail for one such substance; asbestos (Selikoff and Hammond,
1968),(7) which is shown to occur as an air pollutant (Selikoff et
al., 1972)(8) and which commonly occurs as fibers in the lung tissues of individuals from the general population (e.g., Langer, et al.,
1971;(9) Pooley et al., 1970, 1976).(10,11)

B.    Inorganic Particles and Disease

     Exposure to inorganic dusts in the workplace is capable of
producing disease that may cause disability or premature death.
These facts have been known since antiquity, and have been the subject of early extensive treatises (e.g., Agricola, 1556).(12)
Pneumoconiosis, a term that is recent in origin, was recognized
first as a dust disease of the lungs (Zenker, 1867).(13)   Indeed,
it was not until the early 20th century that the most common of the
dust diseases (silicosis) began to be understood on a sound basis
(Collis, 1915).(14)   Since this time, a number of other dust diseases have been recognized as related to exposure to inorganic
agents.   These have been reviewed extensively [Rosen, 1943;(15)
Holt, 1957;(16) Hunter, 1969;(6) Aponte, 1970;(17) Langer and
Mackler, 1972(18)].   Interestingly, not only have these diseases
been reported in the areas where the materials are mined, but also
in workplaces where milling, processing, and even use of the materials occur.

     Not all inorganic dusts produce only lung scarring; some dis-
seminate throughout the host, producing reactions in extra-pulmonary
organs, as is the case with silica (Holt, 1957).(16).   In addition to
scar-tissue development, a number of inorganic dusts have been
implicated in the etiology of malignant neoplasms.   During the last
25 to 30 years, a number of inorganic particles have been implicated
as the agent (or agents) responsible for malignant neoplasms in the
workplace:   chromium ores (Mackle and Gregorius, 1948);(19) heavy
metals, especially lead, zinc, and copper (Breslow, 1954); (20) hematite ore, in the presence of free silica and other silicates (Lamy,
et al., 1959;(21) talc (Kleinfeld et al., 1967);(22) uranium ore
(Holaday, 1969).(23)   Perhaps the best studied inorganic agent is
asbestos.   It is of particular importance because it is now used
throughout the world, in thousands of products, so that it pervades
all society (IARC, 1977).(24)   To appreciate this great preoccupation
with asbestos, one must understand its disease potential.

C.    Asbestos Exposure and Human Disease

Asbestos has been identified as a biologically active agent in relatively recent times. Asbestos fiber was first recognized as a potent fibrogenic agent capable of producing a fatal lung scarring with intensity and severity, as observed in cases of silicosis, when Cooke, in 1927(25) noted several cases of fibrosis among asbestos workers. Several years later, there were two separate reports of primary bronchogenic carcinoma in individuals with asbestosis (Lynch and Smith, 1935, U. S. A.; (26) Gloyne, 1935, U. K.).(27) These observations were regarded as "curiosities" in that they may have been merely coincidental occurrences; i.e., asbestos and lung cancer. However, Wedler, in 1943(28,29) later reported several autopsy series in which the occurrence of lung cancer among asbestos workers was far in excess of a similar matched autopsy series among individuals from the general population presumed to have not been exposed to asbestos. With the work of Doll in 1955(30), a firm epidemiological basis was established for the occurrence of lung cancer in workmen exposed to asbestos fiber.

In 1960, Wagner et al.(31) reported that a tumor, heretofore considered rare, frequently occurred among asbestos-exposed workers in the Northwest Cape Province of South Africa. They reported the occurrence of pleural mesothelioma, which they suggested was a risk not only among occupationally exposed asbestos workers, but to individuals who merely lived in the area where asbestos was being mined and milled. Similar tumors were reported to have occurred intra-abdominally in factory workmen in the United Kingdom (Keal, 1960).(32) In addition to mesotheliomas, Selikoff et al. in 1964(33) reported the occurrence of excess gastrointestinal tumors among asbestos-exposed workmen as well. Less than 15 years ago, data accumulated suggesting that occupational exposure to asbestos fiber resulted in excess risk to asbestosis, pleural and peritoneal mesothelioma, lung cancer, and gastrointestinal cancer.

In addition to workmen incurring increased neoplastic risk, it appeared that individuals indirectly exposed to asbestos were also among the "at risk" population. Several studies of shipyard workers on the European continent demonstrated that asbestos disease carried over to all trades, rather than being confined to the insulation categories (or "laggers") (Harries, 1968;(34) Bohlig et al., 1970; (35) Stumphius, 1971;(36) Edge, 1976).(37)  To add to these worrisome observations, a number of papers also reported the occurrence of asbestos-related tumors among individuals who merely lived in the environment of an asbestos plant (Wagner, et al., 1960; (31) Newhouse and Thompson, 1965;(38) Lieben and Pistawka, 1967).(39)  Also, individuals who merely lived within a short distance of the workplace where asbestos was being processed or used, and members of the households of asbestos workers also incurred increased neoplastic risk (Anderson et al., 1976).(40)

One can readily understand why asbestos has been investigated
so intensively.  The literature concerning this material has so increased in the last decade that extensive review papers and bibli-
ographies have been written (Harington, 1967;(41) IARC Monographs,
1972, 1977;(42,24) Harington et al., 1975).(43)   Indeed, asbestos
has become one of the important 20th century carcinogens.

D.   Asbestos Studies in Animals

Utilizing a variety of animal species including substrains and
colonies: rat, mouse, rabbit, guinea pig, gerbel, hamster; and different routes of administration, such as oral, inhalation, intrapleu-
ral, intratracheal, intraperitoneal, subcutaneous, all asbestos
fiber varieties have produced malignant tumors in animals (Tables
14-21, reference 24).   All asbestos varieties have induced mesotheliomas, and most have produced other carcinomas.(43)   Doses, exposure intensities, fiber types, and species of animals have been
varied to establish carcinogenicity and dose-response curves for
each fiber type.(24)

E.   *In Vitro* Studies of Asbestos

As the number of animal studies has grown, so have *in vitro*
test systems.  Most of these systems have dealt with relative toxicity of the fiber types and their ability to stimulate fibroblast
growth and form scar tissue.  Membrane systems (hemolysis) have provided a rough index of cytotoxicity, which appears to correlate well
with relative fibrogenicity of the fibers.(43)   However, little relevance has been gained concerning carcinogenicity.  Cell systems
have concentrated on hemolysis of mature erythrocytes, alveolar
macrophage systems (viability, lysosomal enzyme changes, phagocy-
totic properties, etc.), other cell lines, especially dividing cells;
organ culture involving specific tissues, e.g., tracheal transplant;
and others; e.g., Davis, 1967;(44) Koshi et al., 1968;(45) Bey and
Harington, 1971;(46) Allison, 1971, 1972;(47,48) Miller and Harington, 1972).(49)   Whereas the animal studies determined the fibrogenicity and carcinogenicity of the fiber types, so the *in vitro*
test systems were oriented toward determination of mechanisms.   An
extensive review of these papers may be found in Harington et al.(43)

F.   Status Concerning Asbestos Activity

There continue to be many clinical and epidemiological studies
concerning asbestos disease in workmen, an extensive literature
concerning experimental carcinogenesis in animal models, and an
ever growing literature in the area of mechanisms of interaction of
asbestos fiber in cellular systems, all reflecting the importance
of asbestos as a diverse and complex agent in human disease, and a
widespread environmental contaminant.  Significant quantitative and
qualitative questions remain including the relative hazards associated with each of the asbestos fiber types, and those mechanisms
leading to disease.

## II.  ASBESTOS AS A MATERIAL

A.  The Nature of Asbestos

Asbestos is the name given to a group of naturally occuring
silicate mineral fibers in the serpentine and amphibole series.
Normally, only six of these fibrous silicates are recognized as
asbestos, although some rare forms of other mineral fibers may be
used as well, e.g., fibrous clays (Whittaker, 1960).(50)  The most
commonly used fiber in the United States is the serpentine mineral
chrysotile, sometimes referred to as white asbestos.  Five amphibole silicate fibers make up the other common varieties:  actinolite,
amosite (brown asbestos), anthophyllite, crocidolite (blue asbestos),
and tremolite.  The mineral nature of asbestos is extensively reviewed in Speil and Leineweber, 1969;(51) and in the IARC Monograph,
1977.(24)

1.  Atomic Structure - Chrysotile has been shown to be a
curled sheet silicate that spirals around a central capillary.  This
has been determined on the basis of X-ray diffraction, single-crystal
X-ray crystallographic, transmission electron microscopic, and selected area electron diffraction studies (Bates et al., 1950; (52)
Jagodzinski and Kunze, 1954;(53) Whittaker, 1956;(54) Zussman et
al., 1957;(55) Kalousec and Muttart, 1957;(56) Bates, 1959;(57)
Maser, et al., 1960; (58) Whittaker, 1960, 1963;(50,59,60) Huggins
and Shell, 1965;(61) Clifton et al., 1966; (62) Yada, 1967, 1971;
(63,64) Langer et al., 1974).(65)  These investigators determined
the structure of chrysotile to be the magnesium analog of kaolin in
which planar-linked silica tetrahedra face an adjoining brucite sheet
composed of magnesium ions coordinated octahedrally with oxygens
and hydroxyl groups.  Two of the three apical oxygens in the silica
sheet replace the hydroxyl groups in the brucite sheet to complete
the chrysotile structure.  The distance between these adjacent
sheets are on the order of 7.3 angstroms, with symmetry repetition
every 14.6 angstroms.  The curvature of chrysotile is a function of
the structural mismatch of the larger brucite sheet "stretched over"
the smaller silica sheet to structurally satisfy the cation accom-
modations.  There are several structural types that characterize the
crystallography of chrysotile, the most important of which occurs in
the monoclinic system and is called clinochrysotile (Zussman et al.,
1957).(55)

The structure of the amphibole minerals is more complex.  These
minerals are termed inosilicates, occurring as double chains of
linked silica tetrahedra that are cross-linked with bridging cations.
The amphibole chain is formed by coplanar sharing of two of the three
oxygens at the base of the silica tetrahedra to form an infinite
chain axis.  The double chain is completed by the third basal oxygen
that is shared between two opposite-facing, single-chain structures.
These basic units make up the asbestos fiber axis (Deer et al.,

1967; (66) Whittaker; (50) Ernst, 1968; (67) Speil and Leineweber. (51)
The different amphibole asbestos fibers possess the same basic
structure, with small modifications brought about by chemical variation.   The cations within this structure alter interplanar spac-
ings and the angle at which the adjacent units are stacked within
the structure (referred to as the beta angle, forming the inclined
plane of the monoclinic structure).

   2.   Fiber Unit - Electron micrographs demonstrate that single
chrysotile fibers (called fibrils) are formed as hollow tubes (the
internal capillaries surrounded by the spiraling sheet).   These
structures have been demonstrated many times.   Studies of their
dimensional characteristics indicate that the single fibril may
range considerably with diameters ranging from 100-600 Angstroms
(e.g., Langer and Pooley, 1973; (63) Langer et al., 1974). (65)
Bundles of individual fibrils form the chrysotile fiber.   These may
range in diameter and in length, from millimeters to centimeters.

   Amphibole asbestos fibers appear to consist of single crystals,
twinned crystals, and stack-faulted fibers, in which the width distribution tends to be different.   It has been observed that the
different amphibole varieties behave differently when comminuted to
form width distributions that are unique and characteristic for each
mineral species (Timbrell et al., 1970, 1971; (69,70) Timbrell,
1972). (71)   These studies demonstrated that crocidolite forms the
shortest and thinnest fibers, followed by amosite, followed by
anthophyllite.   The log normal distribution of such width distribution appears to center at about 0.12 μ and smaller for crocidolite,
0.16 μ for amosite, and a polymodal distribution, greater than 0.20 μ
for anthophyllite.   The importance of such characteristics will be
discussed in the section on inhalation potential.   However, all of
the amphibole fibers appear generally as straight rods when examined by electron microscopical techniques, with diffraction contrast
figures resulting from flexing of the structure under the electron
beam; curved fibers are noted as well. (65)   It has been suggested
that some of the internal structures of amphiboles, a fine, 20-50
Angstrom internal lamellar structure parallel to the fiber axis, may
reflect twinning which imparts the unusual optical and tensile
strength characteristic of the fiber (Seshan and Zoltai, 1976). (72)

   3.   Chemistry - The empirical chemical composition of chrysotile is $Mg_3Si_2O_5(OH)_4$.   Although magnesium predominantly occupies
the octahedral site within the structure, it is also common to have
iron, nickel, and manganese substituting within this site up to several tenths of a percent.   Occasionally, aluminum may substitute for
silicon in structure, and fluorine may occupy several of the hydroxyl positions.   In the Canadian chrysotile samples, originating
from ultramafic rock types, the high iron content may be attributable to intergrowths of the mineral magnetite within the chrysotile

fiber bundle.  Serpentine deposits that originate from silicified dolomites tend to have high calcium oxide content, reflecting inter-growth of carbonate minerals.  Other trace metals that may have bio-logical importance are nickel, chromium, and cobalt, which have been identified in concentrations up to several thousand parts per million in chrysotiles originating from ultramafic rocks.  The chemistry of chrysotile has been discussed at length in several papers:  Pundsack, 1956;(73) Pundsack and Reimschussel, 1956;(74) Nagy and Faust, 1956;(75) Brindley and Zussman, 1957;(76) Gaze, 1965;(77) Harington, 1965;(78) Speil and Leineweber;(51) and Table 1.(24)

The chemistry of the amphibole asbestos minerals is far more complex than the chrysotile mineral.  Generally, it may be described by the structural chemical formula:(67)

$$W_{0-1} \, X_2 \, Y_5 \, (Si_4O_{11})_2 \, (O,OH,F)_2$$

For anthophyllite, no cations occupy the W structural site, and the X and Y cation sites are theoretically filled with magnesium.  There is limited substitution of iron for magnesium in the structure, and some limited substitution of aluminum for silicon.  Amosite has no cations in the W site also, and contains almost total iron in the X and Y sites.  Some magnesium does substitute for iron, as well as manganese.  Actinolite and tremolite, both forming the end members of a solid solution series, may contain some calcium, sodium, or potassium in the W site, in limited amounts.  The X site is filled with calcium and the Y site with magnesium and iron (for actinolite the iron is greater than the magnesium, for tremolite the magnesium is greater than iron).  Manganese may occur in these sites as well. Crocidolite may have traces of calcium and potassium in the W site, contain sodium in the X cation site, and iron in the Y site.  Antho-phyllite may contain traces of aluminum which substitutes for sili-con in the basic chain structure.  Crocidolite may contain substantial amounts of magnesium and occasionally traces of aluminum as well. Originating from different rock sources, there are a number of different trace metals that may be associated with the amphibole asbestos varieties, again a function of provenance and geological origin.  This is reviewed in Whittaker;(50) Ernst;(67) Speil and Leineweber;(51) and in Tables 5, 6, 7.(24)

It is of interest to note that both chrysotile and the amphi-bole asbestos varieties may be contaminated with hydrocarbon traces, originating either from the geologic environment at the time of min-eral formation (or migration of hydrocarbons after rock formation) or hydrocarbon contamination from processing and storage (Gibbs, 1969, 1970;(79,80) Commins and Gibbs, 1969;(81) Gibbs and Hui, 1971).(82)  In addition to these sorbed hydrocarbons, occasionally impurities from the metals encountered during processing might con-taminate these samples as well (Ayer and Lynch, 1967;(83) Baddolet, 1952;(84) Baddolet and Edgerton, 1961(85)).

4.   Surface Charge - Chrysotile asbestos has a surface layer
of magnesium hydroxide groups bonded to the silica layer through
the sharing of oxygens.  The surface hydroxyl layer, having protons
outermost, imparts a net positive charge to the fibril surface.
Zeta potential measurements show a surface charge of +40 to +100 mv
from pH 4 through 8.(73)  The amphibole asbestos fibers tend to
have surface layers composed predominantly of silica, with oxygens
on the surface rendering a negative charge.  Surface charge measurements of these fibers have been studied as a function of pH, ionic
strengths, and differing cation concentrations of the media (Prasad
and Pooley, 1973).(86)  The negative range of zeta potential for
the amphiboles is similar to that of quartz, but smaller in magnitude.

5.   Mineral Stability - It is known that chrysotile asbestos
possesses a chemical stability only in liquid media with pH centered
at 10.8.  Contact with solutions below this pH value results in
magnesium loss from the fiber (Hargreaves and Taylor, 1946).(87)
This instability has been noted in the mineralogical literature and
was demonstrated to take place when the fiber was retained in residence in living tissues (Morgan and Holmes, 1970;(88) Langer et
al., 1970, 1972;(89,90) Morgan et al., 1975).(91)   Chemical degradation of the amphibole minerals *in vivo* has also been observed,
mostly by electron microprobe characterization of fibers in tissues.

III.   FACTORS TO BE CONSIDERED IN ASBESTOS CARCINOGENESIS

A.   Fiber Types and Malignant Disease in Humans

Currently, all asbestos fiber types have been associated with
malignant diseases: chrysotile exposure; e.g., McDonald and
McDonald, 1976,(92) amosite exposure;(8,9) and anthophyllite exposure (Meurman et al., 1974).(93)  A detailed summary, reflecting
the world literature concerning human populations studied, is provided in Table 22.(24)

Exposure to all asbestos fiber types, with the exception of
anthophyllite, has been observed to be associated with mesothelioma
(both pleural and peritoneal); all asbestos fiber types have been
implicated as an agent with bronchogenic carcinoma; chrysotile,
crocidolite, and amosite have been associated with excess gastrointestinal cancers.  In addition to these tumors, chrysotile and/or
the amphibole fibers are implicated in excess malignancies of the
trachea, kidney, and central nervous system among insulation workers
who use all fiber types.  In addition to implication of all fibers
with many tumor types, multiple primary tumors also have been found
in single individuals exposed to asbestos.(94)

Multiple tumors in the same individual and in different individuals point to the fact that asbestos fibers disseminate once in-

haled and/or ingested. (*95,96,97,98,99,100,101,102*).  Such information and data point to the fact that a number of different organs
exist as targets for asbestos, as well as at least two major cell
types (epithelial and mesenchymal cells).

B.    Fibers in Tissues

A number of studies have been made demonstrating the presence
of asbestos fibers in the lung and extra-pulmonary tissues, of
workemn exposed to asbestos fiber. (*11,89,90,102,103,104,105,106*)
Most of these studies demonstrated the prevalence of submicroscopic
fibers in relation to those that may be observed by light microscopy.  More importantly, asbestos fibers were found in greater
abundance in individuals exposed to the material in the work environment, as compared with those in the general population (which
tended to have fewer and smaller fibers).

C.    Retention of Fibers

The presence of fibers in tissues, many years after cessation
of exposure, points to retention for long periods of time.  Retention rates experimentally determined appear to be related to the
animal model, route of administration, and fiber type involved in
exposure.  For example, rats exposed to milligram amounts of crocidolite by inhalation were observed to retain about 35%, with about
9% left 30 days later. (*107*)  In inhalation studies in rats by
Wagner et al., 1974(*108*) amphibole minerals (crocidolite and amosite) were retained, as much as 26% of the original amount being
present 18 months after cessation of exposure; however, up to 59%
of the original dosage of the larger anthophyllite fiber was retained.  Elimination rates for chrysotile were not calculated because extremely low concentrations were found as compared to the
amphibole fibers.  Since it is known that the chrysotile fiber de-
grades *in vivo*, it tends to become lost in this manner, thus com-
plicating retention estimation.

D.    Dose Response and Latent Period

Utilizing human studies in retrospective-prospective epidemiological studies, it has become apparent that the different malignant tumors possess different latent periods between first onset of
exposure to dust and clinical appearance of disease.  Lung cancer
appears to peak after some 25-30 years from onset of exposure to
the mineral dust; pleural mesothelioma, 25-30 years; peritoneal
mesothelioma, 35-40 years. (*109,110,111*)  Latent period is also influenced by dose, in that the latent period for the above disease
increases as the intensity of exposure decreases.  This was observed
for factory workers exposed to amosite. (*8,9*)  In this latter study,
holding all other factors equal, demonstrable neoplastic risk was
also found to decrease as the exposure decreased and the latency
period increased; that is, those individuals exposed for short time

periods had a significantly decreased attributable risk to neoplastic disease which, when it occurred, appeared only after a greatly extended time period.

It is of interest to note that several investigators, in experimental animal systems, have produced data suggesting that a dose-response exists for lung scarring, but not for tumor production.(112)  This was also suggested by Gold in 1970(113) who correlated the number of asbestos bodies in lung tissue with severity and extent of fibrosis, but no such correlation existed in individuals with tumors.  Importantly, an "excess" dose which may produce asbestosis in animal or man, may produce death in the organism before neoplastic change can occur.  Thus, competitive risk between asbestosis and cancer suggests that high exposures may result in asbestosis, whereas lower exposures would produce an increased life span, and a long enough latent period for the tumors to become manifest.

On the basis of examination of the best cohort studies available, coupled with exposure data, Schneiderman, in 1974(114) concluded that a zero cancer response may exist only at a zero exposure level.

E.    Cofactors in Disease

On the basis of a number of epidemiological studies of asbestos workers, it has been demonstrated that those individuals who smoke cigarettes and are exposed to asbestos incur a significantly elevated risk of developing lung cancer.(7,115,116,117)  Indeed, the risk of bronchogenic carcinoma has been demonstrated to be greater than 90 times more for the cigarette-smoking asbestos worker than for a noncigarette-smoking individual from the general population who does not work with asbestos.  Cofactors in the induction of tumors in animals have been investigated in a number of laboratory studies as well.(118,119,120)  As in the human studies, it has been demonstrated that polycyclic aromatic hydrocarbons, in addition to asbestos exposure, greatly enhances tumor risk in living organisms.

The bronchogenic carcinomas in cigarette-smoking asbestos workmen are positioned unlike the bronchogenic carcinomas found in cigarette smokers; first, they tend to occur more peripherally and not in the main bronchus or bronchi of the individual; the tumor cell type tends to be more undifferentiated and of the more virulent "oat cell" variety.

F.    Size, Shape Characteristics

Fiber size, including both diameter and length, influences the relative "toxicity" of the dust indirectly and directly.  Particle

size affects many important properties to be considered in the biological activity of dusts:  stability of the aerosol; inhalation
potential; site of reaction; migration potential; type of cellular
response; and surface area.

1.    Aerosols - Small asbestos fibers form stable aerosols in
the work environment.  Asbestos fibers are aerodynamically stable
because their falling speed is primarily determined by fiber diameter.(121)  Fiber diameters for the asbestos minerals tend to be
in the tenth micron range, which compares with falling speeds of
spherical particles in the submicron size range; therefore, asbestos
fibers tend to form stable aerosols, thereby increasing inhalation
potential and dosage.

2.    Inhalation Potential - As asbestos dust persists in the
work environment, the inhalation potential is increased.  Depending upon the concentration of the dust, the duration of exposure,
and the individuality factors involved; e.g., physiology of the
individual, etc.; the risk associated with each dust appears to
be primarily related to particle size.(122)

3.    Site of Reaction - With smaller particle size (primarily
length) there is deeper penetration to the alveolar spaces and
greater retention by means of both diffusion and inertial impaction
mechanisms.(71)  This latter study demonstrated that long fibers
(>8μm) that come to rest in the trachea and tracheal bronchial tree
are by and large eliminated, or cause fibrosis, whereas the smaller
fibers (<8μm) penetrate to the alveolar spaces and are retained.
It is of interest to note that the smallest fibers are those that
reach the mesothelial lining of both the visceral and parietal pleural surfaces.

4.    Migration Potential - Small fibers tend to be those that
migrate and that are found in extra-pulmonary organs.(102)  These
observations have been made by other investigators as well, suggesting that small fibers migrate more efficiently than large ones.

5.    Type of Cellular Response - A number of investigations
has demonstrated that the longer asbestos fibers tend to come to
rest in the upper and middle bronchial tree, whereas the majority
of shorter fibers lodge in the alveolar spaces.  Long and short
fibers in the tracheal bronchial tree tend to be eliminated in
greater amounts than those that come to rest in the more peripheral
areas.  Complete phagocytosis of short fibers and incomplete phagocytosis of long fibers, which Kuschner and Wright(123) have termed
"frustrated phagocytosis," occurs.  This incomplete phagocytosis may
lead to "leaking" of lysosomal enzymes and cell death, followed by
collagen development.  Observations, on both an experimental and a
human basis, have demonstrated that asbestosis tends to occur with

long fibers.(*124*)   Although peribronchiolar fibrosis is observed in
humans (long fibers only?) the characteristic scar pattern developed
involves septal cells as well.   Long and short fibers are implicated, although some investigators consider long fibers more potent.
Long fiber activity has carried over into the carcinogenesis area
in that some investigators consider long fibers responsible for
carcinogenesis as well.(*125,126*)   Indeed, a number of experimental
pathology studies utilizing short fiber have reported no responses
in laboratory animals, thereby dismissing short fiber ( < 5μ in
length) as biologically innocuous.(*124,127,128,129,130,131*)   It is
of interest to note that each of these investigators produced short
asbestos fiber by vigorous mechanical methods (e.g., ball-milling)
which may have significantly altered the fiber surface and biological properties.(*132*)

     Indeed, a number of workers has demonstrated short fibers to
be extremely active in a number of animal models.(*133,134,135*)
These investigators produced short fibers using special techniques
that prevented surface destruction.   They remarked that most of the
disease processes were intracellular in nature and required small
fibers at the onset.   Pott et al., 1972(*136*) and Pott and Friedrichs, 1972(*112*) noted the importance of short fibers in terms of
human carcinogenesis.   Suzuki and Churg, in 1969(*137*) noted cellular response with chrysotile fibers less than one micron in length.
These were also phagocytized by attached epithelial cells and were
observed to be present in alveolar septa where fibrosis and thick-
ened membranes indicated marked activity.   Wagner, in 1968(*138*), and
Wagner and Berry in 1969(*139*) produced more mesotheliomas with a
superfine chrysotile fiber (92% <6μ in length) than with any other
fiber used experimentally.   Indeed, this group reports that the
smaller the fiber, the greater its carcinogenic potential.(*135*)

     These investigations are supported in part by human data that
suggests that the finer crocidolite fiber encountered in the Northwest Cape Province of South Africa produces more mesotheliomas as
compared with similar fibers in the Transvaal of South Africa.(*71*)
This feature seems to support the concept that small fibers are
active in terms of carcinogenic potential.

G.    Structure of the Fiber Bundle

     It has been proposed that the physical character of asbestos
fiber is responsible for its biological acitvity; i.e., its poly-
filamentous character.(*140*)   Chrysotile asbestos was examined in
various states and it was concluded that only when chrysotile was
used in fiber bundle form did it possess biological activity.   However, monofilamentous fibrous glass has been demonstrated to produce tumors in animals;(*125*) chrysotile reduced to single fibrils
by vigorous mechanical methods produced no response in animals;(*127,
124*) which may be explained by alteration of its surface activity;

(132) "monofilamentous" chrysotile asbestos fibers used by Gross
and Hanley in 1973(140) to demonstrate lack of activity was produced by extreme heat, and thus dehydroxylated and recrystallized
into an entirely different mineral phase.(132,51)

1.    Surface Area - It has been estimated that several of the
asbestos types, especially chrysotile, may be comminuted until surface areas reach 90-100 square meters per gram of material.   Since
the surface of the alveolar spaces is about 100 square meters, vast
interaction phenomenon can be possible.   Large surface areas with
small particle sizes provide great potential for cellular interaction.

2.    Fiber Chemistry - It has been demonstrated that chrysotile
asbestos is markedly unstable in an acid environment and readily
releases magnesium in aqueous media with pH less than 10.8.(141,
142,143,144)   The in vivo degradation of asbestos has been documented as well, with magnesium loss from both chrysotile and amphibole fibers observed.(90)   Thus, fiber chemistry may play a significant role in carcinogenesis.

3.    Magnesium - Magnesium may be an important ion in controlling such reactions as cell membrane lysis (especially the red cell).
For example, sialic acid groups protrude on the surface of the cell,
with carboxyl units outermost.   These units are hydrophilic, with a
high net negative charge.   It was postulated that magnesium ion,
lost from asbestos fibers, interacts with these carboxyl groups and
by pulling on the oppositely charged glycoproteins, cross-links several of these groups at the surface, forming channels that tend to
increase the passive permeability of both potassium and sodium ions
far in excess of the normal transport system.(145)   This induces an
osmotic force within the cell, causing sodium and water accumulation,
cellular swelling and bursting.   Such an effect, it seems to us,
might not necessitate removal of magnesium from the fiber.   In fact,
magnesium structurally confined by the fiber crystalline matrix would
have the ability to stereochemically interact at membrane surfaces
at a higher effective concentration.   Experimentally, the membrane
system, hemolysis, is used to relate to cytotoxicity.(45,146)   Fiber
type and hemolytic activity are apparently related to the mesothelioma yield as observed in chrysotile-exposed rats by Wagner, in
1973.(135)   The direct relationship between these membrane studies
and carcinogenesis is presently unknown.

Macnab and Harington, in 1967(148) suggested that the relative
activities observed for the asbestos fiber types may be related to
their magnesium concentrations.   Using chelating agents specifically
for magnesium, treated fibers were observed to be far less hemolytic
than untreated fibers.   The leaching of magnesium from the fiber
also greatly decreased the hemolytic potency.   The use of several

varieties of chelating agent, calcium specific versus magnesium specific, demonstrated again the importance of magnesium in membrane interaction.(48)   A number of adsorbed chemical agents have been used to antagonize the hemolytic response.(146,148,149,150) Again, these investigations suggested the importance of magnesium. However, these chelation and adsorption studies do not preclude more complex surface mechanisms such as those involving silicate or hydroxyl groups.

  4.   Iron - A number of investigators have considered iron and several of its compounds as possibly being involved in carcinogenesis.  Some have suggested that iron plays a role in enzyme blockage, in interference with the immune system, and in upsetting iron-sensitive cellular energy dynamics and enzymatic transformations through interference with iron$^{+2}$: iron$^{+3}$ equilibrium.(151,152,153) As is the case with magnesium, the iron contents of the various asbestos fibers range greatly, and those iron-rich fibers tend to keep this cation structurally bound when in biological residence. The low iron content of certain biologically quite active fibers speaks against its being the only factor in carcinogenesis.

  5.   Silicon - The question may be posed whether silicon as a silicate entity is a chemical carcinogen.  Several investigators consider this unlikely in that silicon is normally present in man at concentrations that are detectable.(154)  However, exposed silica surfaces (whic can exist in amphibole asbestos minerals, and in chrysotile that has been degraded by organic acids in vivo) may act as powerful hydrogen-bonding agents.(155)   Nash et al. suggested that hydrogen donors, especially those of the phenol configuration, can be extremely damaging to living cells.  Silicic acid, as well as other weak acids, may act as hydrogen donors.

  6.   Hydroxyl Groups - The concept of hydrogen donors in the form of "phenolic-like" groups as damaging to living cells as discussed by Nash et al. may be the fundamental, or at least initial approach to understanding biological interaction of asbestos, which inevitably contains active surface or interlayer hydroxyl groups in the crystalline structure.  Pundsack(73) estimated that 7% of the total hydroxyl groups of chrysotile were on the surface of the fiber. Allison(145) described such hydroxyls as phenolic-like in activity, and we have found that these surface hydroxyls interact with a number of organic compounds to reduce or oxidize them.(132)  We have observed chemisorption, free radical and acid-base interactions at the surface of the fiber which suggest that the surface of chrysotile is amphoteric (as befits magnesium hydroxide).  Such reactions are attributed to surface activity related to the phenolic groups.  Both phenomena vary greatly as a function of the pretreatment of the fiber (especially heating and other manipulations which alters the surface configuration of the phenolic groups).  These

reactions occur with other magnesium silicates and amphiboles, usually to a much smaller degree, which can be accounted for at least qualitatively by the stereochemical and electronic presentation of the Mg-OH groups. Such reactions have been seen at highly reactive catalytic surfaces, e.g., for zeolites.

7. Trace Metals - As indicated previously, most of the asbestos fibers contain significant quantities of trace metals (ranging up to several thousand ppm). It is of interest to note that the concept of nickel, chromium, and cobalt activity, implicated early in asbestos carcinogenesis research as one of the mechanisms of action, is now less important. The idea lost favor mainly because of experiments wherein the same number of tumors were produced in animals utilizing fibers with and without detectable amounts of trace metals. (139,135) However, the role of trace metals may be important, and can be considered in the category of iron.

8. Adsorbed Hydrocarbons - A number of studies has suggested that the adsorbed hydrocarbons on the surfaces of the asbestos fibers are responsible for their carcinogenic properties. Again, this theory cannot account entirely for the general phenomenon of asbestos carcinogenesis, since tumors were produced in animals utilizing fiber with and without adsorbed hydrocarbons. (139,147,156) However, this concept should not be discarded since it represents many experimentally substantiated synergistic carcinogenesis studies, which parallels strikingly the asbestos-cigarette smoking lung cancer incidence in man. Furthermore, in the light of the very active chemical redox reactions observed by us and others, it is clear that the benzopyrene-asbestos synergism may be less important than interactions with more potent electron donors and acceptors, exogenous and endogenous.

It is also of interest to consider the interference of asbestos with repair mechanisms in this regard, so that the presence of the active fiber would (a) prolong the insult of a proximate carcinogen; or (b) inhibit repair processes.

The potential carcinogenicity of the hydrocarbons adsorbed on asbestos has led many investigators to study these surface compounds. Polycyclic aromatic hydrocarbons such as phenanthrene, perylene, anthracene, and the carcinogen benzpyrene, adsorb on the surface of chrysotile. (156) Adsorption of various organic polymers has been studied extensively by Schnitzer et al. (150) Indeed, specific polymers adsorb more readily to the surface of chrysotile (through interaction with the "phenolic" surface groups) whereas, others prefer the oxide surface of the amphibole asbestos fibers. Those polymers that theoretically inactivate the surface hydroxyls or magnesium by their adsorption also reduce hemolytic potency.

9.    Surface Sorption Properties - It has been noted that asbestos fibers; e.g., chrysotile, can adsorb five times more protein
from human serum than many other mineral species; e.g., quartz.(147)
The adsorption of specific substances at the surface of asbestos is
well known.   The physisorption of benzene, ethanol, hexane, and other
organic liquids has been reported, with polar molecules possessing
a greater affinity for chrysotile as compared to the amphiboles.
This subject has been investigated by Gorski and Stettler.(157)
This aspect can be independent of those discussed here; for example,
by causing an imbalance in cellular components.

        One cannot readily distinguish between true surface phen-
omenon, or physical-chemical interaction.   It is known, for example,
that proteins may be denatured at the surface of quartz particles
by interacting with the surface oxide groups with the hydrogens on
the amine groups of the proteins.(158)   This mechanism of interaction may take place at the surface of the amphibole asbestos
fibers, or at the surface of chemically degraded chrysotile.   It
has been reported that silicon may be chelated directly from the
surface by serum proteins, causing possible changes in the organic
materials.(159)   Indeed, these investigators consider the surface
of silica compounds as the key to biological interaction.   In addition, such oxide surfaces provide secondary amide-hydrogen bonding
to amino acids.(160)   The extent of this interaction in terms of
carcinogenesis is presently unknown.   In addition, direct adsorption of substances including "tumor inhibitors" has been proposed
by Oppenheimer et al.(161) and by Bischoff and Bryson.(154)

        Asbestos fibers adsorb a number of organic compounds.
These organic compounds are both endogenous to the organism and exogenous, derived from pollutants.   These materials tend to be non-
polar for the amphibole asbestos types and polar for the serpentine
asbestos variety.   The mineral surfaces can act as solid-state cata-
lysts and may reduce and/or oxidize these compounds, creating altered forms.   It has been suggested that the denaturation of proteins may produce materials that are antigenic to the host, iniat-
ing an immune response.   Protein or polysaccharide adsorption may
simply cause an undesirable concentration gradient or stereochemical
effect (e.g., membrane configuration).   Adsorption of other biochemical substrates such as those leading to hemosiderin deposition
may interfere with iron-dependent energetics (redox).   It has been
reported that silicotic nodules contain substances rich in gamma
globulin.(162)   As in the present instance, no specific antigen or
immunological factor has been observed for the asbestos minerals.

        In addition to the surface-controlled chemical phenomena,
there appears to be chemisorption which may involve specific components of the organic compounds, producing alteration to specific
sites of the organic molecule.   Again, these reactions may involve

either oxidation or reduction reaction.  Some surfaces may behave
amphoterically and may change with time as chemical degradation of
the surface proceeds, as is the case for chrysotile. (132)

## IV.  ASBESTOS ACTIVITY:  CHRYSOTILE AS A MODEL

Chrysotile may comminute to particles that are only several
hundred angstroms in diameter and a few thousand angstroms in
length.  The aerosol formed by such particles is extremely stable,
durable in the environment, and has associated with it a high inhalation potential.  The inhalation of such small fibers would
produce deposition in the alveolar spaces and the peripheral areas
of the respiratory tract.  Such fibers may have only to migrate a
short distance to reach the mesothelial surfaces of the lung and
the parietal pleura.  The fibers could be easily available to reaction to form both mesotheliomas and the peripheral lung carcinoma characteristic of asbestos exposure.  In addition to its presence in the deep regions of the lung, chrysotile may migrate to
other organs for interaction.  We have observed fibers in liver,
spleen, testicle, brain, and intestinal tissue (Langer et al., unpublished results).

Small particle sizes suggest that these fibers are easily
phagocytized and removed from the lung tissue; hence, the levels
of chrysotile observed in lung tissues (even in highly dosed experimental animals) are often very much less than observed in similar animals exposed to the amphibole fibers.  Also, the chemical
activity of chrysotile is such that one would suspect that both
phagocytosis and chemical degradation would account for a significant loss of fiber from the lung.

This very process of chemical degradation of chrysotile, however, may provide several major mechanisms for cellular interaction.
Once phagocytized by cells within the lung, the surface of chrysotile structure may readily oxidize and/or reduce organic compounds
present within the cell.  Release of magnesium may follow phenolic-
like hydroxyl group interaction, causing alteration of membrane
geometry, and cause lysis.  Denaturing of proteins, alteration of
macromolecules of various kinds, or adsorption of proteins involved
in immunological processes also may take place on the surface of
the mineral.  Trace metals may be released, or trace iron within
the structure be present, causing interference with enzyme systems
(especially those that are governed by iron equilibrium).

Chrysotile asbestos offers continuous interaction throughout
its chemical degradation ("phenolic" interaction at the surface,
oxidation-reduction reaction, magnesium release, iron and trace
metals release, silicic acid release) or even a reaction with macromolecules, merely providing a "passive" mechanism for alteration.

Indeed, all these processes may take part in its biological activity.

The greater membrane activity of chrysotile versus amphibole asbestos is, we hypothesize, a more complex event than any single potential interaction. With chrysotile, interaction may proceed through sequential layers: proton or hydrogen radical; hydroxyl ion or radical; oxide (Mg-O) ion or radical; magnesium ion; silicon-oxygen or hydroxyl group; silicon ion or radical; cation or anion substitutions (Fe, F$^-$). The various reactions through such layer stripping have extreme potential biological ramifications, especially when combined with the stereochemical control that can occur at its well-defined crystalline surfaces.

Amphibole fibers possess all of these molecular possibilities, in an entirely different sequence and chemical range.

These factors, coupled with factors that are related to the host conditions of work and the presence of other agents that might act synergistically with the fiber, underscore the complexity of the problem. Investigators in this field cannot help to amplify the observations of Bryson and Bischoff(159) who said:

> "Considering the extent to which silicates comprise
> man's environment on this planet, and bearing in
> mind the silicate-induced diseases (including
> cancer) had been recognized since antiquity, the
> sparsity of animal experimentation concerned with
> silicate carcinogenesis is striking and deplorable."

Asbestos research has gone beyond the "sparse" stage and has been increasingly detailed and focused. The problem is not so much the lack of experimentation as the complexity of mechanisms of carcinogenesis.


## REFERENCES

1.  Silverberg, E. and Holleb, A., Cancer Statistics, American Cancer Society, New York, 1972, 1971.

2.  Haddow, H. A., Health Page 23, summer 1970.

3.  Boyland, E., Prog. Exp. Tumor Research 11, Page 222, 1969.

4.  Saffioti, U., Evaluation of Environmental Carcinogens: Ad Hoc Committee on the Evaluation of Low Levels of Chemical Carcinogens, Report to the Surgeon General, USPHS, April 1970.

5.    Pott, P., _Chirurgical Observations_, Hawkes, Clarke and Collings,
      London, U.K., 1976.

6.    Hunter, D., _The Diseases of Occupations_, English University
      Press, London, 1969.

7.    Selikoff, I. J., Hammond, E. C. and Churg, J., J. American
      Medical Association _204_, Page 106, 1968.

8.    Selikoff, I. J., Nicholson, W. J. and Langer, A. M., Arch.
      Environmental Health _25_, Page 1; Selikoff, I. J., Hammond, E.
      C. and Churg, J., Ibid, Page 183, 1972.

9.    Langer, A. M., Selikoff, I. J. and Sastre, A., Arch. Environ.
      Health _22_, Page 348, 1971.

10.   Pooley, F. D., Oldham, P., Chang-Hyum, U. M. and Wagner, J. C.,
      _Pneumoconiosis_, H. A. Shapiro, Editor, Oxford University Press,
      London, Page 108, 1970.

11.   Pooley, F. D., Environmental Research _12_, Page 281, 1976.

12.   Agricola, G., _De Re Metallica_, Translated by H. and L. Hoover,
      Dover Publishing Company, New York, 1956.

13.   Zenker, F. A., Dtsch. Arch. Klin. Med. _2_, Page 116, 1867.

14.   Collis, E. L., Public Health _28_, Page 252; _29_, Page 11, 1915.

15.   Rosen, G., _The History of Miners' Disease - A Medical and
      Social Interpretation_, Shuman Co., New York, 1943.

16.   Holt, P. F., _Pneumoconiosis_, Ed. Arnold Pub., London, 1957.

17.   Aponte, G. E., _Laboratory Diagnosis of Diseases Caused by
      Toxic Agents_, F. W. Sunderman and F. W. Sunderman, Editors,
      W. H. Green, St. Louis, Page 484, 1970.

18.   Langer, A. M. and Mackler, A. D., _Encyclopedia of Geochemistry
      and Environmental Sciences_, R. Fairbridge, Editor, Van Nostrand-
      Reinhold, New York, Page 730, 1972.

19.   Mackle, W. and Gregorius, F., Public Health Reports _63_, Page
      1114, 1948.

20.   Breslow, L., American J. Public Health _44_, Page 171, 1954.

21.   Lamy, P., Senault, R., Sadoul, P., Huttin, R. and Guillerm, J.,
      J. Franc. Med. Chir. Thoraciques _13_, Page 283, 1959.

22.  Kleinfeld, M., Messite, J., Kooyman, O. and Zaki, M. H., Arch.
     Environmental Health 14, Page 663, 1967.

23.  Holaday, D., Health Phys. 16, Page 547, 1969.

24.  International Association for Research on Cancer, Monograph
     Series on the Evaluation of Carcinogenic Risk of Chemicals
     to Man 14, Asbestos. WHO, Lyon, 1977.

25.  Cooke, W. E., British Medical Journal 2, Page 1024, 1927.

26.  Lynch, K. M. and Smith, W. A., American J. Cancer 24, 56, 1935.

27.  Gloyne, S. R., Tubercle 17, Page 550, 1935.

28.  Wedler, H. W., Deutsch Med. Wschr. 69, Page 575, 1943.

29.  Wedler, H. W., Deutsch Arch Klin. Med. 191, Page 189, 1943.

30.  Doll, R., British J. Ind. Medicine 12, Page 81, 1955.

31.  Wagner, J. C., Sleggs, C. A. and Marchand, P., British J.
     Industrial Medicine 17, Page 260, 1960.

32.  Keal, E. E., Lancet, Page 1211, 3 December 1960.

33.  Selikoff, I. J., Churg, J. and Hammond, E. C., J. American
     Medical Association 188, Page 22, 1964.

34.  Harries, P. G., Annual Occupational Hygiene 11, Page 135, 1968.

35.  Bohlig, H., Dabbert, A. F., Dolquen, P., Hain, E. and Hinz, I.,
     Environmental Research 3, Page 365, 1970.

36.  Stumphius, J., British J. Industrial Medicine 28, Page 59, 1971.

37.  Edge, J. R., Environmental Research 11, Page 244, 1976.

38.  Newhouse, M. and Thompson, M., Annals New York Academy Science
     132, Page 579, 1965.

39.  Lieben, J. and Pistawka, H., Arch. Environmental Health 14,
     Page 559, 1967.

40.  Anderson, H. A., Lilis, R., Daum, S. M., Fischbein, A. S.
     and Selikoff, I. J., Annual New York Academy Science 271,
     Page 311, 1976.

41.  Harington, J. S., Prevention of Cancer, R. W. Raven, and F.
     J. C. Roe, Editors, Butterworth, London, Page 207, 1967.

42. International Association for Research on Cancer, <u>Biological Effects of Asbestos</u>,Bogovski et al.,Editors, WHO, Lyon, 1972.

43. Harington, J. S., Allison, A. C. and Badami, D. V., Adv. in Phar. and Chemo., 1975.

44. Davis, J. M. G., British J. Exp. Pathology <u>48</u>, Page 379, 1967.

45. Koshi, K., Hayashi, H. and Sakabe, H., Industrial Health <u>6</u>, Page 69, 1968.

46. Bey, E. and Harington, J.S., J.Exp.Medicine <u>133</u>, Page 1149, 1971.

47. Allison, A. C., Arch. Internal Medicine <u>128</u>, Page 131, 1971.

48. Allison, A. C., <u>Biological Effects of Asbestos</u>, <u>IARC Monographs</u>, Bogovski et al., Editors, Lyon, Page 89, 1972.

49. Miller, K. and Harington, J. S., British J. Experimental Pathology <u>53</u>, Page 397, 1972.

50. Whittaker, E. J. W., Acta Cryst. <u>13</u>, Page 291, 1960.

51. Speil, S. and Leineweber, J. P., Environmental Research <u>2</u>, Page <u>166</u>, 1969.

52. Bates, T. F., Sand, L. B. and Mink, J. F., Science <u>111</u>, Page 512, 1950.

53. Jagodzinski, H. and Kunze, G., Neu. Jahrb. f. Mineral. <u>4</u>, Page 95; <u>6</u>, Page 113, 1954.

54. Whittaker, E. J. W., Acta Cryst. <u>9</u>, pp. 855, 862, 865, 1956.

55. Zussman, J., Brindley, G. W. and Conner, J. J., American Mineral.<u>42</u>, Page 133, 1957.

56. Kalousec, G. L. and Muttart, L. E., Ibid Ref. 55, Page 1.

57. Bates, T. F., American Mineral. <u>44</u>, Page 78, 1959.

58. Maser, M., Rice, R. V. and Klug, H. P., American Mineral. <u>45</u>, Page 680, 1960.

59. Whittaker, E. J. W., Chemical Engineering News <u>9</u>, <u>30</u>, 1963.

60. Whittaker, E. J. W.,"Asbestos," <u>Fibre Structure</u>, Butterworths, London, Page 594, 1963.

61. Huggins, C. W. and Shell, H. R., American Mineral. <u>50</u>, Page 1058, 1965.

62. Clifton, R. A., Jr., Huggins, C. W. and Shell, H. R., American Mineral. 51, Page 508, 1966.

63. Yada, K., Acta Cryst. 23, Page 704, 1967.

64. Yada, K., Proceedings Conference Physics and Chemistry Asbestos, Louvain University, Belgium, Pr. 2-3, 1971.

65. Langer, A. M., Mackler, A. D. and Pooley, F. D., Environmental Health Persp. 9, Page 63, 1974.

66. Deer, W. A., Howie, R. A. and Zussman, J., Rock-Forming Minerals. Chain Silicates 2, Longmans, London, 1967.

67. Ernst, W. G., Minerals, Rocks and Inorganic Materials. Amphiboles: Chrystal Chemistry Phase Relations and Occurrence, Springer-Verlag, New York, 1963.

68. Langer, A. M. and Pooley, F. D., Biological Effects Asbestos, IARC Meeting, Bogovski et al., Editors, Lyon, Page 119, 1973.

69. Timbrell, V., Pooley, F. D. and Wagner, J. C., Pneumoconiosis, H. Shiparo, Editor, Oxford University Press, London, Page 65, 1970.

70. Timbrell, V. and Rendall, R. E. G., Powder Technology 5, Page 279, 1971.

71. Timbrell, V., Inhalation and Biological Effects of Asbestos, T. Mercen et al., Editors, Thomas, Publishers, Springfield, Illinois, Page 429, 1972.

72. Seshan, K. and Zoltai, T., Personal Communication, 1976.

73. Pundsack, F. L., J. Physical Chemistry 59, Page 892, 1955; 60, Page 361, 1956.

74. Pundsack, F. L., and Reimschussel, G., J. Phys. Chem., 60, Page 1218, 1956.

75. Nagy, B. and Faust, G. T., American Mineral 41, Page 817, 1956.

76. Brindley, G. W. and Zussman, J., American Mineral 42, Page 461, 1957.

77. Gaze, R., Annals New York Academy Science 132, Page 23, 1965.

78. Harington, J. S., Annals New York Academy Science 77, Page 458, 1965.

79. Gibbs, G. W., American Ind. Hygiene Association Journal 30, Page 458, 1969.

80.  Gibbs, G. W., Pneumoconiosis, H. A. Shapiro, Editor, Oxford
     University Press, New York, Page 165, 1970.

81.  Commins, B. T. and Gibbs, G. W., British J. Cancer 23, Page 358,
     1969.

82.  Gibbs, G. W. and Hui, H. Y., American Industrial Hygiene
     Association Journal 32, Page 519, 1971.

83.  Ayer, H. E. and Lynch, J. R., Inhaled Particles and Vapours
     II, C. N. Davies, Editor, Oxford, Pergamon Press, Page 511, 1967.

84.  Baddolet, M. S., Canadian Min. Metall. Trans. 55, Page 185, 1952.

85.  Baddolet, M. S. and Edgerton, N. W., Canadian Min. Metall.
     Bulletin 64, Page 56, 1961.

86.  Prasad, N. A. and Pooley, F. D., J. Applied Chemical Bio-
     technology 23, Page 675, 1973.

87.  Hargreaves, A. and Taylor, W. H., Mineral Magazine 27, Page 204, 1946.

88.  Morgan, A. and Holmes, A., Pneumoconiosis, H. Shapiro, Editor,
     Oxford University Press, London, Page 52, 1970.

89.  Langer, A. M., Rubin, I. B. and Selikoff, I. J., Pneumoconiosis,
     I. Webster, Editor, Oxford University Press, London, Page 57, 1970.

90.  Langer, A. M., Rubin, I. B., and Selikoff, O. J. and Pooley,
     F. D., J. Histochem. and Cytochem. 20, pp. 723 and 735, 1972.

91.  Morgan, A., Evans, J. C., Evans, R. J., Hounam, R. F., Holmes,
     A. and Doyle, S. G., Environmental Research 10, Page 196, 1975.

92.  McDonald, A. D. and McDonald, J. C., Review Franc. Mal. Resp.
     4, Page 25, 1976.

93.  Meurman, L. O., Kiviluoto, R. and Hakama, M., British J. Ind.
     Medicine 31, Page 105, 1974.

94.  Dohner, V. A., Beegle, R. G. and Miller, W. T., American Rev.
     Res. Dis. 112, Page 181, 1975.

95.  Westlake, G. E., Spjut, H. J. and Smith, M. N., Laboratory
     Investigations 14, Page 2029, 1965.

96.  Holmes, A. and Morgan, A., Nature, London 215, Page 441, 1967.

97.  Karacharova, V. N., Olshvang, R. A. and Kogan, F. M., Byull.
     Eksp. Biol. Medicine 67, Page 117, 1969.

98. Friedrichs, K. H., Hilscher, W. and Sethi, S., Int. Arch. Arbeit Med. 28, Page 341, 1971.

99. Morgan, A., Holmes, A. and Gold, C., Environmental Research 4, Page 558, 1971.

100. Morgan, A., Holmes, A. and Lally, A., Physics and Chemistry Asbestos Minerals, Pr. 2-8, Louvain University, Belgium, 1971.

101. Cunningham, H. M. and Pontefract, R. D., Nature, London 249, Page 177, 1973.

102. Langer, A. M., Environmental Health Perspective 9, Page 229, 1974.

103. Pooley, F. D., British J. Industrial Medicine 29, Page 146, 1972.

104. Pooley, F. D., Biological Effects Asbestos, IARC Monog., Bogovski et al., Editors, WHO, Lyon, Page 222, 1973.

105. Fondimare, A. and Desbordes, J., Environmental Health Perspect. 9, Page 147, 1974.

106. Sebastien, P., Fondimare, A., Bignon, J., Monchaux, G., Desbordes, J. and Bonnaud, G., Inhaled Particles and Vapours, IV., W. Walton, Editor, Pergamon, New York, 1977.

107. Evans, J. C., Evans, R. J., Holmes, A., Hounam, R. F., Jones, D. M., Morgan, A. and Walsh, M., Environmental Research 6, Page 180, 1973.

108. Wagner, J. C., Berry, G., Skidmore, J. W. and Timbrell, V., British J. Cancer 29, Page 252, 1974.

109. Selikoff, I. J., Hammond, E. C. and Churg, J., Pneumoconiosis, H. Shiparo, Editor, Oxford University Press, London, Page 180, 1970.

110. Newhouse, M., Berry, G., Wagner, J. C. and Turok, M., British J. Industrial Medicine 29, Page 134, 1972.

111. Selikoff, I. J., Annals New York Academy Science 271, Page 448, 1975.

112. Pott, F. and Friedrichs, K. H., Naturwissensch. 59, Page 318, 1972.

113. Gold, C., Unpublished report presented at Asbestos Meeting, Cardiff, PRU-MRC, April, 1970.

114. Schneiderman, M. A., Environmental Health Perspective 9, Page 207, 1974.

115. Doll, R., J. Royal Stat. Society 134, Page 133, 1971.

116. Berry, G., Newhouse, M. and Turok, M., Lancet 2, Page 476, 1972.

117. Hammond, E. C. and Selikoff, I. J., Biological Effects Asbestos, IARC Monograph, Bogovski et al., Editors, Lyon, Page 312, 1973.

118. Miller, L., Smith, W. E. and Berliner, S. W., Annals New York Academy Science 132, Page 489, 1965.

119. Vosamaë, A., Annual Report, IARC, Page 46, 1971.

120. Pylev, L. N., Vop. Oncology 40, 1972.

121. Timbrell,V., Annals New York Academy Science, 132,Page 255, 1965.

122. Klösterkotter, W. and Robock, K., American Industrial Hyg. Association Journal 35, Page 659, 1975.

123. Kuschner, M. and Wright, G., Proceedings Symposium Occupational Exposure to Fibrous Glass, HEW-PHS, Page 151, 1976.

124. Klösterkotter, W., International Conference Biological Effects Asbestos, Dresden, Holstein and Anspach, Editors, DDR, 449, 1968.

125. Stanton, M. F. and Wrench, C., J. National Cancer Institute 48, Page 797, 1972.

126. Stanton, M. F., Biological Effects Asbestos, IARC Monograph, Bogovski et al., Editors, 289, 1973.

127. Reeves, A. L., Puro, H. E. and Smith, R. G., Environmental Research 8, Page 178, 1974.

128. Vorwald, A. J., Durkan, T. M. and Pratt, P. C., Arch. Indust. Hygiene 3, Page 1, 1951.

129. Timbrell, V. and Skidmore, J. W., International Conference Biological Effects Asbestos, Anspach and Holstein, Editors, Dresden, DDR, Page 52, 1968.

130. Webster, I., Pneumoconiosis, H. Shapiro, Editor, Oxford University Press, London, Page 209, 1970.

131. Hilscher, W., Sethi, S., Friedrichs, K. H. and Pott, F., Naturwissensch. 57, Page 356, 1970.

132. Langer, A. M., Wolff, M. S., Rohl, A. N. and Selikoff, I. J., J. Toxicology and Environmental Health, 1977.

133. Holt, P. F., Mills, J. and Young, D. R., J. Pathology and Bacteriology 87, Page 15, 1964.

134. Davis, J. M. G., British J. Exp. Pathology 45, Page 634, 1964.

135. Wagner, J. C., Berry, G. and Timbrell, V., British J. Cancer 28, Page 173, 1973.

136. Pott, F., Huth, F. and Friedrichs, K. H., Zentralbl. Bakteriol. Hyg., 155, Page 463, 1972.

137. Suzuki, Y. and Churg, J., American J. Pathology 55, Page 79, Environmental Research 3, Page 107, 1969.

138. Wagner, J. C., International Conference Biological Effects of Asbestos, Anspach and Holstein, Editors, Dresden, DDR, 223, 1968.

139. Wagner, J. C. and Berry, G., British J. Cancer 23, Page 567, 1969.

140. Gross, P. and Hanley, R. A., Arch. Environmental Health 27, Page 240, 1973.

141. Clark, S. G. and Holt, P. F., Annual Occupational Hygiene 3, Page 22, 1960.

142. Faust, G. T. and Nagy, B., American Mineral. 41, 819, 1965.

143. Monkman, L. J., Physics and Chemistry of Asbestos, 1971.

144. Atkinson, A. W. and Rickards, A. L., Physics and Chemistry of Asbestos, Abstract Pr. 3-1, Louvain University, Belgium, 1971.

145. Allison, A. C., The Regulation of Proliferation in Animal Cells, Cold Spring Harbor Press, New York, 1974.

146. Harington, J. S., Miller, K. and Macnab, G., Environmental Research 4, pp. 95 and 118, 1971.

147. Wagner, J. C., Recent Results Cancer Research, 39, Page 37, 1972.

148. Macnab, G. and Harington, J. S., Nature, London, 214, Page 522, 1967.

149. Schnitzer, R. J., Bunesco, G., Arch. Environmental Health 20, Page 481, 1970.

150. Schnitzer, R. J. Bunesco, G. and Baden, V., Annual New York Academy Science 172, Page 757, 1971.

151. Richmond, H. G., British Medical Journal 1, Page 947, 1959.

152. Kunze, J., Shahab, L. Henze, K. and David, H., Acta Biol. Med. Germ. 10, Page 602, 1963.

153. Flowers, E., American Industrial Hygiene Association Journal 35, Page 724, 1975.

154. Bryson, G. and Bischoff, F., Fed. Proceedings 23, Page 106, 1964.

155. Nash, T., Allison, A. C. and Harington, J. S., Nature, London 210, Page 259, 1966.

156. Wagner, J. C., Hygiene Standard for Airborne Amosite Asbestos Dust, from Comm. Report, BOHS 6, 1970.

157. Gorski, C. H. and Stettler, L. E., American Industrial Hygiene Association Journal 36, Page 292, 1975.

158. Scheel, L. D., Smith, B., Van Riper, J. and Fleisher, E., Arch. Industrial Hygiene 9, Page 29, 1954.

159. Bryson, G. and Bischoff, F., Prog. Exp. Tumor Research 9, Page 77, 1967.

160. Holt, P. F. and Osborne, S. G., British J. Industrial Medicine 10, Page 152, 1953.

161. Oppenheimer, B. S., Oppenheimer, E. T., Stout, A. R., Danishefsky, I. and Eirich, F. R., Science 118, Page 783, 1953.

162. Vigliani, E. C. and Pernis, B., Pneumoconiosis, A. Orenstein, Editor, Little, Brown & Co., Boston, Page 395, 1960.

*CHAPTER 4*

CARCINOGENICITY OF NICKEL SUBSULFIDE IN FISCHER RATS
AND SYRIAN HAMSTERS AFTER ADMINISTRATION BY VARIOUS ROUTES

F. William Sunderman, Jr., Ronald M. Maenza, Patricia R. Alpass,
John M. Mitchell, Ivan Damjanov and Peter J. Goldblatt

Departments of Laboratory Medicine and Pathology
University of Connecticut School of Medicine
Farmington, Connecticut   06032

I.   INTRODUCTION

The carcinogenicity of nickel compounds in industrial workers
and in experimental animals has been comprehensively reviewed in
several publications. (*1-5*)  Increased incidences of cancers of the
lung and nasal cavities have been documented by epidemiological
investigations of nickel refinery workers in Wales, (*6,7*) Canada, (*8,0*)
Norway, (*10*) and Russia. (*11*)  One of the present authors (Sunderman)
maintains a tabulation of respiratory cancers that have occurred in
workers who were exposed to nickel compounds in industrial operations.
As of January 1977, this tabulation included 447 cases of lung cancer and 142 cases of cancers of the nose and paranasal sinuses.  In
addition to increased risk of respiratory tract cancers, increased
risk of laryngeal cancers has been found in Norwegian nickel refinery
workers, (*10*) and increased risk of gastric carcinomas and soft tissue
sarcomas have been reported in Russian nickel refinery workers. (*11*)
Three cases of renal cancer occurred among 225 Canadian workers who
were involved in electrolytic refining of nickel. (*8*)  Since renal
cancer is rare, it seems possible that the renal cancers in these
workers might have been related to occupational exposures to nickel
compounds.  To date, the identity of the nickel compounds that induce cancers in nickel workers remains uncertain, although principal
attention is currently focused upon (a) insoluble dusts of nickel
subsulfide ($Ni_3S_2$) and nickel oxides ($NiO$; $Ni_2O_3$); (b) the vapor of
nickel carbonyl ($Ni(CO)_4$); and (c) soluble aerosols of nickel sulfate
or chloride ($NiSO_4$, $NiCl_2$). (*2,4,12*)

57

Cancers have been induced in experimental animals by administration of several nickel compounds by a variety of routes, as
summarized in Table 1.  Pulmonary carcinomas have developed in rats
following inhalation of $Ni(CO)_4$ and $Ni_3S_2$ (16,17,26) and carcinomas
of the cranial sinuses have developed in cats following implantation
of $Ni_3S_2$ discs.(23)  In most of the studies that are listed in
Table 1, the malignant neoplasms developed locally at the site of
the exposure, injection or implantation.  However, Stoner et al.(28)
have recently observed pulmonary carcinomas in mice that received
repeated intraperitoneal injections of nickel acetate; therefore,
it appears likely that certain nickel compounds may induce tumors
at sites that are distant from the point of primary contact.  In
the present study, the possibility of developing additional experimental models of nickel carcinogenesis has been explored by admini-
stering $Ni_3S_2$ to hamsters and rats by several previously untested
routes.  $Ni_3S_2$ was selected for use in this study, since Payne,(30)
Gilman,(31) and Sunderman and Maenza(32) have found that $Ni_3S_2$ is
the most highly carcinogenic of the nickel compounds that have been
evaluated in experimental animals.


## II.   MATERIALS AND METHODS

The experimental animals were 113 male hamsters of the Syrian
LVG/LAK strain and 103 male albino rats of the Fischer 344 strain.
The hamsters and rats were obtained from Charles River Breeding
Laboratories, North Wilmington, Massachusetts, and were approx-
imately two months old at the time that the carcinogenesis tests
were initiated.  The animals were housed, fed, weighed, and examined
as described in previous studies.(33,34)  The $Ni_3S_2$ dust (median
particle diameter 1.4 μm) was provided by INCO Ltd, Toronto, Canada.
The $Ni_3S_2$ dust contained 72% Ni and 28% S by weight.  The $Ni_3S_2$ dust
was analyzed for Al, Co, Cu, Cr, Fe, and Mn by emission spectroscopy
(J. R. Gordon Research Laboratory, INCO Ltd, Clarkson, Ontario,
Canada) and contamination by these metals was found to be less than
0.01% by weight.  The $Ni_3S_2$ dust did not contain detectable NiO or
NiS, based upon X-ray diffraction analyses (Institute of Materials
Science, University of Connecticut, Storrs, Connecticut).

Glycerol ("certified reagent," Fisher Scientific Company,
Pittsburgh, Pennsylvania) was used as the vehicle for local bilateral
applications of $Ni_3S_2$ onto the cheek pouches of hamsters.  The cheek
pouch applications were performed as described by Shklar(35) without
anesthesia, according to the dosages and schedules listed in Table 2.
The requisite amounts of $Ni_3S_2$ were suspended in 0.2 ml of glycerol,
and 0.1 ml of the $Ni_3S_2$-glycerol suspension was carefully painted
over the mucosa of each of the cheek pouches three times weekly, for
the specified number of weeks.  9,10-Dimethyl-1, 1-benzanthracene
(DMBA) (K and K Laboratories, Plainview, New York) was prepared as

TABLE 1

EXPERIMENTAL MODELS OF NICKEL CARCINOGENESIS

| Authors | Animals | Compounds | Routes | Tumors |
|---|---|---|---|---|
| HUEPER[13,14] | Rats & rabbits | Ni dust | Intraosseous & intrapleural | Sarcomas |
| HUEPER[15] | Guinea pigs | Ni dust | Inhalation | Anaplastic & adenocarcinomas (lung) |
| SUNDERMAN, et al.[16,17] | Rats | $Ni(CO)_4$ | Inhalation | Epidermoid, anaplastic & adenocarcinomas (lung) |
| GILMAN[18] | Rats & mice | $Ni_3S_2$, NiO dusts | Intramuscular | Rhabdomyosarcomas |
| HEATH, et al.[19,20] | Rats | Ni dust | Intramuscular | Rhabdomyosarcomas |
| FURST, et al.[21,22] | Rats & hamsters | Nickelocene | Intramuscular | Sarcomas |
| GILMAN[23] | Cats | $Ni_3S_2$ discs | Sinus implants | Epidermoid & adenocarcinomas, sarcomas |
| LAU, et al.[24] | Rats | $Ni(CO)_4$ | Intravenous | Carcinomas & sarcomas |
| FURST & CASSETTA[25] | Rats | Ni dust | Intrathoracic, Intraperitoneal | Mesotheliomas |
| OTTOLENGHI, et al.[26] | Rats | $Ni_3S_2$ | Inhalation | Epidermoid & adenocarcinomas (lung) |
| SOSINSKI[27] | Rats | $Ni_2O_3$ | Intracerebral | Sarcomas & meningiomas |
| STONER, et al.[28] | Mice | Ni acetate | Intraperitoneal | Adenocarcinomas (lung) |
| JASMIN & RIOPELLE[29] | Rats | $Ni_3S_2$ | Intrarenal | Adenocarcinomas |

TABLE 2

CANCER INCIDENCE IN SYRIAN HAMSTERS
FOLLOWING ADMINISTRATION OF $Ni_3S_2$

| Group | Route | $Ni_3S_2$ mg/dose | Dosage Schedule | Mortality Ratios | Cancers at site | Distant Metastases |
|-------|-------|-------------------|-----------------|------------------|-----------------|--------------------|
| A | Intra-muscular | Vehicle Controls (NaCl) | 1x | 14/14 | 0/14 | |
| B | " | 5 | 1x | 11/15 | 5/15[a,b] | 2/4 |
| C | " | 10 | 1x | 17/17 | 12/17[c,d] | 8/12 |
| D | Buccal Pouch | Vehicle Controls (glycerol) | 3x/wk, 18 wk | 6/6 | 0/6[e] | |
| E | " | Positive Controls (DMBA) | " | 4/4 | 4/4[g,h] | 0/4 |
| F | " | 1 | " | 6/6 | 0/6 | |
| G | " | 2 | " | 5/7 | 0/7 | |
| H | " | Vehicle Controls (glycerol) | 3x/wk, 36 wk | 14/15 | 0/15 | |
| I | " | 5 | " | 11/15 | 0/15[i,j] | |
| J | " | 10 | " | 12/13 | 0/13[i] | |

---

[a] $P < 0.05$ *vs* group A, computed by $\chi^2$ test.

[b] Rhabdomyosarcoma (1), fibrosarcomas (2), undifferentiated sarcomas (2).

[c] $P < 0.005$ *vs* group A, computed by $\chi^2$ test.

[d] Rhabdomyosarcomas (5), fibrosarcomas (2), undifferentiated sarcomas (3).

[e] One hamster had an abdominal lymphoma.

[f] Dimethylbenzanthracene (1 mg/dose).

[g] $P < 0.02$ *vs* group D, computed by $\chi^2$ test.

[h] Squamous cell carcinomas (4).

[i] All hamsters had papillary hyperplasia of buccal mucosa.

[j] One hamster had a pleural mesothelioma.

an 0.5% (w/v) solution in glycerol, and 0.1 ml of the DMBA-glycerol solution was painted over the mucosa of each of the cheek pouches of hamsters in a "positive control" group (group E).  The glycerol vehicle was likewise applied to the cheek pouches of hamsters in "vehicle control" groups (groups A and H).

For parenteral administrations to hamsters and rats, $Ni_3S_2$ dust was suspended in sterile NaCl solution (140 mmole/liter) or in glycerol, and injected as a single dose in a volume of 0.2 to 0.5 ml, using a 1 ml tuberculin syringe with 25-gauge needle, according to the dosages listed in Table 3.  Intramuscular (*im*) injections of $Ni_3S_2$ in saline were made deep into the lateral musculature of the right hind limb at the midlength of the thigh.  Intratesticular injections of $Ni_3S_2$ in saline were made into the center of the right testis.  For hepatic administration of $Ni_3S_2$, rats were anesthetized with diethyl ether and the abdomen was opened by midline incision.  A needle was inserted into a mesenteric vein and threaded into the portal vein.  After injection of 0.5 ml of $Ni_3S_2$-saline suspension, bleeding from the mesenteric vein was controlled with "gel-foam;" the abdominal musculature was sutured with silk thread and the skin incision was closed with surgical clips.  For submaxillary gland administration, rats were anesthetized with diethyl ether and the skin over the right submaxillary gland was incised.  After direct intraglandular injection of 0.2 ml of $Ni_3S_2$-glycerol suspension, the skin over the submaxillary gland was closed with surgical clips.

The hamsters and rats were housed in separate animal rooms, and were isolated from other experimental animals throughout the study.  Two rats died within two months after the initiation of the tests, and these rats were excluded from computations of tumor incidences.  Animals that survived 24 months after the initiation of the tests were killed.  All of the animals were autopsied and their tissues were examined by light microscopy.  Classification of sarcomas was based upon the histological criteria of Stout and Lattes.(*36*)

### III.  RESULTS

The results of carcinogenesis tests in Syrian hamsters are summarized in Table 2.  No sarcomas occurred at the injection site in 14 control hamsters (group A) that received a single *im* injection of 0.5 ml of NaCl solution.  The incidence of sarcomas at the injection site was 5/15 (33%) in hamsters of group B that received 5 mg *im* of $Ni_3S_2$, and 12/17 (71%) in hamsters of group C that received 10 mg *im* of $Ni_3S_2$.  Distant metastases (lung, mediastinal lymph nodes, and/or liver) occurred in 10/16 (63%) of the sarcoma-bearing hamsters.

TABLE 3

CANCER INCIDENCE IN FISCHER RATS
FOLLOWING ADMINISTRATION OF $Ni_3S_2$

| Group | Route | $Ni_3S_2$ mg/rat | Mortality Ratios | Cancers at site | Distant Metastases |
|-------|-------|------------------|------------------|-----------------|--------------------|
| K | Intramuscular | Vehicle Controls (NaCl) | 16/20 | 0/20 | |
| L | " | 10 | 22/23 | 22/23[a,b] | 17/22 |
| M | Submaxillary gland | 2.5 | 8/11 | 0/11 | |
| N | Liver | Vehicle Controls (NaCl) | 5/6 | 0/6 | |
| O | " | 5 | 10/13 | 0/13[c] | |
| P | Testis | Vehicle Controls (NaCl) | 9/18[d] | 0/18[d] | |
| Q | " | 10 | 17/19[d] | 16/19[d,e,f] | 3/16[d] |

[a] $P < 0.0005$ vs group K, computed by $\chi^2$ test.

[b] Rhabdomyosarcomas (15), fibrosarcomas (2), undifferentiated sarcoma.

[c] One rat had distinct hyperplastic hepatic nodules, and one rat had a carcinoma of the abdominal wall.

[d] Preliminary data. Rats in groups P & Q have been followed for only 18 months after injection.

[e] $P < 0.0005$ vs group P, computed by $\chi^2$ test.

[f] Rhabdomyosarcomas (3), fibrosarcomas (10), giant cell sarcoma (3).

No tumors developed in the cheek pouches, oral cavity, or gastro-intestinal tracts of 21 hamsters in the "vehicle control" groups (groups D and H) that were given repeated cheek pouch applications

of the glycerol vehicle. Squamous cell carcinomas of the cheek
pouches were present in 4/4 (100%) of hamsters in the "positive
control" group (group E) that received multiple applications of
dimethylbenzanthracene (DMBA) in glycerol. No malignant neoplasms
occurred in the cheek pouches, oral cavity, or gastrointestinal
tracts of hamsters in any of the groups (groups F, G, I, and J)
that were treated with multiple applications of $Ni_3S_2$-glycerol
suspension in the cheek pouches. Focal or generalized papillary
hyperplasia of the buccal mucosa was found in all of the hamsters
in groups I and J that received $Ni_3S_2$ applications in the cheek
pouches at dosages of 5 or 10 mg, three times weekly for 36 weeks.
Such hyperplastic changes were not observed in any of the corresponding controls (group H). The only malignant neoplasms that were
found in groups D to J were (a) an abdominal lymphoma involving the
liver and intestines of a hamster of group D; and (b) a pleural
mesothelioma in a hamster of group I.

The results of carcinogenesis tests in Fischer rats are summarized in Table 3. No tumors occurred at the injection site in
control rats in groups K, N, or P that received the NaCl vehicle
solution by intramuscular, intrahepatic, or intratesticular routes.
Sarcomas developed at the injection site in 22/23 (97%) of rats in
group L that were given an $im$ injection of 10 mg of $Ni_3S_2$. This
is consistent with results of a previous study(34) in which carco-
mas occurred at the injection site in 28/30 (93%) of rats that were
given a single $im$ injection of 2.5 mg of $Ni_3S_2$, and in 29/30 (97%)
of rats that received a single $im$ injection of 5 mg of $Ni_3S_2$. In
rats in group L, the incidence of distant metastases was 17/22 (77%).

No malignant neoplasms occurred in the submaxillary gland of
rats of group M that received a single local injection of $Ni_3S_2$, or
in rats of group 0 that received a single intrahepatic injection of
$Ni_3S_2$ via mesenteric and portal veins. However, one rat in group 0
had distinct microscopic foci of hepatocellular hyperplasia, and
another rat in group 0 developed a sebaceous carcinoma of the abdominal wall.

Rats in groups P and Q have only been followed for 18 months
after the intratesticular injection, and the 11 presently surviving rats in group P, and two presently surviving rats in group Q
will not be killed until 24 months after the injection. However,
the difference in tumor incidences in these two groups is already
highly significant (P<0.0005 by $\chi^2$ test). Sarcomas of the testis
have developed in 16/19 (84%) of $Ni_3S_2$-treated rats (group Q), and
pulmonary metastases were found in 3/16 (19%) of the sarcoma-bearing
rats. Excepting the sarcomas at the injection sites in groups L and
Q and the carcinoma of the abdominal wall of a rat in group 0, no
other malignant tumors were found in any of the experimental groups
of rats (groups K to Q).

## IV.  DISCUSSION

This investigation has demonstrated that $Ni_3S_2$ is highly carcinogenic in Syrian hamsters following a single *im* injection.  The
59% incidence of tumors in hamsters that received 10 mg of $Ni_3S_2$
(group C) may be compared to (a) a tumor incidence of 14% (4/29)
in Syrian hamsters that received a single *im* injection of 25 mg of
nickelocene; and (b) a tumor incidence of 4% (2/50) in Syrian hamsters that received 5 *im* injections of 5 mg of Ni dust at monthly
intervals, as previously reported by Furst and Schlauder.(22)  The
carcinogenicity of $Ni_3S_2$ has not been previously tested in hamsters
following administration by any route.  The lack of malignant neoplasms in the cheek pouches, oral cavities or gastrointestinal
tracts of hamsters in groups G to J that received multiple buccal
applications of $Ni_3S_2$ is remarkable, in view of the very large total
dosages of $Ni_3S_2$ that the hamsters received.  Thus, hamsters in
group J were given 10 mg of $Ni_3S_2$ for 108 applications, comprising
a total dosage of approximately 1.1 g of $Ni_3S_2$.

This study has also indicated that Fischer rats are very susceptible to development of sarcomas of the testes following a single
intratesticular injection of $Ni_3S_2$.  It is particularly notable that
rhabdomyosarcomas of the testis were found by 18 months in 3/19 (16%)
of $Ni_3S_2$-treated rats, since the rat testis is normally devoid of
striated muscle cells.  As previously mentioned, this portion of the
study is still in progress, and the final results will be subsequently reported.  Negative results were obtained in the carcinogenesis tests of $Ni_3S_2$ following administration to rats by the
intrahepatic route (*via* the portal venous system), and by injection
into the submaxillary gland.  On the basis of the present study, as
well as previous investigations that have been cited in Table 1,
rodents appear to be more susceptible to $Ni_3S_2$-carcinogenesis in
muscle, lung, kidney, and testis than in buccal mucosa, gastrointestinal tract , salivary gland, and liver.  This speculation is
consistent with a recent report by Bruni(37) that primitive meso-
dermal stem cells ("satellite cells") may be particularly susceptible to malignant transformation by $Ni_3S_2$.

## V.  SUMMARY

In an endeavor to expand the variety of experimental models for
study of nickel carcinogenesis, nickel subsulfide ($Ni_3S_2$) was
administered to rodents by five previously untested routes.  In two
groups of Syrian hamsters, $Ni_3S_2$ induced multiple sarcomas at the
sites of single *im* injections (5 or 10 mg of $Ni_3S_2$).  In contrast,
$Ni_3S_2$ did not induce any malignant tumors of the cheek pouches,
oral cavity or gastrointestinal tract, despite multiple local
applications to the cheek pouches of several groups of hamsters in
total dosages as large as 1.1 g of $Ni_3S_2$.  In a group of Fischer

rats, single intratesticular injections of $Ni_3S_2$ (10 mg) induced many testicular sarcomas. In contrast, no malignant tumors developed in two groups of rats that received single injections into the submaxillary gland (2.5 mg of $Ni_3S_2$) or into the liver (5 mg of $Ni_3S_2$ *via* the portal venous system).

## ACKNOWLEDGEMENTS

This investigation was supported by grants from (a) U. S. Energy Research and Development Administration (E-(11-1)-3140); (b) National Institute of Environmental Health Sciences (ES-01337); and (c) International Nickel Company Ltd. The authors are grateful to Dr. Leif Washer, Dr. Leslie Cutler, Dr. Louis Renzoni, and Mrs. Elizabeth Metchell for valuable assistance.

## REFERENCES

1.  Anonymous, "Nickel and Nickel Compounds," in IARC Monographs on the Evaluation of the Carcinogenic Risk of Chemicals to Man, Lyon, International Agency for Cancer Research 11, pp. 75-112, 1976.

2.  Sunderman, F. W., Jr., and Mastromatteo, E., "Nickel Carcinogenesis," in NAS Monographs on Medical and Biological Effects of Environmental Pollutants, Nickel, U. S. Academy Science, pp. 144-188, Washington, D. C., 1975.

3.  Sunderman, F. W., Jr., Annual Clin. Lab. Science 3, Page 156, 1973.

4.  Sunderman, F. W., Jr., Prev. Med. 5, Page 279, 1976.

5.  Fishbein, L., J. Tox. Environmental Health 2, Page 77, 1976.

6.  Doll, R., Morgan, L. G. and Speizer, F. E., British J. Cancer 24, Page 623, 1970.

7.  Doll, R., Mathews, J. D. and Morgan, L. G., British J. Industrial Medicine, in press.

8.  Sutherland, R. B., Report Ontario Dept. Health, pp. 1-153, 1953.

9.  Matromatteo, E., J. Occup. Med. 9, Page 127, 1967.

10.  Pedersen, E., Høgetveit, A. C. and Andersen, A., Intern. J.
     Cancer 12, 1973.

11.  Saknyn, A. V. and Shabynina, N. K., Gig. Trud. Prof. Z. Vol.
     14(11), Page 10, 1970.

12.  Høgetveit, A. C. and Barton, R. T., J. Occup. Med. 18, Page
     805, 1976.

13.  Hueper, W. C., Texas Rep. Biol. Med. 10, Page 167, 1952.

14.  Hueper, W. C., J. National Cancer Inst. 16, Page 55, 1955.

15.  Hueper, W. C., Arch. Path. 65, Page 600, 1958.

16.  Sunderman, F. W., Donnelly, A. J., West, B. and Kincaid, J. F.,
     Arch. Ind. Health 20, Page 36, 1959.

17.  Sunderman, F. W. and Donnelly, A. J., American J. Pathology 46,
     Page 1027, 1965.

18.  Gilman, J. P. W., Cancer Research 22, Page 158, 1962.

19.  Heath, J. C. and Daniel, M. R., British J. Cancer 21, Page 768,
     1967.

20.  Heath, J. C. and Webb, M., British J. Cancer 21, Page 768, 1967.

21.  Haro, R. T., Furst, A., Payne, W. W. and Falk, H., Proceedings
     American Association Cancer Research 9, Page 28, 1968.

22.  Furst, A. and Schlauder, M. C., Proceedings West. Pharmacol.
     Society 14, Page 68, 1971.

23.  Gilman, J. P. W., Personal Communication to F. W. Sunderman,
     Jr., 1970.

24.  Lau, T. C., Hackett, R. L. and Sunderman, F. W., Jr., Cancer
     Research 32, Page 2253, 1972.

25.  Furst, A. and Cassetta, D., Proceedings American Association
     Cancer Research 14, Page 31, 1973.

26.  Ottolenghi, A. D., Haseman, J. K., Payne, W. W., Falk, H. L.
     and MacFarland, H. N., J. National Cancer Institute 54, Page
     1165, 1975.

27.  Sosinski, E., Neuropt. Pol. 13, Page 479, 1975.

28. Stoner, G. D., Shimkin, M. B., Troxell, M. C., Thompson, T. L. and Terry, L. S., Cancer Research 36, Page 1744, 1976.

29. Jasmin, G. and Riopelle, J. L., Lab. Invest. 35, Page 71, 1976.

30. Payne, W. W., Proceedings American Association Cancer Research 5, Page 50, 1964.

31. Gilman, J. P. W., Proceedings Sixth Canadian Cancer Research Conference, pp. 209-223, 1965.

32. Sunderman, F. W., Jr. and Maenza, R. M., Res. Commun. Chemical Path. Pharmacol. 14, Page 319, 1976.

33. Sunderman, F. W., Jr., Lau, T. J. and Cralley, L. J., Cancer Research 34, Page 92, 1974.

34. Sunderman, F. W., Jr., Kasprzak, K. S., Lau, T. J., Minghetti, P. P., Maenza, R. M., Becker, N., Onkelinx, C. and Goldblatt, P. J., Cancer Research 36, Page 1970, 1976.

35. Shklar, G., Prog. Exp. Tumor Research 16, Page 518, 1972.

36. Stout, A. P. and Lattes, R., Atlas Tumor Pathology, Armed Forces Institute Pathology, Washington, D. C., Series 2, Fascicle 1, pp. 1-197, 1967.

37. Bruni, C., Proceedings American Association Cancer Research 17, Page 178, 1976.

*CHAPTER 5*

THE TOPICAL EFFECTS OF NICKEL SUBSULFIDE
ON RENAL PARENCHYMA*

Gaëtan Jasmin
and
Béla Solymoss

Départment de Pathologie
Faculté de Médecine
Université de Montréal

## I.  INTRODUCTION

Earlier investigations have shown that nickel subsulfide ($Ni_3S_2$) is a potent carcinogen when injected intramuscularly in rats.(1,2) More recently we found that intrarenal injection of this metal salt causes malignant tumors in the rat kidney.(3,4)  Interestingly, these animals become plethoric soon after application of the carcinogen and the reaction subsides after removal of the injected kidney.(5)  The early cellular changes mainly involve the distal tubule lining cells with typical inclusions in the nuclei and the mitochondria.(6)  So far, these events are only demonstrable in the rat, and there is, as yet, no clear-cut evidence that they are interrelated. In the present paper, we shall report these and other pertinent findings regarding the topical effects of $Ni_3S_2$ on the kidney parenchyma.

---

*

This work was supported by a grant from the Medical Research Council of Canada (No. MA-1827).

## II.   MATERIALS AND METHODS

Our investigations were performed with finely powdered $Ni_3S_2$ kindly supplied by Dr. L. Renzoni (International Nickel Company, Toronto, Ontario).  The particles were gold coated on a glass cover slip ($\simeq$ 100 Angstroms) and examined under a JSM-50A scanning microscope with an accelerating voltage of 20 kv; their mean diameter approximated 2.5 μ (Figure 1).  They consisted in 73% Ni and 27% S. The metal salt was suspended in normal saline or glycerin, homogenized in a Polytron, and administered at the dose levels and by the routes indicated in the tables.  The technique used for intrarenal injection is illustrated in Figure 2.  Briefly, the right kidney was exteriorized through a costo-lumbar incision, under ether anesthesia, and 5 mg of $Ni_3S_2$ was injected into each pole with a 23-gauge needle.  To prevent reflux of the metal suspension into the abdominal cavity, the needle was slowly withdrawn while gentle pressure was applied to the kidney.

Female Sprague-Dawley rats (Canadian Breeding Farms & Laboratories Ltd., St. Constant, Quebec) were used in most experiments, but optimal results were obtained with a Fischer-344 inbred strain. The animals (40-60 days old) were housed in appropriate cages under controlled room temperature with free access to Purina laboratory chow and tap water.  They were killed by exsanguination; the techniques employed for the hematologic and microscopic studies have been described elsewhere.(4)

## III.   OBSERVATIONS

### Routes of Administration

The carcinogenicity of $Ni_3S_2$ in relation to the site of application is reported in Table 1.  Injection of the metal salt into the rat gastrocnemius muscle produced rhabdomyosarcomas; the tumor incidence could be increased by treatment with a myotrophic steroid.(7)

When injected into each pole of the kidney, $Ni_3S_2$ elicited renal carcinomas which propagated in the abdominal cavity, often with metastasis in the lungs.  This effect was only demonstrable in rats; other species tested (mice, hamsters, and rabbits) were found unresponsive in this respect.  The liver parenchyma, on the other hand, was insensitive to the topical action of the carcinogen.

When injected intravenously, $Ni_3S_2$ tended to accumulate in the lungs, causing fibrotic nodules with no evidence of neoplastic changes, even after one year.  One animal so treated developed myeloid leukemia and several others showed mammary carcinomas.

TABLE 1

CARCINOGENICITY OF NICKEL SUBSULFIDE ($Ni_3S_2$) INJECTED AT DIFFERENT SITES IN RATS

| $Ni_3S_2$ Treatment | No. of affected rats | Primary tumors* Type | Primary tumors* Average time of appearance (days) | Tumor extension** | Other tumors** |
|---|---|---|---|---|---|
| Intramuscular (10 mg in 0.2 ml saline into gastrocnemius m) | 5/15 | Rhabdomyosarcomas | 176 ± 10 | Lungs (2) | |
| Intrarenal (5 mg in 0.05 ml glycerin into each pole) | 11/20 | Renal carcinomas | 302 ± 28 | Mesentery (6) Lungs (5) Liver (2) | Mammary adenomas and/or carcinomas (2) |
| Intrahepatic (5 mg in 0.05 ml glycerin into two separate lobes) | 0/8 | | | | |
| Intravenous (10 mg in 1 ml saline into jugular vein) | 0/20 | | | | Myeloid leukemia(1) Mammary adenomas and/or carcinomas (8) |

* Animals treated with the control vehicle showed occasional mammary nodules but no tumors.

** Figures in parentheses indicate number of rats.

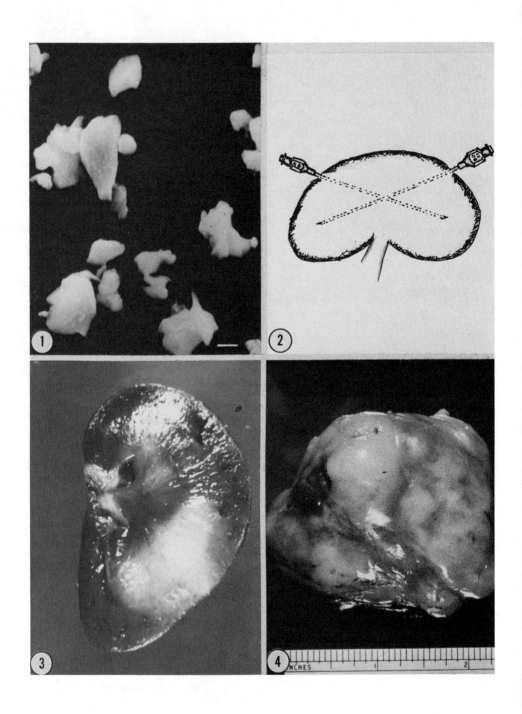

## Morphology of the Renal Tumors

These tumors often developed after eight months, and in some instances, they were found within six months.

The neoplastic growth was fairly well demarcated in the early stages. It invaded the renal parenchyma by contiguity (Figure 3) and extended through the hilar region or bulged on the surface of the kidney. Some tumors reached four to five cubic centimeters and weighed over 100 gm (Figure 4). After routine staining, several neoplasms showed a spindle-cell arrangement, creating somewhat the impression of mesenchymal growth (Figure 5). Staining of thin sections with periodic acid-silver methenamine delineated the ana-plastic carcinoma cells (Figure 6) and outlined the flexuous, trab-ecular, or tubular arrangements. An epithelial pattern was usually exhibited by friable tumors, and this was also apparent in the lung and liver metastases (Figures 7 and 8).

Ultrastructurally, the neoplastic cells often showed surface specialization with numerous villi and junctional complexes similar to those of immature nephrons (Figures 9 and 10). The number of organelles varied greatly from cell to cell, and usually there were large, swollen mitochondria, a few cisternae of rough ER, abundant polysomes, lipid vacuoles, and dense bodies. The nuclei were irreg-ular in shape with marginal chromatin and a prominent nucleolus.

---

Figure 1

Scanning Electron Micrograph of $Ni_3S_2$ Dehydrated Powder
The particles are rather clumpsy, measuring 0.8 to 2.5 $\mu$, mean diameter. Gold coated.

Figure 2

Technique used for Implanting 5 mg of $Ni_3S_2$
In Each Pole of the Kidney

Figure 3

Gross Appearance of the Renal Carcinoma at an Early Stage
The neoplasm rapidly expands into the cortical tissue.

Figure 4

A Large Renal Tumor, Averaging 5 cm in Diameter,
Developed Within 6 Months
Some normal parenchymal tissue is still visible at the periphery.

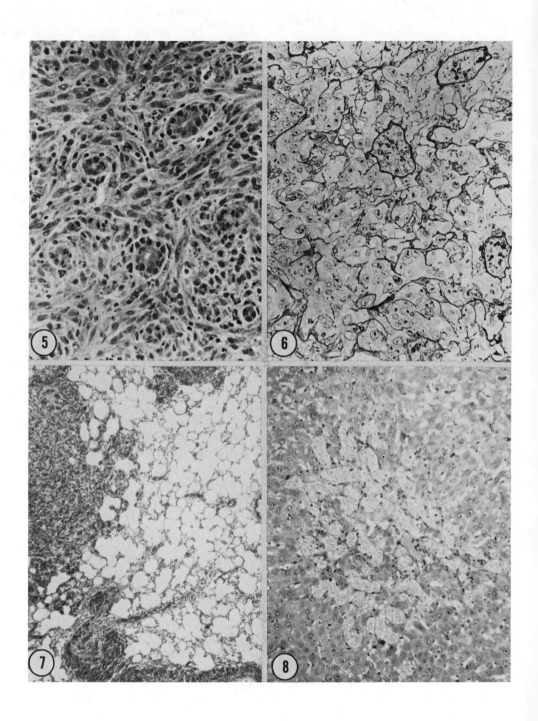

Figure 5

Poorly-differentiated, Spindle-like Tumor Cells
Preexistent renal tubules are engulfed by neoplastic tissue.
HPS X400

Figure 6

Thin Section Stained with Periodic Acid-silver Methenamine
Shows anaplastic carcinoma cells delineated by membrane-like
formations.   X500

Figure 7

Metastatic Pulmonary Nodules in the Vicinity of the Broncheoli
HPS X40

Figure 8

Well-differentiated Metastatic Carcinoma Cells in the Liver Tissue
HPS X125

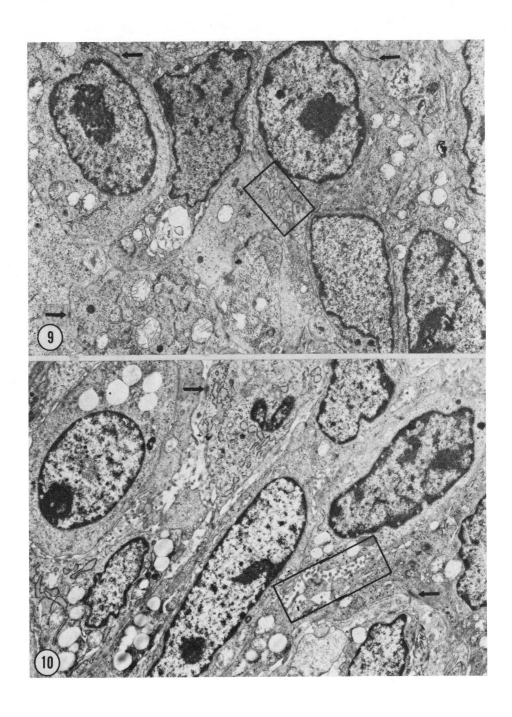

## Early Cellular Changes

The renal parenchyma displayed mononuclear cell infiltration about the metal particles with scar-tissue formation and an eventual increase in basophilia of the tubular lining cells. Electron microscopy revealed seemingly swollen nuclei with dilated cisternae, clumped chromatin, and segregated nucleolus components. The typical membrane-limited inclusion bodies that were found occasionally were presumably composed of metal-bound nucleoproteins (Figure 11). Crystalline, filamentous structures were a constant feature in mitochondria of the basal region of the tubular cells (Figures 12 and 13). These inclusions exhibited a whole range of patterns depending upon their sectioning plane, and in all likelihood, they were derived from the same structural protein. Their genesis was probably related to a dysfunction of the renal tubular cells. Other divalent metals also elicit similar mitochondrial changes, but as shown later, they do not cause erythrocytosis or neoplastic alterations.

While investigating these changes at the subcellular level, we undertook a systematic study of the effects of $Ni_3S_2$ upon various cell fractions of kidney homogenates. After one month, the metal salt was concentrated in the nuclear fraction with smaller amounts being found in the mitochondria, microsomes, and cytosol (Table 2). It virtually disappeared from the fractions after four months, except of course in the scar tissue.

## Erythrocytosis

The plethoric condition was usually apparent in all animals after one month. This phenomenon was associated with increased hematocrit, hemoglobin, erythrocyte, and circulating erythrocyte mass values and

---

Figure 9

Electron Micrograph of Primary Tumor Cells
Showing microvilli (framed), junctional complexes (arrows), swollen mitochondria, vacuoles, and a few cisternae of ER. The cytoplasm contains numerous polysomes and microfilaments.
X11,000

Figure 10

Tumor-cell Propagation in the Mesentery
In addition to the features illustrated in Figure 9, numerous lipid vacuoles can be seen.
X11,000

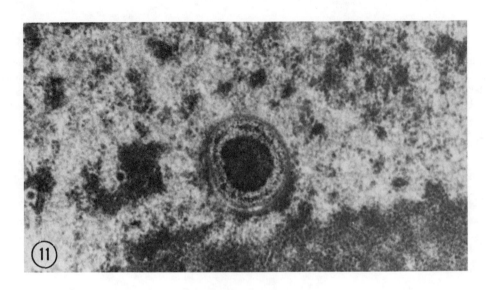

Figure 11
Intramuscular Inclusion Body Found During Early Stages of Tumor
Induction
This membrane-limited formation encloses a dense, granular material
suspected of being a nickel-protein complex.
X35,000

with a normal plasma volume.(5)  The reaction seemed unrelated to
the site of injection in the kidney parenchyma or to the dosage of
$Ni_3S_2$.  Table 3 shows the dose-response relationship and indicates
that already 0.25 mg of  $Ni_3S_2$ is sufficient to produce hematologic
changes, but a minimum of 3 mg are necessary for the production of
renal tumors.  It should be noted that normalization of the blood
values coincides with the time of development of the renal tumors.
As shown in Table 4, ablation of the treated kidney reverses the
erythrocytic reaction within one month; the presence of a humoral
factor released by the nickel-injected kidney is further supported
by transmission of this phenomenon in parabiotic rats.(8)  Ery-
thropoietin dosage studies performed with an *in vivo* biologic technique have revealed a modest but statistically significant elevation
of this hormone two to eight weeks following intrarenal injection
of $Ni_3S_2$.(9)  Finally, we should mention that administration of
nickel monosulfide or various divalent metals under similar experimental conditions does not elicit erythrocytosis or renal carcinomas.(4)

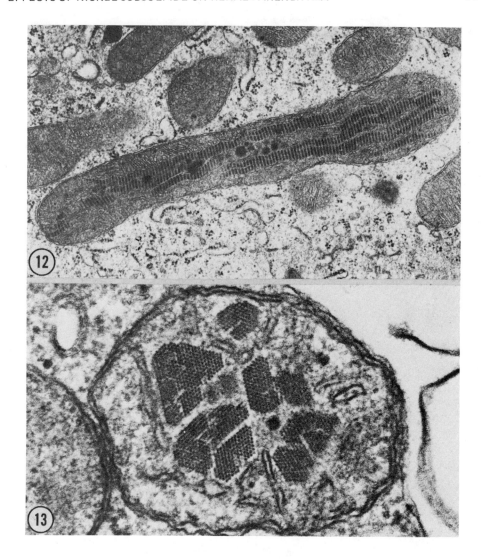

Figure 12
Typical Mitochondrial Crystalline Inclusions Observed in the Basal
Region of the Distal Tubular Cells One Month after $Ni_3S_2$ Treatment
X28,000

Figure 13
A Mitochondrial Crystalline Inclusion Similar to the One in
Figure 12, but in a Transverse Section.  Note the hexagonal arrange-
ment of the composite filaments.
X80,000

TABLE 2

DISTRIBUTION OF $Ni_3S_2$ IN SUBCELLULAR FRACTIONS FROM KIDNEY
HOMOGENATES AFTER INTRARENAL INJECTION IN RATS*

(Nickel content: μg/g kidney)

| Subcellular fractions | Controls | +1 min. | +1 month | +2 months | +4 months |
|---|---|---|---|---|---|
| Nuclear | 5.0 | - | 311.5 | 115.1 | 8.3 |
| Mitochondrial | 0 | - | 4.3 | 3.5 | 1.8 |
| Microsomal | 0 | - | 2.5 | 0 | 0.4 |
| Cytosol | 0.7 | - | 1.8 | 4.5 | 0 |
| Total | 5.7 | 2x7040.0 | 320.1 | 123.1 | 10.5 |

* Each group consisted of 6 female Sprague-Dawley rats.  A glycerin-metal
suspension (5 mg) was injected into each pole of the right kidney (total
nickel content = 7.3 mg).  The kidneys were removed at the indicated time
intervals; in the +1 min group, the kidney was extracorporally injected
to assess the recovery of the metal.  Kidneys were paired and homogenized,
with the nickel content in subcellular fractions being measured by the
atomic absorption method of Nomoto and Sunderman (Clin. Chem., 16: 479, 1970).
The results represent the mean of 3 determinations.

TABLE 3

DOSE-RESPONSE RELATIONSHIP IN Ni$_3$S$_2$-TREATED RATS*

| Ni$_3$S$_2$ treatment | Hemogram after injection of nickel (Mean ± SE) | | | | | | | | Tumor incidence in 12 months |
| | 1 month | | 3 months | | 8 months | | 12 months | | |
| | Hgb[1] | RBC[2] | Hgb | RBC | Hgb | RBC | Hgb | RBC | |
| 0.25 mg/one pole | 17.6±1.6 | 9.02±.75 | 19.3±2.6 | 10.75±.97 | 14.4±0.5 | 7.27±.35 | 13.1±0.3 | 6.98±.14 | 0/6 |
| 0.25 mg/each pole | 16.9±1.4 | 8.91±.69 | 19.8±1.8 | 10.07±.81 | 14.7±0.3 | 7.35±.19 | 14.0±0.2 | 7.47±.15 | 0/6 |
| 0.5 mg/one pole | 15.3±0.2 | 8.12±.06 | 19.4±1.7 | 10.79±.89 | 13.8±0.4 | 6.94±.27 | 12.4±0.1 | 6.85±.12 | 0/6 |
| 0.5 mg/each pole | 18.2±1.7 | 8.54±.79 | 22.8±1.7 | 11.45±.43 | 14.2±1.4 | 6.84±0.8 | 13.9±0.2 | 7.18±.18 | 0/6 |
| 1 mg/one pole | 15.7±0.6 | 8.44±.21 | 18.9±1.4 | 9.50±.61 | 14.4±0.1 | 7.27±0.1 | 14.2±0.3 | 7.39±.16 | 0/5 |
| 1 mg/each pole | 18.2±1.0 | 8.66±.36 | 20.9±1.5 | 10.87±.24 | 15.5±0.9 | 7.72±.43 | 13.0±1.0 | 6.83±.43 | 0/5 |
| 3 mg/one pole | 19.9±1.5 | 10.09±.87 | 22.9±2.4 | 11.52±.48 | 18.2±0.2 | 9.73±.97 | 13.7±0.4 | 7.34±.27 | 1/5 |
| 3 mg/each pole | 18.4±1.4 | 8.77±.56 | 17.6±.46 | 9.18±.23 | 14.9±0.4 | 7.39±1.0 | 13.6±0.2 | 7.11±.25 | 2/5 |
| 5 mg/one pole | 16.1±0.2 | 8.83±.51 | 19.2±.05 | 9.30±.29 | 14.4±0.1 | 7.12±.16 | 11.3±2.0 | 6.89±.77 | 5/8 |
| 5 mg/each pole | 17.1±1.4 | 9.53±.63 | 20.4±1.8 | 10.63±.46 | 13.6±1.2 | 6.88±.61 | 13.7±0.2 | 7.20±.32 | 5/8 |
| 5 mg/one pole of both kidneys | 18.9±1.3 | 9.63±.99 | 21.0±2.6 | 10.84±1.04 | 15.3±1.5 | 9.13±1.01 | 14.6±.26 | 7.93±.18 | 4/6[3] |

* Each group consisted of 5-8 female Sprague-Dawley rats averaging 140±6 g body weight.

[1] Hgb (g/dl). Control rats: 15.2±0.1.

[2] RBC (x10$^6$/mm$^3$). Control rats: 8.0±0.3.

[3] Two of these 4 animals had tumors in each kidney.

TABLE 4

EFFECTS OF NEPHRECTOMY ON THE HEMATOLOGIC CHANGES INDUCED
BY INTRARENAL INJECTION OF $Ni_3S_2$ IN RATS (Mean ± SE)

| Treatment * | Hemogram after 1 month | | Hemogram after 2 months | |
|---|---|---|---|---|
| | Hgb (g/dl) | RBC ($\times 10^6/mm^3$) | Hgb (g/dl) | RBC ($\times 10^6/mm^3$) |
| Glycerin (0.05 ml into each pole) | 15.1 ± 0.3 | 8.0 ± 0.3 | 16.5 ± 0.2 | 7.8 ± 0.3 |
| $Ni_3S_2$ (5 mg in 0.05 ml glycerin into each pole) | 22.2 ± 0.5 | 11.0 ± 0.3 | 25.6 ± 0.6 | 12.4 ± 0.4 |
| $Ni_3S_2$ + removal of the injected kidney 1 month later | 21.1 ± 1.0 (before removal) | 10.1 ± 0.5 (before removal) | 16.3 ± 0.3 (after removal) | 7.8 ± 0.2 (after removal) |

* Each group consisted of 6 female Sprague-Dawley rats averaging 110±10 g body weight.

IV.   CONCLUSIONS

The present studies indicate that nickel subsulfide exerts typical toxic effects when introduced topically into the renal parenchyma.  In addition to the nuclear and mitochondrial changes observed in the distal tubular lining cells, this metal salt elicits erythrocytosis and renal metastatic carcinomas in rats.  All these pathologic alterations are not necessarily interrelated, but most probably result from severe disorders in cellular protein synthesis.

*REFERENCES*

1.   Gilman, J. P. W., Cancer Research 22, Page 158, 1962.

2.   Jasmin, G., Bajusz, E. and Mongeau, A., Revue Canadienne de Biologie 22, Page 113, 1963.

3.   Jasmin, G., J. Microscopie 17, Page 68a, 1973.

4.   Jasmin, G. and Riopelle, J. L., Laboratory Investigations 35, Page 71, 1976.

5.   Jasmin, G. and Solymoss, B., Proceedings Soc. Exp. Biol. Med. 148, Page 774, 1975.

6.   Jasmin, G., J. Microscopie et Biol. Cel. 23, Page 54a, 1975.

7.   Jasmin, G., British J. Cancer XVII, Page 618, 1964.

8.   Jasmin, G., (unpublished data).

9.   Solymoss, B. and Jasmin, G., Exper. Haematology (in press).

CHAPTER 6

LUNG TUMOR RESPONSE IN MICE TO METALS AND METAL SALTS*

M. B. Shimkin, G. D. Stoner, and J. C. Theiss

University of California, San Diego
La Jolla, California 92093

I.  SUMMARY

Two studies tested the ability of metals and their salts to
produce lung tumors in strain A mice.  Of 13 compounds examined,
lead subacetate, manganous sulfate, molybdenum trioxide, and
nickelous acetate elicited a weakly carcinogenic response following
intraperitoneal injection.  Nine metallic compounds were negative.
There was no evidence of cocarcinogenic effect between metals and
the chemical carcinogen , 3-methylcholanthrene.  On the basis of
these and other data, recommendation is made for further investigations in metal carcinogenesis.

II.  INTRODUCTION

In our laboratory, chemicals are assayed for carcinogenic activity by the pulmonary tumor response in mice.  The method, introduced in 1940, was detailed in 1975, and its applications to carcinogenesis bioassay were summarized.[1]

Briefly, the method is as follows:  Mice of susceptible inbred
strains, especially strain A, are exposed to the chemical.  Within
12 weeks, if the chemical is a carcinogen, the lungs of the animals
will show a significant increase in the number of tumors.  The
tumors are pearly white, spherical masses easily recognized by the
naked eye and of monotonously uniform adenomatous appearance under
the microscope.  The tumors arise from type 2 pneumocytes of the
alveolar epithelium.  During the earlier period of growth, the

*  Supported in part by Contract No. NIH-NO1-CP-33232.

tumors are morphologically benign, but with time, become malignant in appearance, invading contiguous tissues and in a small proportion of cases, metastasizing to distant sites. Untreated mice also develop lung tumors, but considerably later and in much smaller numbers, usually one per mouse.

The induction of lung tumors in mice is one of the rapid *in vivo* methods available for studies in carcinogenesis. It also provides a quantitative measure of the reaction, since the number of tumors is related to the dose of the carcinogen.

The pulmonary tumor response is evoked by a wide variety of chemical carcinogens such as the polycyclic hydrocarbons, the carbarmates, and alkylating agents. It is evoked with aflatoxin, but with other hepatocarcinogens, the response is weak and follows large, repeated doses of azo dyes or aminofluorenes. We have not observed positive responses with carbon tetrachloride or chloroform, hepatotoxins that do evoke hepatomas in mice and rats. The lung tumor response is uniformly negative to steroid hormones. Inhibition of the immune systems of the animal will produce a modest increase in tumors.

We have applied the lung tumor bioassay to some metal salts, and have explored the effect of metal ores on carcinogenesis with polycyclic hydrocarbons. The investigations are summarized in this report.


### III.   EXPERIMENT 1

This experiment was reported in detail by Stoner et al.(2) in 1976. Strain A mice, in groups of 20, 6 to 8 weeks old and weighing 18-20g, were injected intraperitoneally thrice weekly, for 6 to 24 injections, with 13 metallic compounds. The maximum tolerated dose, and 1:2 and 1:5 dilutions were used for each compound. Controls consisted of mice injected with the vehicles, and untreated mice. Mice given a single intraperitoneal injection of urethane served as positive controls.

The animals were killed 30 weeks after the first injection and the carcinogenic effect assayed by the number of lung tumors. The results as previously published(2) are presented in Table 1, summarizing only the highest tolerated dose.

A statistically significant increase in the average number of lung tumors per mouse was elicited with 4 of the 13 compounds: lead subacetate, manganous sulfate, molybdenum trioxide, and nickelous acetate. All the positive responses, however, were weak.

TABLE 1

STRAIN A MOUSE LUNG TUMOR RESPONSE TO SELECTED METAL SALTS

| Compound | LT/mouse |
|----------|----------|
| Cadmium (II) Acetate | 0.40 |
| Calcium (II) Acetate | 0.58 |
| Chromium (III) Sulfate | 0.63 |
| Cobalt (II) Acetate | 0.79 |
| Cupric (III) Acetate | 0.56 |
| Iron (II) 2,4-pentanedione | 0.60 |
| Lead (II) Subacetate | 1.47* |
| Manganous (II) Sulfate | 1.20* |
| Molybdenum (III) Trioxide | 1.13* |
| Nickelous (II) Acetate | 1.26* |
| Stannous (II) Chloride | 0.50 |
| Vanadium (III) 2,4-pentanedione | 0.79 |
| Zinc (II) Acetate | 0.78 |
| | |
| Untreated Controls | 0.28 |
| Solvent Controls | 0.46 |
| Urethane Controls | 21.60 |

* Significant (p<0.05) from solvent controls.

VI. EXPERIMENT 2

This experiment was performed and reported in detail in 1940. (3)
Pulverized ores of arsenopyrite (46% inorganic arsenic), chromite
(39-60% chromium oxide), quartz.(silicon oxide), or thorite (48-70%
thorium oxide) were suspended in saline and injected intravenously
in Strain A mice, 50 per group. The mice tolerated 5 mg of the
materials, except for quartz, with which 1 mg was the maximum dose.
As controls, 30 mice were injected intravenously with 2.5 mg of a
carcinogenic soot, and 75 mice were kept as untreated animals.

The mice were killed at 3, 4.5, and 6 months after injection.
Although particles of ore were visible in the lungs, and the lungs

contained chronic inflammatory reactions, no increase in primary
pulmonary tumors was elicited. The number of lung tumors was
significantly increased in mice injected with the carcinogenic
soot. The results are summarized in Table 2 and Figure 1.


TABLE 2


LUNG TUMORS IN MICE 26 WEEKS AFTER SINGLE INTRAVENOUS INJECTION
OF PULVERIZED ORES

| Compound | Dose (mg) | LT/mouse |
|---|---|---|
| Arsenopyrite | 5 | 0.45 |
| Chromite | 5 | 0.57 |
| Quartz | 1 | 0.48 |
| Thorite | 5 | 0.24 |
| Untreated Controls | | 0.53 |


## V.   EXPERIMENT 3


Concurrently with Experiment 2, mice injected with pulverized
ores of arsenopyrite, chromite, quartz, or thorite were injected
intravenously with 0.1 mg of 3-methylcholanthrene dispersed in
horse serum. Thirty animals were injected only with the carcinogenic hydrocarbon, as controls.

The mice were killed at 3 and 4.5 months. All had multiple
pulmonary tumors, for an average of 12 to 28 per mouse. There was
no significant difference between the numbers of tumors in mice
that received the ores a week before the carcinogen.

The results of Experiment 3 are summarized in Table 3, and in
Figure 1. Single intravenous injections of ores did not induce
pulmonary tumors, nor enhance the tumors induced by methylcholanthrene. Thus, they were, by this test procedure, neither carcinogenic nor cocarcinogenic.

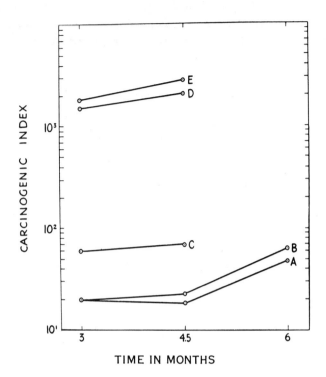

Figure 1
Response of Lungs of Strain A Mice to Intravenously Injected Ores
and Soot

A.  Single injection of 5.0 mg of arsenopyrite, chromite, or
    thorite, or 1.0 mg of quartz.

B.  Untreated controls.

C.  Single injection of 2.5 mg of unextracted soot.

D.  Injection of ores as in A, 0.1 mg of methylcholanthrene a
    week later.

E.  Single injection of 0.1 mg of methylcholanthrene.

Carcinogenic Index - percentage of mice developing pulmonary
tumors times average number of tumors per positive animal.

TABLE 3

LUNG TUMORS IN MICE 18 WEEKS AFTER SINGLE INTRAVENOUS INJECTION
OF PULVERIZED ORES, AND A WEEK LATER, 0.1 mg 3-METHYLCHOLANTHRENE

| Compound | LT/Mouse |
|----------|----------|
| Arsenite | 12.1 |
| Chromite | 20.8 |
| Quartz | 22.0 |
| Thorite | 22.1 |
| Controls | 27.8 |

## VI.   DISCUSSION

Review of the subject of metal carcinogenesis by Sunderman(4)
in 1971 indicates that seven compounds have been found to elicit
sarcomas at the site of parenteral injection into experimental
animals:  beryllium, cadmium, chromium, cobalt, iron, nickel, and
zinc.   Iron carcinogenesis, however, seems to have been limited to
parenteral injection of iron-dextran complexes.   Lead and selenium
were the only elements that produced malignant tumors following
oral administration.

Schroeder et al. (5,6) studied the effect of metal salts added
at levels of 5 ppm to the drinking water of Swiss mice.   Specifically, cadmium, chromium, lead, nickel, tin, vanadium, and zinc
did not increase the number of lung tumors.

The discrepancy between our results and those reported by
Sunderman(4) and by Schroeder et al.(5,6) could be due to differences in results of administration and of the experimental animals
used.

It is important to resolve the different reports on metal carcinogenesis by systematic long-term studies in which several species
and several routes of administration are employed.

The resolution of the uncertainties that exist are of both
theoretical and of practical importance.   Some of the elements

reported as carcinogenic are essential nutritional requirements in trace amounts:  chromium , cobalt, selenium, and zinc.(7)

It should be established by additional data whether there are chemicals that at high doses injected parenterally produce indubitable neoplasms and at trace amounts are essential nutrients involved in normal physiological functions.  Positive, unambiguous data would require conceptual and interpretative modifications in the applications of the Delaney clause to food-additive legislation and of the no-threshold Mantel-Bryan model(8) to carcinogenesis.

## REFERENCES

1.  Shimkin, M. B. and Stoner, G. D.,"Lung Tumors in Mice:  Application to Carcinogenesis Bioassay," Advanced Cancer Research 21, pp. 1-58, 1975.

2.  Stoner, G. D. et al. "Test for Carcinogenicity of Metallic Compounds by the Pulmonary Tumor Response in Strain A Mice," Cancer Research 36, pp. 1744-1747, 1976.

3.  Shimkin, M. B. and Lester, J. "Induced Pulmonary Tumors in Mice. III.  The Role of Chronic Irritation in the Production of Pulmonary Tumors in Strain A Mice," J. National Cancer Institute 1, pp. 241-254, 1940.

4.  Sunderman, F. W., "Metal Carcinogenesis in Experimental Animals," Food Cosmet. Toxicology 9, pp. 105-120, 1971.

5.  Schroeder, H. A., Balassa, J. J. and Vinton, W. H., "Chromium, Lead, Cadmium, Nickel and Titanium in Mice:  Effect on Mortality, Tumors and Tissue Levels," J. Nutrition 83, pp. 239-250, 1964.

6.  Schroeder, H. A. and Balassa, J. J., "Arsenic, Germanium, Tin and Vanadium in Mice:  Effects of Growth, Survival and Tissue Levels," J. Nutrition 92, pp. 245-252, 1967.

7.  Underwood, E. J., Trace Elements in Human and Animal Nutrition, Edition 3, Academic Press, New York, 1971.

8.  Mantel, N. and Schneiderman, M. A., "Estimating 'Safe' Levels, A Hazardous Undertaking," Cancer Research 35, pp. 1379-1386, 1975.

*CHAPTER 7*

OCCUPATIONAL CANCER IN MEN EXPOSED TO METALS*

Lorne Houten,** Irwin D. J. Bross
Enrico Viadana, Geraldine Sonnesso

Department of Biostatics
Roswell Park Memorial Institute
Buffalo, New York

## I.  INTRODUCTION

In this paper we shall investigate the incidence of cancer in men employed in occupations which expose them to metals or to metal compounds.

The relationship between occupational exposure and excess risk of cancer has been recognized for more than 200 years.  The extent of the contribution of the workplace to the cancer picture is, however, only now beginning to be fully appreciated.  A thorough survey of the relevant literature may be found in Houten et al.(1)

The purpose of this investigation is to screen several metal-related occupations and to determine what cancers are associated with them, and to suggest possible etiological relationships.  Further, this study will suggest for which occupations further studies would likely be of importance to the protection of the public health.

* This investigation was supported in part by Public Health Service Research Grant No. CA-11531 from the National Cancer Institute and the National Institute for Occupational Safety and Health Contract HSM-99-73-5.

** Current address:  Department of Research Medicine, University of Pennsylvania, School of Medicine, Philadelphia, Pennsylvania.

## II.  PROCEDURES

The men considered in this study were patients admitted to the
Roswell Park Memorial Institute for Cancer Research at Buffalo, New
York during the years 1956 to 1965.  Before diagnosis, the men were
interviewed.  Among other information recorded were the patient's
age, lifetime occupational history including length of time employed in the occupation, smoking history, and place of birth.  For
the purpose of this study, the men were classified by occupation or,
when the occupation was insufficiently specific, by industry and
occupation.

The occupations considered were:  blacksmiths; boilermakers;
electricians; fabricated-metal workers; filers, grinders and
polishers; furnacemen, smeltermen and pourers; machinists; mechanics
and repairmen; millwrights; mine workers; metal molders; painters;
plumbers and pipe fitters; primary metal workers; tinsmiths and
coppersmiths; toolmakers, diemakers, and setters; and welders and
flame cutters.  Workers in the primary metal industry were subdivided into laborers (unskilled workers), operatives (semiskilled
workers), and foremen.  Fabricated-metal workers were subdivided
into laborers and operatives.

The cancers considered were buccal cavity (lip, tongue, other
mouth, and pharynx); esophagus; stomach;. liver; pancreas; colon and
rectum; nose; larynx; lung (including trachea and bronchi); bladder;
kidney; prostate; testes; melanoma; skin (other than melanoma);
leukemia; lymphoma; multiple myeloma; and brain.

A measure of elevated risk for a given occupation at a given
cancer site was given by the calculation of the relative risk.
Relative risk is a quantity used in epidemiological research that
measures the chance that an individual exposed to the occupational
hazard will have the disease in question relative to the chance that
an individual not exposed to the hazard will have the disease.

The calculation of relative risks requires the selection of a
control (comparison) population which represents the relative proportion of the occupational group in question in the population as
a whole.  In addition, a population not exposed to the occupational
hazard must be chosen.  For further explanation of the relative
risk concept see MacMahon et al. (2)

For the purpose of this study, we chose as the control population those Roswell Park patients who proved not to have neoplastic
disease.  Men engaged in clerical occupations were chosen as the
unexposed group.  This choice was motivated by our desire to have a
sizable and relatively homogeneous occupational group for which
occupationally associated cancer rarely has been reported.  Sample

cases were calculated for other choices; however, the basic conclusions were unchanged; i.e., occupations whose risks were high
under one choice were high under others.

The sample was subdivided by age into two groups; namely,
ages 14-59, and 60 and over.  Relative risks were calculated within
each age group.  The complete figures may be found in Houten et
al.(1)  To minimize the effect of the differences in age between
the population of cases and that of controls, an age-adjusted
relative risk was calculated for each occupation and cancer site.
The adjustment was performed using the Cochran-Mantel-Haenzel
method (see Fleiss(3)).  This age-adjusted relative risk is the
statistic reported in this paper.

For four sites (buccal, larynx, lung, and bladder) for which the
cancer incidence is known to be related to smoking habits, smoking-
adjusted relative risks to the age-adjusted risks were calculated.
We compared the smoking-adjusted risks to the age-adjusted risks,
and we concluded that although the numbers varied slightly, the
patterns remained constant; that is, that high risks remained high,
and low risks remained low.  As a result, we can conclude that it is
unlikely that the high risks reported at these sites are the result
of differential smoking habits between occupations.

It is always a difficult problem to decide which results should
be reported.  The most conservative solution would be to report only
those results for which the number of cases is large (defined for
our purpose as at least five), the relative risks are high and the
elevation is statistically significant at the 5% level.  Less reliable would be those situations in which the sample size is large
and the relative risk elevated but not statistically significant at
the 5% level.  Then there are those cases in which the risk is elevated but the number of cases is smaller.  We have chosen to report
all of these.  We feel that this is justified since (1) this is a
screening study; (2) we have explained to the reader that some results may be more reliable than others; and (3) that it is possible
that the combination of several results, each individually of lesser
reliability may yield interesting and important information.

### III.  DISCUSSION OF THE OCCUPATIONS AT RISK

In this section, we shall be referring to the figures in Table 1.

Blacksmiths show a highly elevated risk for cancer of the prostate, the highest statistically significant increase in the study.
They also show an elevated risk for stomach on a smaller sample size.

Boilermakers howed greatly elevated risks for kidney and elevated risks for bladder and lung, all on small samples.

TABLE 1

RELATIVE RISKS FOR METAL-RELATED OCCUPATIONS

|                         | No. Cases | Relative Risk |
|-------------------------|-----------|---------------|
| **Blacksmiths**         |           |               |
| Prostate                | 5         | 6.7*          |
| Stomach                 | 2         | 3.6           |
| **Boilermakers**        |           |               |
| Lung                    | 3         | 4.4           |
| Kidney                  | 2         | 32.5          |
| Bladder                 | 2         | 3.2           |
| **Electricians**        |           |               |
| Lung                    | 20        | 2.1*          |
| Buccal and Larynx       | 21        | 1.5           |
| Bladder                 | 6         | 1.8           |
| Testes                  | 3         | 2.6           |
| Esophagus               | 2         | 2.2           |
| **Operatives in Fabricated Metal** |  |           |
| Bladder                 | 13        | 2.1*          |
| Kidney                  | 4         | 3.1           |
| Pancreas                | 2         | 2.8           |
| **Laborers in Fabricated Metal** |    |             |
| Buccal                  | 13        | 1.8           |
| Esophagus               | 2         | 3.0           |
| **Filers, Grinders and Polishers** | |            |
| Stomach                 | 5         | 2.1           |
| **Furnacemen, Smeltermen and Pourers** | |        |
| Bladder                 | 9         | 2.4*          |
| Lung                    | 13        | 1.6           |
| Leukemia                | 4         | 2.3           |
| Esophagus               | 3         | 4.0           |

\*  Statistically significant at the p >.05 level.

| Table 1 (Continued) | No. Cases | Relative Risk |
|---|---|---|
| **Machinists** | | |
| Leukemia | 8 | 2.9* |
| Buccal and Larynx | 31 | 1.5 |
| Prostate | 7 | 2.4 |
| Kidney | 4 | 3.9 |
| Nose | 4 | 3.8 |
| Testes | 4 | 2.4 |
| Esophagus | 3 | 2.2 |
| Brain | 2 | 14.2 |
| Melanoma | 2 | 2.4 |
| | | |
| **Mechanics and Repairmen** | | |
| Prostate | 27 | 2.1* |
| Stomach | 15 | 1.6 |
| Nose | 9 | 1.9 |
| Pancreas | 7 | 2.0 |
| | | |
| **Millwrights** | | |
| Stomach | 7 | 5.5* |
| Bladder | 5 | 1.8 |
| | | |
| **Mine Workers** | | |
| Leukemia | 6 | 2.2 |
| Prostate | 6 | 2.0 |
| Melanoma | 3 | 6.8 |
| Esophagus | 3 | 2.0 |
| | | |
| **Metal Molders** | | |
| Stomach | 5 | 2.9* |
| Lung | 16 | 1.6 |
| Esophagus | 3 | 3.0 |
| Kidney | 2 | 3.9 |
| | | |
| **Painters** | | |
| Esophagus | 7 | 3.0* |
| Stomach | 8 | 2.4* |
| Lung | 42 | 1.7* |
| Prostate | 9 | 1.9 |
| Bladder | 16 | 1.6 |
| Kidney | 4 | 2.6 |
| Melanoma | 2 | 3.2 |

* Statistically significant at the p > .05 level.

| Table 1 (Continued) | No. Cases | Relative Risk |
|---|---|---|
| **Plumbers and Pipe Fitters** | | |
| Lung | 17 | 1.6 |
| Bladder | 7 | 1.6 |
| Nose | 4 | 5.1 |
| Stomach | 4 | 2.5 |
| Kidney | 3 | 4.8 |
| **Operatives in Primary Metal** | | |
| Stomach | 7 | 2.9* |
| Prostate | 7 | 2.2 |
| Leukemia | 7 | 2.2 |
| Buccal | 6 | 2.0 |
| Lung | 28 | 1.5 |
| Pancreas | 3 | 3.5 |
| Kidney | 3 | 2.5 |
| **Laborers in Primary Metal** | | |
| Stomach | 8 | 2.4* |
| **Foremen in Primary Metal** | | |
| Prostate | 3 | 5.4 |
| Stomach | 2 | 4.8 |
| **Tinsmiths and Coppersmiths** | | |
| No reportable risks | | |
| **Toolmakers, Diemakers and Setters** | | |
| Larynx | 6 | 1.8 |
| Multiple Myeloma | 4 | 4.8 |
| Esophagus | 3 | 3.8 |
| Testes | 3 | 2.9 |
| Prostate | 3 | 2.1 |
| **Welders and Flame Cutters** | | |
| Stomach | 3 | 2.5 |

* Statistically significant at the p >.05 level.

Electricians showed a statistically significant increased risk for cancer of the lung and an elevated risk for other respiratory sites, buccal cavity, and larynx. There were also elevated risks for bladder, esophagus, and testes.

Operatives in the fabricated-metal industry had a significant risk for cancer of the bladder, as well as an increase of cancer of the pancreas and of the kidney. Laborers in the fabricated-metal industry showed increases for cancer of the buccal cavity and the esophagus.

Filers, grinders, and polishers of metals had an increased risk in cancer of the stomach.

Furnacemen, smeltermen, and pourers showed a significant increased risk in cancer of the bladder. Men in this occupation also showed increases in cancer of the lung and esophagus, and leukemia.

Machinists showed increased risk for more than half the sites investigated. These men exhibited a significant increase in the risk of leukemia, the highest relative risk observed for this malignancy in this study. Cancer of the brain was strikingly increased, albeit on a very small sample. In addition, there were elevated relative risks in cancer of the buccal cavity, larynx, prostate, kidney, nose, testes, esophagus, and for malignant melanoma.

Mechanics and repairmen exhibited a significantly elevated risk of cancer of the prostate, as well as increases in cancer of the stomach, pancreas, and nose.

Millwrights showed a significant increased risk in cancer of the stomach, and a moderately increased risk in cancer of the bladder.

Workers in the mining industry (operatives and laborers combined) exhibited a very high relative risk in malignant melanoma, albeit on only three cases. In addition, men working in this industry had increased risk of leukemia, and of cancer of the esophagus and prostate.

Metal molders had significantly elevated risk of cancer of the stomach. They also exhibited elevated risks in cancer of the lung, kidney, and esophagus.

Painters (interior and exterior combined) showed one of the largest number of elevated risks reported in this study. They had significantly increased risk of cancer of the esophagus, stomach, and lung. In addition, malignant melanoma and cancer of the prostate, bladder, and kidney were elevated.

Both laborers and operatives in the primary metal industry showed a significantly increased risk in cancer of the stomach. Foremen in this industry also had an elevated stomach cancer risk. Operatives and foremen both exhibited an elevated risk of cancer of the prostate. In addition, the operatives who would probably be most directly exposed to the hazards, had elevated risk of cancer of the lung, pancreas, kidney, buccal area, and of leukemia.

Plumbers and pipe fitters had a substantial increase in risk in cancer of the kidney and nose on small sample sizes. The risk of cancer of the lung, bladder, and stomach were also elevated.

Tinsmiths and coppersmiths had no reportable elevated risk.

Toolmakers, diemakers, and setters had increased risk of cancer of the larynx, prostate, esophagus, and testes. In addition, men in these occupations showed a substantial increased risk of multiple myeloma. Although there were only four cases, the unique appearance of an elevated risk in this rare malignancy is sufficiently intriguing to suggest further investigation.

Welders and flame cutters showed an increased risk of cancer of the stomach.

## IV.   ANALYSIS BY CANCER SITE

Table 2 shows the results of the study arranged by cancer site. We shall discuss several implications of this table.

Elevated risk of cancer of the stomach was reported in more than half the occupations considered. The risk was significantly elevated in one-fourth of the occupations. One possible nonoccupational explanation of this observation is that many of the industrial workers in western New York are of Slavic or other eastern European descent. The incidence of stomach cancer in eastern Europe is considerably higher than it is in the United States. In order to control in part for this factor, we calculated relative risks of stomach cancer for the American-born subsample. When the sample sizes of American-born workers were sufficiently large to permit the calculations, the high relative risk remained elevated. The elevated stomach cancer rates, therefore, cannot be ascribed to the influence of foreign-born patients. This does not eliminate the problem, however, as genetic factors may be at work, and since American-born men of eastern European descent may retain old-world dietary habits.

No other site showed more than two significantly elevated occupations; however, six cancers (prostate, lung, bladder, buccal (including pharynx and larynx), and kidney, were reported in at least one-fourth of the occupations surveyed; thus, the virtue of having

reported all results can be appreciated.  The important influence
of occupational exposure on the incidence of cancer at rarer sites
such as esophagus and kidney would likely have been missed if a
more conservative approach had been taken.  It is therefore probable that a larger sample study would add melanoma, nose, and pancreas to the list of sites of cancer frequently influenced by
occupational exposure.

TABLE 2

NUMBER OF OCCURRENCES OF ELEVATED RISKS
(By Cancer Site)

| | Elevated Risk (Statistically Significant) | Elevated Risk (5 Cases) | Elevated Risk (2 Cases) |
|---|---|---|---|
| Stomach | 5 | 7 | 11 |
| Prostate | 2 | 6 | 8 |
| Lung | 2 | 6 | 7 |
| Bladder | 2 | 6 | 7 |
| Leukemia | 1 | 3 | 4 |
| Esophagus | 1 | 1 | 8 |
| Buccal and Larynx | | 5 | 5 |
| Kidney | | | 7 |
| Pancreas | | 1 | 3 |
| Nose | | 1 | 3 |
| Melanoma | | | 3 |
| Testes | | | 3 |
| Multiple Myeloma | | | 1 |
| Brain | | | 1 |

## V.   CONCLUSIONS

We have shown that metal-related occupations may be associated with high risks in as many as 14 different types of cancer.  While this screening study could not elucidate the nature of the specific agents responsible for the increased risk, further studies are indicated to investigate the role of metals as well as solvents and other chemicals, combustion products and dusts, or combinations of these agents in the etiology of these occupational cancers.

## REFERENCES

1.    Houten, Lorne, Bross, I. D. J. and Viadana, E., Occupational Cancer, National Institute for Occupational Safety and Health, 1977.

2.    MacMahon, B. and Pugh, T., Epidemiology, Little, Brown & Co., 1970.

3.    Fleiss, Joseph, Statistical Methods for Rates and Proportions, Wiley Interscience, 1973.

CHAPTER 8

INFIDELITY OF DNA SYNTHESIS

AS RELATED TO MUTAGENESIS AND CARCINOGENESIS

Lawrence A. Loeb, Michael A. Sirover, and Shyam S. Agarwal

The Institute for Cancer Research
Fox Chase Cancer Center
Philadelphia, Pennsylvania  19111

## I.   INTRODUCTION

The interactions of oncogenic viruses, ultraviolet radiation, and chemical carcinogens with DNA *in vivo* have been thoroughly documented.(*1-3*)  To investigate the mechanism by which carcinogens induce stable and inheritable alterations in the nucleotide sequences that contain the cells' genetic information, we have asked how the cell accurately copies DNA, and whether chemical carcinogens perturb this fidelity.  This has involved a study of the copying *in vitro* of polynucleotides by DNA polymerases and the determination of the effects of mutagens and carcinogens on the accuracy of this copying.

In this communication, we shall consider the evidence for somatic mutations as a basis for malignant initiation and tumor progression as well as a new screening test for identifying potential mutagens and carcinogens, based on their capacity to decrease the fidelity of *in vitro* DNA synthesis.

## II.   SOMATIC MUTATIONS AS THE BASIS OF MALIGNANCY

This theory is based on the hypothesis that tumors arise as a consequence of permanent alterations in the base sequences within the DNA of normal somatic cells.  Cells that contain the altered base sequences that determine the neoplastic potential are presumed to possess proliferative advantages over adjoining normal cells. With this proliferative advantage, a mutant cell gives rise to a mass of cells that may be clinically observed as a tumor.  During

103

the proliferation of mutant cells, there is continuous selection
of cells that have the capability to escape the organism's
mechanisms that control growth and differentiation; thus, the
emerging tumor consists primarily of "undifferentiated-like" cells.
Furthermore, tumor cells acquire the ability to infiltrate locally
and to metastasize to distant sites.  It is not known how many mutations in a cell are needed to initiate this process; whether the
mutations are recessive or dominant; whether they involve structural
genes or regulatory genes; whether they represent additions of
genetic information, deletions of information, or alterations of
existing information.  On the basis of age-related mortality from
all cancers in humans, it has been calculated that at least two,
and probably as many as five to six mutational events occur during
oncogenesis.(4)  With respect to hereditary childhood cancers, a
two-mutation hypothesis has been suggested in which the first mutation is in the germ line.(5)  Theoretically, mutations can occur
spontaneously during DNA replication or DNA repair, and have been
shown to be brought about by exogeneous environmental agents including chemicals, viruses and radiation.  The overriding evidence
that malignancy is inherited at the cellular level has been the
driving force behind the theory of somatic mutations.  The arguments
for and against the somatic mutation hypothesis are summarized in
Table 1.  The direct proof of the somatic mutation hypothesis would
be to document changes in the base sequence of DNA; however, this
is usually considered beyond current methods of resolution in eucaryotic cells.

     In addition, we have been concerned whether there is a cascad-
ing or errors in DNA synthesis during tumor progression.(6)  This
concern seems reasonable when one considers the phenotypic changes
that become manifest during malignancy, even though there is no
definitive evidence at the moment that malignant cells have a greater
mutation rate than do normal cells.  Tumor progression, as described
by Foulds,(7) is the process by which malignant cells become progressively anaplastic.  It is usually manifested by a continuous
evolvement of new tumor variants as indicated (a) by the appearance
of new antigenic determinants; (b) by increasing numbers of chromosomal aberrations; (c) by the ability of tumor cells to progressively circumvent the host's mechanisms for the control of DNA replication and cell proliferation; and (d) by the ability of tumor cells
to become more resistant to therapeutic agents.  One possible mechanism by which DNA synthesis in malignant cells could become less
exact than in normal cells would be if the enzymes functioning in
base selection are altered so as to permit frequent mistakes during
DNA synthesis.  The concept of a cascading increase in mutations as
a result of random mutations producing enzymes with altered abilities
in base selection is diagrammed in Figure 1.

Alterations in base sequences can arise through several mechanisms. With respect to the polymerization step, there are two general possibilities; the first is the modification of DNA. As a result, the polymerase will insert a base complementary to the modified base on the template, even though it may be biologically incorrect. The second mechanism is through alteration in the DNA polymerase itself, so that this altered polymerase now inaccurately copies DNA. In order to consider these possibilities, we have studied the way in which DNA polymerases select and incorporate complementary deoxynucleotides *in vitro* and determined factors that alter the fidelity of *in vitro* DNA synthesis. In our initial studies, we focused on DNA polymerases(8) since these enzymes function in base selection,(9) and assays can be designed that measure misincorporation at a frequency as low as one in a million.(10,11)

TABLE 1

SOMATIC MUTATION AS THE BASIS FOR MALIGNANCY

| | Evidence For | Evidence Against |
|---|---|---|
| 1. | Agents causing malignancy interact with DNA, e.g., Chemical carcinogens and Radiation | Also interact with RNA & Protein Induce latent viruses Suppress host immune responses |
| 2. | Oncogenic viruses are integrated into host DNA | All cells with integrated oncogenic viruses are not malignant. |
| 3. | Most chemical carcinogens are mutagens | Not all mutagens are carcinogens. |
| 4. | Malignant phenotype is permanent and heritable at the cellular level | Does not exclude stable epigenetic changes. Reversal of the neoplastic state to a normal or quasinormal state has been reported. |
| 5. | Malignancy is frequently characterized by chromosomal aberrations | May be an epiphenomenon. Significant number of neoplasms in early stages do not exhibit any karyotypic abnormality. |
| 6. | Defective DNA repair in patients of Xeroderma pigmentosum is associated with malignancy. | May be an unique example. |
| 7. | Single autosomal dominant lesions are associated with malignancy, e.g., Retinoblastoma, Familial polyposis of the colon and Bilateral medullary carcinoma of thyroid. Certain autosomal recessive mutations predispose to malignancy, e.g., Bloom's syndrome Fanconi's anemia and Ataxia telangiectasia | Both dominant and recessive mutations could make individuals susceptible to neoplastic change rather than causing it by themselves. |

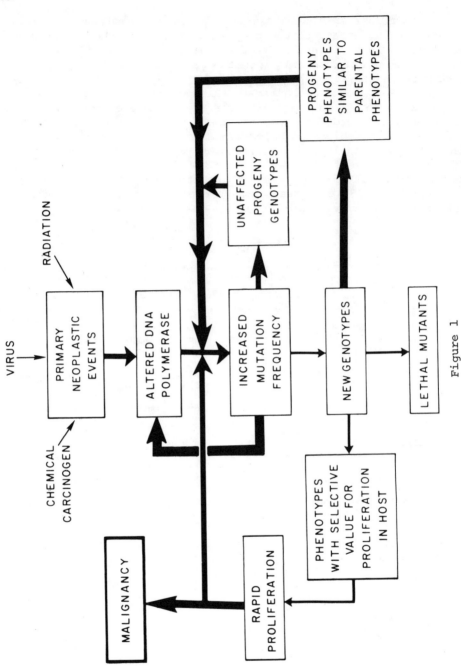

Figure 1

Model for the Cascading of Errors in DNA Synthesis During Tumor Progression

III.   MEASUREMENTS OF THE FIDELITY OF DNA SYNTHESIS

Ideally, one desires to measure the accuracy by which DNA
polymerases copy native DNA templates, and to determine the frequency of base selection in the newly synthesized product.  Alternately, the frequency of incorrect base selection may be quantitated, using synthetic polynucleotides containing only one or two
nucleotide species.  For example, with poly d(A-T) as a template,
our assay(12) measures the incorporation of the complementary
nucleotides, dATP and dTTP (one labeled with [$\alpha$-$^{32}$P], and a noncomplementary nucleotide, either dGTP or dCTP (labeled with [H$^3$]).
The assay is so designed that the specific activity of the complementary nucleotide is about 20 dpm per picomole, while that of
the noncomplementary nucleotide is about 10,000 dpm per picomole.
The frequency of mistakes; i.e., the error rate, is determined from
the ratio of H$^3$ to $^{32}$P in the reaction product.  A list of the
error rates of some DNA polymerases is given in Table 2.  The DNA
polymerases purified from bacteria are highly accurate in base
selection.(10,11)  There is considerable evidence to support the
hypothesis that this accuracy is at least in part determined by an
associated proofreading 3' → 5'-exonuclease.(20)  Fragmentary evidence suggests that homogeneous DNA polymerases from eucaryotic
cells are also accurate in base selection,(20) even though these
enzymes lack any associated 3' → 5'-exonucleolytic activity.(21)
In contrast, the DNA polymerases from RNA tumor viruses have a much
higher frequency of misincorporations(12,19) and these homogeneous
enzymes also lack any associated 3' → 5'-exodeoxynuclease activity.(22)


IV.   MISINCORPORATIONS REPRESENT SINGLE-BASE SUBSTITUTIONS
        AND ARE CATALYZED BY DNA POLYMERASE

The availability of homogeneous preparations of avian myeloblastosis virus (AMV) DNA polymerase and the frequent misincorporation
by this enzyme has permitted detailed analysis of the kinetics of
incorporation of complementary and noncomplementary nucleotides.
Using poly d(A-T) as a template, the error frequency of AMV DNA
polymerase is approximately 1 in 1,000 for dCMP incorporation.  The
incorporation on noncomplementary nucleotides (dCTP or dGTP) requires the presence of the complementary nucleotides, a divalent
metal cation, template, and enzyme.(12)  These requirements suggest
that the incorporation of noncomplementary nucleotides is indeed
catalyzed by the DNA polymerase.  Using [$\alpha$-$^{32}$P] labeled noncomplementary nucleotides, nearest neighbor analyses of the product of
the reaction have been carried out with a variety of polynucleotide
templates.(23,24)  After enzymatic hydrolysis of the product, greater
than 95% of the incorporated $^{32}$P is recovered as the complementary
nucleoside 3'-monophosphate; thus, the noncomplementary nucleotides
are incorporated in phosphodiester linkage and are present as single-

TABLE 2

FIDELITY IN COPYING POLYNUCLEOTIDE TEMPLATE

| Source of DNA Polymerase | Template | Non-Complementary Nucleotide Incorporated | Error Rate | Reference |
|---|---|---|---|---|
| Procaryotic DNA Polymerases | | | | |
| E. coli Polymerase I | poly[d(A-T)] | dGTP | 1/100,000 | (11) |
| Bacteriophage T₄ | poly[d(A-T)] | dCTP | 1/12,000 | (13) |
| Eucaryotic DNA Polymerase | | | | |
| Sea Urchin Nuclei | poly[d(A-T)] | dCTP | 1/12,000 | (14) |
| Calf Thymus (3S) | poly(A).oligo(dT) | dCTP | 1/180,000 | (15) |
| Human Lymphocyte (6S-8S) | poly[d(A-T)] | dCTP | 1/20,000 | (16) |
| RNA Polymerase | | | | |
| E. coli | poly[d(A-T)] | dCTP | 1/2,400 | (17) |
| E. coli | poly[d(A-T)] | dGTP | 1/42,000 | (17) |
| Reverse Transcriptases | | | | |
| Avian myeloblastosis virus | poly(A).oligo(dT) | dCTP | 1/300-800 | (12) |
| Avian myeloblastosis virus | poly(dA).oligo (dT) | dCTP | 1/200-600 | (12) |
| Rous Sarcoma Virus | poly (C).oligo d(G) | dATP | 1/900 | (18) |
| Rauscher Leukemia Virus | poly(A).oligo d(T) | dCTP | 1/400 | (19) |

base substitutions.  Moreover, with poly d(A-T) as the template,
the incorrect nucleotide, dCMP, invariably substitutes for dTMP,
while dGMP is found in place of dAMP.

Three types of experiments indicate that the incorporation
of both complementary and noncomplementary nucleotide is catalyzed
by AMV DNA polymerase, itself.  First, homogeneous AMV DNA polymerase was rechromatographed; there was a constant ratio of incorrect to correct nucleotide incorporation observed across the
polymerase peak.(12)  Secondly, inhibition of AMV DNA polymerase
by o-phenanthroline, a metal chelator with a high affinity for zinc,
inhibits proportionately the incorporation of complementary and
noncomplementary nucleotides.(25)  Third, and most importantly,
three temperature-sensitive DNA polymerases have been purified from
avian sarcoma virus mutants.  With each of these mutant polymerases,
incorporation of noncomplementary nucleotides is temperature-
sensitive.(18)  These combined results establish unambiguously that
viral DNA polymerases themselves catalyze the incorporation of noncomplementary nucleotides.


V.   INFLUENCE OF ENVIRONMENTAL AGENTS
ON THE FIDELITY OF DNA SYNTHESIS

To determine whether exogeneous agents influence the fidelity
of DNA synthesis, a number of chemicals have been added to polymerase assays.  The results of some of these studies are summarized
in Table 3.  Base selection does not depend upon the length of the
initiator, structure of the template, or the sequence of nucleotides
in the template.  The fidelity of DNA synthesis was invariant with
respect to the presence of a large number of chemicals; although in
many situations, synthesis was inhibited at high concentrations.
Denaturation of the polymerase by heat, urea (4 M) or ethanol (20%)
did not alter the ratio of incorporation of incorrect to correct
nucleotides.  So far, only a restricted number of changes decreased
the fidelity of DNA synthesis (Table 3); use of different polymerases (see Table 2); change in nucleotide substrate concentrations;(25) alkylation of the template;(26) use of different metal
activators(27) and the addition of nonactivating metals.(24)  With
AMV DNA polymerase, substitution of an incorrect pyrimidine for a
correct pyrimidine, or an incorrect purine for a correct purine
occurs at a frequency of 1/300 to 1/2500, while the insertion of a
purine in place of a pyrimidine is a much less frequent event.  In
addition, at nonsaturating substrate concentrations, the frequency
of misincorporation is proportional to the ratio of correct to incorrect nucleotides in the reaction.(25)  Thus, it will be interesting to observe if similar alterations in the relative concentrations
of deoxynucleoside triphosphates in cells affect mutation rates or
if a cell has mechanisms to excise incorporated noncomplementary
nucleotides.

TABLE 3

EFFECTS OF EXOGENOUS AGENTS ON THE FIDELITY OF DNA SYNTHESIS
WITH AMV DNA POLYMERASE

| No Effect on Fidelity | Increased Mistakes |
| --- | --- |
| Template | Type of Incorrect Nucleotide |
| Initiator | Ratio of Correct to Incorrect Nucleotide Substrate |
| pH (6-8) | |
| Temperature (15-41°C) | Alkylation of Template |
| Urea (0-4 M) | Different Metal Activators for DNA polymerase |
| Monovalent Cations | Non-activating metal mutagens or carcinogens |
| Anions | |
| Caffeine | |
| Ethanol | |

The biological consequence of the stable interactions of chemical carcinogens with DNA is only beginning to be defined. Alkylation of the template-primer, poly (dA).oligo (dT), with the carcinogen, β-propiolactone, resulted in an enhanced frequency of misincorporation when the modified template was copied by AMV DNA polymerase and sea urchin nuclear DNA polymerase.(26) This system may serve as a prototype to explore the effect of template modifications on the fidelity of DNA synthesis. This is particularly important, since mounting evidence suggests that many covalent interactions of carcinogens with DNA may not be excised in cells prior to DNA replication. Using different templates for modification, it may be possible to determine which template modifications cause base substitutions.

VI.   EFFECT OF METAL CATIONS ON THE FIDELITY OF DNA SYNTHESIS

We have previously reported that substitution of $Mn^{2+}$ or $Co^{2+}$ for $Mg^{2+}$ as the added divalent metal cation alters the fidelity of DNA synthesis.(27,28) For example, with poly (rC) as a template and $Mg^{2+}$, AMV DNA polymerase incorporated one molecule of dAMP for every 1400 molecules of dGMP polymerized.(28) The error frequency is invariant with respect to $Mg^{2+}$ concentration (0.12 to 16 mM). However, in the same experiment with 1 mM $Mn^{2+}$, the error rate is greater: 1/800. Furthermore, the incorporation of the correct but not the incorrect nucleotide is progressively decreased at inhibitory concentrations of $Mn^{2+}$. At 5 mM $Mn^{2+}$, the frequency of noncomplementary nucleotide incorporation approaches 1/30, and most misincorporations occur as a single-base substitution. Similar increases in infidelity using $Mn^{2+}$ and unequal substrate concentrations has recently been recorded by Mizutani and Temin[29] using different viral DNA polymerases as well as *E. coli* DNA polymerase I. These authors point out that fidelity of DNA synthesis can be markedly affected by changes in the environment of the enzyme. Our results suggest that these changes may be related to the biological consequences of the agents. For example, decreases in fidelity observed *in vitro* with $Mn^{2+}$ is in accord with its mutagenic effects in bacteria.[30]

Beryllium is a known chemical carcinogen. Also, $Be^{2+}$ is unable to substitute for $Mg^{2+}$ during catalysis.[24] Yet, this nonactivating metal cation decreases the fidelity of DNA synthesis in the presence of $Mg^{2+}$. Preincubation experiments have suggested that the beryllium forms a stable complex with the polymerase at a noncatalytic site. Glycerol gradient centrifugation dissociates the polymerase-Be complex and restores the initial error frequency of the polymerase. It may be possible for a carcinogen to interact weakly with a polymerase and yet induce base substitutions in DNA. Therefore, modifications of other components in the DNA replication complex may bring about base substitution in the absence of modification of DNA.

## VII.  INFIDELITY OF DNA SYNTHESIS:  A BIOCHEMICAL SCREENING SYSTEM FOR METAL MUTAGENS AND CARCINOGENS

The experimental results that have been considered on the alteration in the fidelity of DNA synthesis by nonactivating and activating divalent metal cations and the dynamic nature of metal-macromolecular interactions prompted us to ask if mutagenic and/or carcinogenic metals could be identified by alterations in the fidelity of DNA synthesis. So far, 31 metal compounds have been tested in graded concentrations in this cell-free system.[31] The method of analysis and the results are summarized in Figure 2. Twenty-two of these metal salts were tested in a triple-blind study in which the assays, computations, and designation of each unknown compound with respect to fidelity were carried out independently. Compounds which increased infidelity by greater than 30% at two or more concentrations were scored as positive. Metals were designated as carcinogens or mutagens by an evaluation of the literature prior to assessment of their effects on fidelity. An enhancement in the infidelity of DNA synthesis was observed with all of the known mutagens and/or carcinogens tested (Ag, Be, Cd, Co, Cr, Mn, Ni, Pb). The evidence in the literature on the mutagenicity or carcinogenicity of three of the metal cations was considered equivocal. Of these, $Cu^{2+}$ increased misincorporation; $Fe^{2+}$ and $Zn^{2+}$ did not alter fidelity. All other metal salts that were tested were considered to be neither carcinogenic nor mutagenic, and they did not increase misincorporation.

Only a few of the metal salts that did not alter fidelity are listed in Figure 2. If one considers the metals that are questionable as possible mutagens and carcinogens (Cu, Fe, Zn) to have a biological effect that is the opposite of those observed in the fidelity assay, the worst possible situation, the hypothesis that increases in fidelity and mutagenicity/carcinogenicity are independent variables can be rejected with a p = 1.6 x $10^{-4}$ using the data from the entire series.

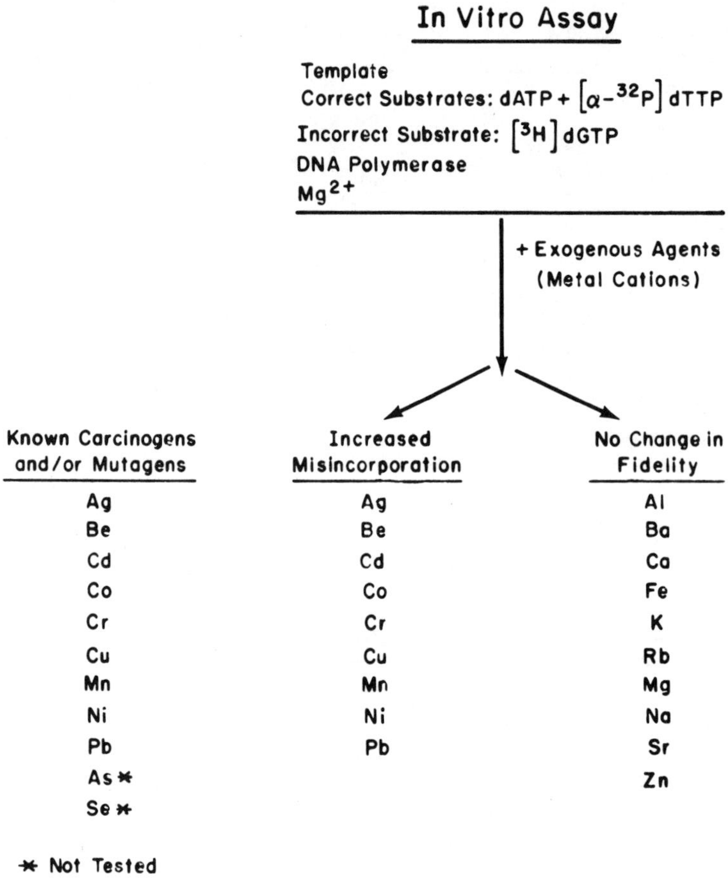

## In Vitro Assay

Template
Correct Substrates: dATP + $[\alpha-^{32}P]$ dTTP
Incorrect Substrate: $[^3H]$ dGTP
DNA Polymerase
$Mg^{2+}$

+ Exogenous Agents
(Metal Cations)

| Known Carcinogens and/or Mutagens | Increased Misincorporation | No Change in Fidelity |
|:---:|:---:|:---:|
| Ag | Ag | Al |
| Be | Be | Ba |
| Cd | Cd | Ca |
| Co | Co | Fe |
| Cr | Cr | K |
| Cu | Cu | Rb |
| Mn | Mn | Mg |
| Ni | Ni | Na |
| Pb | Pb | Sr |
| As ✶ | | Zn |
| Se ✶ | | |

✶ Not Tested

Figure 2

Fidelity Assay Screen for Mutagens and/or Carcinogens

VIII.   ANALYSES WITH OTHER CLASSES OF CARCINOGENS

As an initial approach to using fidelity assays as a biochemical screening procedure for environmental mutagens and carcinogens,
we chose to test metal salts.  We reasoned that an *in vitro* assay
would be particularly suitable for quantitating any labile interactions between metal cations and cellular macromolecules.  Moreover, metals have been identified as carcinogens after occupational
exposure in humans or by extensive animal experimentation.  So far,
studies with bacterial mutagen systems have failed to detect this
class of carcinogens.  We also chose to use AMV DNA polymerase in
these initial studies in that the enzyme could be obtained in homogeneous form, is free of any associated exodeoxynuclease that might
function in excising mismatched nucleotides after incorporation, and
appears to permit mistakes in DNA synthesis.  We would anticipate
that the DNA polymerases from animal cells would be similarly affected since they also lack any exodeoxynuclease activity.

There is no apparent reason that our system should be limited
to metal salts.  Further, the coupling of microsomal activating
enzymes(*3,32*) with this system may provide a means of testing a
wide variety of potential carcinogens.  The concept of detecting
mutagens and carcinogens by a biochemical assay is particularly
attractive since all components in the reaction can be accurately
quantitated.  The correlation between alterations in infidelity
*in vitro* and mutagenicity and carcinogenicity *in vivo* is in accord
with the hypothesis that infidelity during DNA synthesis may cause
mutations.  However, metal cations may have many effects *in vivo*.
Therefore, considerable evidence will be required to document whether
or not metal alterations in the fidelity of DNA synthesis is caus-
ally associated with malignancy.  Irrespective of this biological
underpinning, the correlation between alterations in infidelity and
mutagenicity and/or carcinogenicity indicates the practicality of
using fidelity assays as a screen for evaluating possible mutagens
or carcinogens.

*ACKNOWLEDGEMENTS*

This study was supported by grants from the National Institutes
of Health (CA-11524, CA-12818, and CA-01034) and the National Science
Foundation (BMS73-06751), by grants to this Institute from the
National Institutes of Health (CA-06927 and RR-05539) and by an
appropriation from the Commonwealth of Pennsylvania.

*REFERENCES*

1.  Temin, H. M. and Baltimore, D., Advances in Virus Research 17, Page 129, 1972.

2.  Grossman, L., Advances in Radiation Biology 4, Page 77, 1974.

3.  Miller, E. C. and Miller, J. A., The Molecular Biology of Cancer, Page 377, H. Busch, Editor, Academic Press, New York, 1974.

4.  Cairns, J., Scientific American, 233, Page 64, 1975.

5.  Knudson, A. G., Jr., Hethcote, H. W. and Brown, B. W., Proceedings National Academy Science, USA 72, Page 5116, 1975.

6.  Loeb, L. A., Springgate, C. F. and Battula, N., Cancer Research 34, Page 2311, 1974.

7.  Foulds, L., Cancer Research 14, Page 327, 1954.

8.  Kornberg, A., DNA Synthesis, W. H. Freeman and Co., San Francisco, 1974.

9.  Speyer, J. F., Biochem. Biophys. Research Communications 21, Page 6, 1965.

10. Trautner, T. T., Schwartz, M. N. and Kornberg, A., Proceedings National Academy Science, USA 48, Page 449, 1962.

11. Springgate, C. F. and Loeb, L. A., Proceedings National Academy Science, USA 70, Page 245, 1973.

12. Battula, N. and Loeb, L. A., J. Biol. Chemistry 249, Page 4086, 1974.

13. Hall, Z. W. and Lehman, I. R., J. Mol. Biol. 36, Page 321, 1968.

14. Springgate, C. F., Battula, N. and Loeb, L. A., Biochem. Biophys. Research Commun. 52, Page 401, 1973.

15. Chang, L. M. S., J. Biol. Chem. 248, Page 6983, 1973.

16. Agarwal, S. S. and Loeb, L. A., unpublished results.

17. Springgate, C. F. and Loeb, L. A., J. Mol. Biol. 97, Page 577, 1975.

18. Weymouth, L. A. and Loeb, L. A., unpublished results.

19.  Sirover, M. A. and Loeb, L. A., Biochem. Biophys. Res. Commun.
     61, Page 410, 1974.

20.  Brutlag, D. and Kornberg, A., J. Biol. Chem. 247, Page 241, 1972.

21.  Loeb, L. A., The Enzymes 10, P. Boyer, Editor, Page 173, 1974.

22.  Seal, G. and Loeb, L. A., J. Biol. Chem. 251, Page 975, 1976.

23.  Battula, N. and Loeb, L. A., J. Biol. Chem. 250, Page 4405,
     1975.

24.  Sirover, M. A. and Loeb, L. A., Proceedings National Academy
     Science, USA 73, Page 2331, 1976.

25.  Battula, N., Dube, D. K. and Loeb, L. A., J. Biol. Chem. 250,
     Page 8404, 1975.

26.  Sirover, M. A. and Loeb, L. A., Nature 252, Page 414, 1974.

27.  Sirover, M. A. and Loeb, L. A., Biochem. Biophys. Res. Commun.
     70, Page 812, 1976.

28.  Dube, D. K. and Loeb, L. A., Biochem. Biophys. Res. Commun. 67,
     Page 1041, 1975.

29.  Mizutani, S. and Temin, H. M., Biochemistry 15, Page 1510, 1976.

30.  Orgel, A. and Orgel, L. E., J. Mol. Biol. 14, Page 453, 1965.

31.  Sirover, M. A. and Loeb, L. A., Science 194, Page 1434, 1976.

32.  Ames, B. N., Durston, W. E., Yamasaki, E. and Lee, F. D.,
     Proceedings National Academy Science, USA 70, Page 2281, 1973.

CHAPTER 9

METALS AS MUTAGENS*

C. Peter Flessel

Department of Biology, University of San Francisco
San Francisco, California  94117

Present Address:  Biochemistry Group, Air and Industrial Hygiene
Laboratory, State of California, Department of
Health, 2151 Berkeley Way, Berkeley, California

*SUMMARY*

A number of metals are mutagenic in bacteria or phage.  These
include compounds of arsenic, chromium, copper, iron, manganese,
molybdenum, platinum, and selenium.  Compounds containing aluminum,
antimony, arsenic, cadmium, copper, lead, mercury, nickel, and tellurium have been shown to induce chromosomal aberrations or abnormal
cell divisions in animal or plant cells.  Genetic evidence suggests
that arsenic, chromium, and molybdenum compounds may influence the
accuracy of DNA repair processes in microorganisms.

I.   INTRODUCTION:  MUTATIONS, METALS, AND CANCER

A.  Cancer as a Genetic Disease

The first suggestion that heredity influenced the occurrence
of cancer was made by Hanau who observed, in 1889, that animal
carcinomas could be transplanted between animals of the same genetic
stock more easily than between members of outbred lines.[1,2]  Ten
years later, Loeb, studying endemic cancer in the stockyards of
Chicago, noted that "cattle coming from a certain ranch in Wyoming
were particularly susceptible to cancer of the inner canthus of
the eye," and suggested that "the occurrence of neoplastic growths
were due to a hereditary condition rather than an infection".[2]

---

\*    Mutagens:  Compounds which induce well-characterized heritable
                phenotypic changes in genetically described viruses,
                cell lines, or organisms.

117

Loeb's conception of cancer involved the interplay of internal
(inherited) and external (environmental) factors.  Although it
was usually difficult to separate these factors, "sometimes, as
in cases where there is obviously a clearcut source of chemical
stimulation such as coal tar, external forces predominate".(2)

B.   Environmental Factors and Somatic Cell Mutations

    The hypothesis that external factors might cause cancer by
inducing mutations was first introduced by Boveri in 1895.(3)   The
essence of the theory involved the occurrence of an "abnormal
chromatin-complex.  Every process that brings about this chromatin condition would lead to a malignant tumor.  Certain chromosomes
becoming diseased (owing to an inherited disposition), or a disturbance of these chromosomes by intracellular parasites or external influences that act perniciously on certain chromosomes, may
be considered important in producing tumors."(3)   According to
Strong(2), Williams, in 1908, also suggested "that the cause under-
lying tumor-cell formation may be analogous to the phenomenon known
as mutation".  While both somatic and germ cell lines are susceptible to mutation, the theory as currently applied seeks to explain
cancer primarily in terms of environmentally induced somatic cell
mutations.  Extensive reviews of the theory have been presented by
Burdette in 1955(4), and by Miller and Miller in 1971.(5)   Strong
contemporary support has come from the work of Ames and coworkers(6)
who have shown a ninety percent correlation between organic compounds that are carcinogens and mutagens.

C.   Metal Mutagenesis and Carcinogenesis:   Manganese, A Case History

    The mutation hypothesis will be given credence with respect to
metal carcinogenesis "if it is found that the carcinogenic metals,
more so than the noncarcinogenic ones, can cause chromosome breaks
readily" argued Furst and Haro(7) in 1969.  Soon after, Corbett,
Heidelberger, and Dove(8) attempted to demonstrate the mutagenic
activity of two suspected metal carcinogens, $CaCrO_4$ and $Pb(CH_3COO)_2$.
The genetic test employed the *Escherichia coli* phage T4 in a highly
sensitive manner and proved negative for both compounds.  These
negative results were not attributable to some special property of
the phage since Orgel and Orgel(9) had previously shown T4 to be
sensitive to mutagenesis by manganese chloride.

    Manganese, as a mutagen and a carcinogen, has an interesting
history.  It is probably the best-known metal mutagen.  Mutagenicity was first demonstrated in 1950 by Demerec and Hanson(10) in
bacteria (*Escherichia coli*) 15 years prior to the discovery in
bacteriophage.  Recently, Mn(II) has been shown to induce mutations
in yeast, affecting primarily the mitochondrial genes.(11)   This
later result clarified early observations of Lindegren et al.(12)
that "manganese salts induced respiratory deficiency with great

efficacy", and that "the effect of manganous salts on yeast seems to be due almost exclusively to their effect on *cytoplasmic granules* rather than on the genome".  The failure to recognize the existence of genetic target sites in the mitochondria comprising these cytoplasmic granules accounted for the following conclusion:  "It is commonly said that most mutagens...are carcinogens and it has been inferred that the problem of cancer is related in some way to the structure of deoxyribonucleic acid.  This inference rests on the assumption that gene mutation is an important factor in carcinogenesis.  Many of the effects, however, that are ascribed to gene mutation may be due to the damage to autonomous cytoplasmic granules, and such carcinogens as ultraviolet and X-rays have often been demonstrated to produce stable variations in the extra-chromosomal apparatus.  Reevaluation of ideas relating gene mutation to carcinogenesis may be in order."(12)

Indeed, although effects of metal ions and X-rays on "autonomous cytoplasmic granules" in no way weakens the mutation theory, since mutations in mitochondrial genes are no less mutations than those in nuclear genes, the preceding statement focuses attention on the possible interconnectedness of energy metabolism, mutations, and cancer.  This appears especially prudent in light of current tendencies to separate theories of cancer into metabolic or genetic categories.  Finally, there is now evidence that manganese is a carcinogen in animals.  A weak carcinogenic response has been reported by Furst(13) with manganese diacetyl acetone in rats and by Shimkin et al.(14)  with manganese sulfate in mice.  To these findings should be added the observations of Sunderman(15) that manganese metal antagonizes the carcinogenic effects of nickel subsulfide ($Ni_3S_2$) in rats.

## II.   METAL MUTAGENESIS IN BACTERIA AND BACTERIOPHAGE: ASSAYS AND OBSERVATIONS

Because of their simplicity and sensitivity, as well as economy of use, bacteria and bacterial viruses are the organisms in which most studies of mutagenesis have been carried out.  The question of the relevancy of conclusions drawn from genetic studies in microorganisms to higher organisms is a topic of debate.  The fact remains, however, that the same chemical substance, DNA, serves as the repository of genetic information in bacteria as well as in man. It is hardly surprising that many physical and chemical agents react with the DNA of both procaryotic and eucaryotic cells to produce mutations.  At the very least, the demonstration that a particular substance is a mutagen in bacteria increases our awareness of its potential mutagenicity, and perhaps also carcinogenicity, in higher organisms.

A.    The Ames Assay in Salmonella typhimurium

The extensive correlation compiled by Ames and coworkers[6] compared the carcinogenicity of organic carcinogens in animals, usually rats or mice, with their mutagenicity in strains of Salmonella typhimurium especially sensitive to mutagens.  Of one hundred seventy-four carcinogens tested, one hundred fifty-six (90%) were found to be mutagenic.  Among over 100 noncarcinogens tested, fewer than one in seven showed mutagenic activity.  The Ames assay for mutagenesis consists in treating histidine-requiring (his$^-$) bacteria with the test substances on agar plates.  After incubation, the plates are scored for the presence of histidine-independent colonies (his$^+$ revertants), each the result of a genetic alteration that corrects the defect in histidine biosynthesis.  In many cases, an animal cell extract, obtained from rat liver, is added to the agar to permit the enzymatic activation of precursors to active mutagens.

A number of metal compounds have been shown to be mutagenic in the Salmonella reversion assay.  They include compounds of chromium containing chromate and dichromate [Cr(VI)],[16] iron [Fe(II)],[17] manganese [Mn(II)],[18] platinum [Pt(IV)],[19] and selenium [Se(VI)].[16]

B.    The Rec Assay in Bacillus subtilis

An early study of Weed, 1962[20] implicated copper [Cu(II)] as a mutagen in B. subtilis.  Stable variants with altered colony morphology and transformability were isolated from liquid cultures exposed to copper sulfate.

Recently, a different methodology has been developed by Nishioka [21] to test the potential mutagenicity of fifty-six metal compounds including a number of known or suspected carcinogens.  The assay is based on the fact that bacteria normally possess the capacity to repair physical and chemical lesions in their DNA.  The normal (wild type) strains are designated Rec$^+$, for recombination, which appears to be crucially involved in certain forms of DNA repair.  Recombination deficient strains are called Rec$^-$.  Nishioka has observed that "cells deficient in the repair capacity of DNA lesions (Rec$^-$) are usually killed much more by any DNA-damaging agent than wild (Rec$^+$) cells".  A positive result using the assay does not prove mutagenicity.  However, "when a chemical is more inhibitory for Rec$^-$ than for Rec$^+$ cells, it is reasonable to suspect mutagenicity based on its DNA-damaging capacity".  Compounds giving positive Rec effects were arsenic (AsCl$_3$, NaAsO$_2$, and Na$_2$HAsO$_4$), cadmium (CdCl$_2$), chromium (K$_2$CrO$_4$ and K$_2$Cr$_2$O$_7$), mercury (CH$_3$HgCl and CH$_4$COOHgC$_6$H$_5$), manganese [MnCl$_2$, Mn(NO$_3$)$_2$, MnSO$_4$, and Mn(CH$_3$COO)$_2$], and molybdenum [K$_2$MoO$_4$ and (NH$_4$)$_6$Mo$_7$O$_{24}$].  Among the metal compounds tested which showed no Rec effect were beryllium (BeCl$_2$), cobalt (CoCl$_2$), copper (CuCl and

CuCl$_2$), iron [FeCl$_2$, K$_3$(Fe[CN]$_6$), and K$_4$(Fe[CN]$_6$], lead [PbCl$_2$, Pb(CH$_3$COO)$_2$] and nickel (NiCl$_2$).

## C. Studies in Escherichia coli and Its Phage

The mutagenic actions of manganese(10) and iron(22) salts were first described in *E. coli* by Demerec and coworkers more than a quarter of a century ago. A strain of *E. coli* dependent upon streptomycin for its growth (*E. coli* B/rSd-4) was treated with the metal salts in suspension culture and then plated in the absence of the drug, to select for mutations from streptomycin dependence to non-dependence. Both manganese [Mn(II)] and iron [Fe(II)] salts were found to have mutagenic potencies that compared well with that of nitrogen mustard and radiation under conditions that produced little or no killing. Extensive studies with MnCl$_2$(10) revealed that the mutagenic potency of this compound could be made to vary greatly, depending upon the physiological state of the organism. For example, washing the bacteria before metal treatment with hypertonic solutions of NaCl, KCl, or sucrose increased the mutagenic response. Similar experiments in *Salmonella* showed manganese to be much more strongly mutagenic in exponentially growing as opposed to stationary phase cells.(18) In addition to its mutagenic activity in bacteria, Orgel and Orgel(9) showed that divalent manganese is also mutagenic in the bacteriophage, T4. Treatment of T4 infected *E. coli* with MnSO$_4$ at concentrations of $10^{-2}$M increased the proportion of rII (rapid lysis) mutants from less than 0.04% to about 1%, a factor of at least 25.

The mutagenicity of chromate has also been examined extensively in *E. coli* by several groups. Veniti and Levy(23) demonstrated that Na$_2$CrO$_4$, K$_2$CrO$_4$, and CaCrO$_4$ induced reversion of a tryptophan auxotroph, *E. coli* WP2(trp$^-$), to tryptophan independence. Positive results were first obtained by spotting chromate solutions on agar plates containing lawns of trp$^-$ bacteria and scoring for trp$^+$ revertants. These results were confirmed by treating bacteria in suspension with Na$_2$CrO$_4$, after which the chromate was removed and the mutagenicity and lethality determined independently. Under conditions where 10-30% of the cells survived chromate treatment, the mutation frequency of trp$^+$ revertants was 100-200 times the background level.

A study of metal mutagenesis in *E. coli* WP2(trp$^-$) was also carried out by Nishioka.(21) Suspensions of bacteria were treated briefly with millimolar concentrations of K$_2$Cr$_2$O$_7$, (NH$_4$)$_6$Mo$_7$O$_{24}$, and NaAsO$_2$, which gave 30-40% survival. All three compounds were reported to have given an increase in the frequency of trp$^+$ revertants. However, when tested in a derivative of WP2 lacking a functional RecA (DNA repair) gene, strain CM571 (trp$^-$ RecA$^-$), the three compounds were not mutagenic.

Green, Muriel, and Bridges(24) also investigated chromate
mutagenesis in *E. coli* WP2(trp⁻) by means of a simplified fluctua-
tion test. The assay was positive for $K_2CrO_4$ at concentrations as
low as 0.5 µg/ml. Tindall, Warren, and Skaar(25) have recently
measured the mutagenic effects of metal ions in *E. coli*. In their
study, $K_2CrO_4$ and $K_2Cr_2O_7$ (CrVI) proved mutagenic, inducing revertants in *E. coli* WP₂ as well as exhibiting strong "Rec" effects in
*E. coli*.

D.    The Role of Metabolic Activation

Several mutagenic metal compounds were tested by Nishioka(26)
in the presence and absence of a rat liver enzyme extract (S-9) to
determine the role of metabolic activation in metal mutagenesis.
Chromium (CrVI) compounds that were positive in the standard assay,
were negative in the presence of $NaSO_3$. However, treatment with
$NaSO_3$ plus the enzyme extract caused the chromium compounds to become mutagenic again. Inorganic mercury, which itself was non-
mutagenic, became mutagenic when applied in the presence of the S-9,
indicating the possible formation of organo-mercury compounds.
Also, arsenic compounds were found to be less active in the presence
of the S-9 extract than in its absence.

III.    METAL-INDUCED GENETIC DAMAGE IN HIGHER ORGANISMS

There are a number of studies that indicate that certain heavy
metal salts produce chromosome aberrations or abnormal cell divisions
in higher plants and animals. While such studies generally fail to
demonstrate mutagenesis using the classical criterion (i.e., the
induction of stable, heritable phenotypic changes), they also may be
relevant to the problems of metal carcinogenesis.

A.    Cytological Observations and C-Mitosis

Patton and Allison(27) reported chromosome damage in human cell
cultures exposed to metal salts. Treatment of cells with subtoxic
doses ($10^{-8}$ - $10^{-9}$M) of compounds of arsenic (especially $NaAsO_2$, but
also acetylarsan), antimony (sodium antimonate), and tellurium (ammon-
ium tellurate and sodium tellurite) produced chromosome breaks in
leukocytes and fibroblasts. No chromosomal aberrations were seen with
selected salts of cobalt, nickel, iron, selenium, vanadium, mercury,
or beryllium. However, Komczynski et al.(28) showed that salts of
the iron group (cobalt, nickel, and iron), especially the nitrates,
caused changes in cell nuclei and disturbances in cell division in
roots of the broad bean (*Vicia faba*). Chromosomal disturbances were
observed in *Allium* roots and human leukocytes following treatment
with various organic mercury halogenides.(29) At concentrations of
$10^{-6}$M, methyl mercury chloride, ethyl mercury chloride, methoxethyl
mercury chloride and butyl mercury bromide were all active.

"The most prominent genetic effect of methyl mercury is its interference with the mitotic spindle, causing chromosome doubling or
defective distribution of individual chromosomes during cell division, which leads to daughter cells with one or more missing or
additional chromosomes (C-mitosis)."(30, see also 31) Verschaev et
al.(32) have recently reported genetic damage to lymphocytes obtained from whole blood of human subjects occupationally exposed to
mercury.  Aluminum chloride and cadmium nitrate have been reported
to produce chromosome breaks(33) and chromosome aberrations are
seen in lymphocytes of workers occupationally exposed to cadmium
and lead.(34-36)  Chromosome damage preveiously had been demonstrated
in experimentally induced lead poisoning in animals(37) and plants.(38)

B.    Genetic Assays

     As described above, manganese salts have been shown by
Putrament et al. (11) to induce mutants in yeast (*Saccaromyces
cerevisiae*) affecting primarily the mitochondrial genes.  The mitochondria are believed to have arisen by inclusion of procaryotic
cells during an early stage in the evolution of the eucaryotes.
The specificity of manganese for the mitochondrial genes, taken
together with the ample demonstration of its mutagenic potency in
procaryotes suggests that this metal may have a selective affinity
for procaryote-type genetic structures.

IV.   GENETIC STUDIES ON THE MECHANISMS
OF METAL MUTAGENESIS IN MICROORGANISMS

A.    The Nature of the Mutational Changes

     Genetic studies in microorganisms often permit not only the
identification of mutagens *per se*, but often also give information
about the nature of the mutational changes induced.  In a reversion
test, bacterial strains carrying well-defined mutations are treated
with the suspected mutagen and then plated under selective conditions
that permit only the growth of "wild-type" revertants that have
undergone mutation.  Tester strains used in such assays usually
carry either point mutations, resulting from the substitution of one
base pair for another, or frameshift mutations, resulting from the
deletion of one or two base pairs in their DNA.

     The demonstration that a substance reverts a particular strain
does not always accurately identify the nature of the mutational
change involved because expression of the wild phenotype is sometimes
the result of a suppressor mutation.  Suppressors are secondary mutations that suppress other mutations, even though they may occur
at a site some distance on the DNA from the primary mutational site.
A complete genetic analysis, therefore, requires checking revertants
for suppressors.  In mutagen screening studies, however, such procedures are often omitted.  With this limitation in mind, tentative

conclusions regarding the nature of the genetic changes induced by
metal compounds nevertheless may be drawn.

Manganese (II) salts have been shown to induce both point and
frameshift mutations in microorganisms. The early study of Orgel
and Orgel (9) indicated that manganese sulfate produced primarily
point mutations in the E. coli phage T4. Their analysis showed
that about 90% of the metal ion induced rII (rapid lysis) mutants
were reverted by DNA base analogs, 5-bromodeoxyuridine and 2-amino-
purine. In a more recent study, Scholla et al.(18) showed that
manganous chloride reverted a Salmonella tester strain TA1532,
carrying the his C3076 frameshift mutation. Chromium [Cr(VI) also
appears to induce both frameshift and point mutations, depending on
the strains and assay systems employed. Löfroth and Ames(16) showed
that salts of chromate and dichromate are frameshift mutagens in
Salmonella, reverting strains with the his C3076 and his D3052 mutations as well as strains with the his G46 point mutation which
also carry a resistance transfer factor (R factor). Strains carrying the frameshift mutation his D3052 have a repetitive -C-G-C-G-
C-G-C-G sequence near the site of the histidine mutation, while
strains with the his C3076 mutation appear to have a run of C's at
the site of the mutation.(39) If direct binding of metal ions to
DNA is involved in mutagenesis, then chromate and dichromate apparently show a propensity for GC-rich regions of the bacterial chromosome. The fact that both ions are also capable of reverting point
mutations in strains carrying the R factor could indicate that they
potentiate error-prone DNA repair processes that are known to be
mediated by genes carried by the R factor.

The study of Venitt and Levy(23) on chromate mutagenicity in
E. coli leads to the same conclusion, namely, that chromate facili-
tates mutations in GC-rich regions of the chromosome. Their study
was carried out in a strain of E. coli, WP2(trp⁻), which requires
tryptophan biosynthesis (trpE). Among the 64 triplets comprising
the genetic code, three, UAA, UAG, and UGA, do not represent any
amino acid but instead, are involved in protein chain termination.
Mutations giving rise to one of the three within, instead of at the
end of a gene, lead to premature chain release and are referred to
as nonsense triplets. In the present example, the nonsense mutation
carried by strain WP2 is an ochre triplet, UAA, containing only AT
DNA base pairs at the site of mutation. Venitt and Levy tested
100 chromate-induced trp⁺ revertants and discovered that 98 contained ochre suppressors. In contrast, only about half the spontaneous revertants tested carried a suppressor. Since only 2% of
the metal-induced revertants contained an alteration at the primary
site, it was concluded that chromate did not modify AT base pairs,
but instead, preferentially facilitated mutations in GC-rich regions
of the DNA.

In addition to manganese and chromium, ferrous sulfate also has

been reported to revert the "frameshift" *Salmonella* tester
strains.(*17*)

In contrast, selenium [Se(VI)](*16*) and platinum [Pt(IV)](*19*)
both appear to be point mutagens.  Löfroth and Ames(*16*) reported
low but significant mutagenic activity with selenate [Se(VI)], but
not selenite [Se(IV)], in *Salmonella* strains carrying the base pair
substitution his G46.  Likewise, Rosenberg(*19*) showed that *cis*-
diamino platinum (IV) tetrachloride was mutagenic in *Salmonella*
*typhimurium* TA100, carrying the his G46 mutation and the error-prone
R factor, but was not active in *Salmonella* strains carrying frameshift mutations.  Furthermore, the effect was stereospecific for
the *cis* complex, the *trans* isomer being inactive.

B.   The Genetic Systems Involved:   The Role of DNA Repair

Nishioka(*21*) compared the mutagenic potential of several metal
compounds in bacterial strains altered in their DNA repair capacity.
As described above, treatment of *E. coli* WP2(trp$^-$) with $K_2Cr_2O_7$,
$(NH_4)_6Mo_7O_{24}$, or $NaAsO_2$ increased the frequency of trp$^+$ revertants.
When tested in a derivative of WP2 lacking the DNA repair gene uvrA
(*E. coli* WP2 uvrA$^-$), all three compounds were again mutagenic.  However, when tested in another derivative of WP2 lacking the RecA DNA
repair gene, CM571 (trp$^-$uvrA$^+$RecA$^-$), none of the compounds showed
mutagenic activity.  Apparently, the presence of the RecA function
is essential to mutagenesis by these metals, while the effect of
the uvrA gene is minimal.

The role of arsenic as $NaAsO_2$ in bacterial DNA repair has also
been advanced by Rossman et al.(*40*)  Their studies indicated the
sodium arsenite decreased the survival of ultraviolet-irradiated
*E. coli* WP2, but had no effect on the survival of a RecA mutant,
WP10.  It was postulated that arsenite inhibits a RecA-dependent
step in the repair of uv-induced DNA lesions.

While the exact role of the RecA gene in DNA repair is not
understood, it is known to influence "error-prone" postreplication
repair.(*41*)  This process, which occurs after excision repair synthesis in DNA repair, may involve inaccurate recombinational repair
or a special type of repair replication capable of inserting bases.
The RecA system increases the sensitivity of strains carrying it to
a wide variety of mutagenic agents and its effects may be poten-
tiated by certain metal ions; however, RecA-dependent, error-prone
repair apparently does not occur in higher organisms.(*42*)

V.   CONCLUSIONS

Evidence that metal compounds containing arsenic, chromium,
copper, iron, manganese, molybdenum, platinum, and selenium are

mutagenic in microorganisms has been presented.  In addition, compounds of aluminum, antimony, arsenic, cadmium, copper, lead, mercury, nickel, and tellurium induce chromosomal damage in higher organisms.  Of these metals, arsenic, cadmium, chromium, iron, lead, manganese, and nickel are reported carcinogens in animals or man,(43) while selenium(44) and platinum(19) have been described as cancer-protecting or carcinostatic agents, respectively.

*REFERENCES*

1.    Wells, H. J. American Medical Association 81, Page 1017, 1923.

2.    Strong, L. American Naturalist 60, Page 201, 1926.

3.    Boveri, T., The Origin of Malignant Tumors (M. Boveri, trans.)
      Williams and Wilkins, Baltimore, Page 34, 1929.

4.    Burdette, W., Cancer Research 15, Page 201, 1955.

5.    Miller, E. and Miller, J., The Chemical Mutagens:  Principles
      and Methods for Their Detection, Vol. I, A. Hollaender, Editor.
      Plenum Press, New York, Page 83, 1971.

6.    McCann, J., Choi, E., Yamasaki, E. and Ames, B., Proceedings
      National Academy Science 72, Page 5135, 1975.

7.    Furst, A. and Haro, R., The Jerusalem Symposia on Quantum Chemistry and Biochemistry, Vol. I, E. Bergmann and B. Pullman,
      Editors, The Israel Academy of Sciences and Humanities, Jerusalem, Page 310, 1969.

8.    Corbett, T., Heidelberger, C. and Dove, W., Mol. Pharmacology
      6, Page 667, 1970.

9.    Orgel, A. and Orgel, L., J. Mol. Biology 14, Page 453, 1965.

10.   Demerec, M. and Hanson, J., Cold Spring Harbor Symposia on
      Quantitative Biology 16, Page 215, 1951.

11.   Putrament, A., Baranowake, H., Ejchart, A. and Prazmo, W.,
      J. General Microbiology 62, Page 265, 1975.

12.   Lindegren, C., Nagai, S. and Nagai, H., Nature 182, Page 446,
      1958.

13.   Furst, A., personal communication.

14.   Shimkin, M., Stoner, G. and Theiss, J., this Symposium.

15.   Sunderman, F., this Symposium.

16. Löfroth, G. and Ames, B., Environmental Mutagen Society Abstracts, Annual Meeting, February 13-17, 1977, Colorado Springs, Colorado.

17. Brusick, D., Gletten, F., Japannath, D. and Weeker, U., Mutation Research 38, Page 387, 1976.

18. Scholla, C., Schibler, M., May, J. and Flessel, P. (manuscript in preparation).

19. Rosenberg, B., this Symposium.

20. Weed, L., J. Bacteriology 85, Page 1003, 1963.

21. Nishioka, H., Mutation Research 31, Page 185, 1975.

22. Demerec, M., Wallace, B., Witkin, E. and Bertani, G., Carnegie Institute of Washington (Yearbook) 48, Page 156, 1949.

23. Venitt, S. and Levy, L., Nature 250, Page 493, 1974.

24. Green, M., Muriel, W. and Bridges, B., Mutation Research 38, Page 33, 1976.

25. Tindall, K., Warren, G. and Skaar, P., Environmental Mutagen Society Abstracts, Annual Meeting, February 13-17, 1977, Colorado Springs, Colorado.

26. Nishioka, H., Japanese J. Genetics 50, Page 485, 1975.

27. Paton, G. and Allison, A., Mutation Research 16, Page 332, 1972.

28. Komczynski, L., Nowak, H. and Rejniak, L., Nature 198, Page 1016, 1963.

29. Fiskesjo, G., Hereditas 62, Page 314, 1969; 64, Page 142, 1970.

30. Löfroth, G., Trace Substances in Environmental Health, D. Hemphill, Editor, University of Missouri, Columbia, Page 63, 1973.

31. Ramel, C., Hereditas 61, Page 208, 1969.

32. Verschaeve, L., Kirsch-Volders, M., Susanne, C., Embriel, C., Haustermans, R., Lecomte, A. and Roossels, D., Environmental Research 12, Page 306, 1976.

33. Oehlkers, F., Heredity, Supplement 6, Page 95, 1953.

34.  Bauchlinger, M., Schmid, E., Einbrodt, H. and Dresp, J.,
     Mutation Research 40, Page 57, 1976.

35.  Bui, T., Linsten, J., Norberg, G., Environmental Research 9,
     Page 187, 1975.

36.  Shiraishi, Y., Humangenetik 27, Page 31, 1975.

37.  Muro, L. and Goyer, R., Arch. Pathology 87, Page 660, 1969.

38.  Levan, A., Nature 156, Page 751, 1945.

39.  Ames, B., McCann, J. and Yamasaki, E., Mutation Research 31,
     Page 347, 1975.

40.  Rossman, T., Meyn, S. and Troll, W., Mutation Research 30,
     Page 157, 1975.

41.  Witkin, E., Genetics 79, Page 199, 1975.

42.  Trosko, J. and Chu, E., Adv. in Cancer Research 21, Page 391,
     1975.

43.  Furst, A., this Symposium.

44.  Schrauzer, G., this Symposium.

# Part II

# Metal Compounds in Chemotherapy
# and Related Topics

*CHAPTER 10*


NOBLE METAL COMPLEXES IN CANCER CHEMOTHERAPY*

Barnett Rosenberg

Professor of Biophysics
Department of Biophysics, Michigan State University
East Lansing, Michigan

*ABSTRACT*

Platinum coordination complexes form a new class of active anti-
cancer agents in animals and man. *Cis*-dichlorodiammineplatinum(II),
the most widely investigated drug, is now in experimental clinical
use against a wide variety of cancers in man. The dose-limiting
toxicity in man is renal tubular damage. Hydration of the patient
and the use of osmotic diuretics have minimized this effect and
allowed higher doses with largely improved responses. Combination
chemotherapy with the drug has also produced significant response
rates in a variety of cancers. The mode of action of the drug is
not yet clear, but most likely involves a primary lesion on nuclear
DNA and the stimulation of a host reaction to the cancer. So far,
only square planar and octahedral complexes of platinum, with a
variety of inorganic and organic ligands, have shown marked activity
in animal studies.

---

* This manuscript is, in large part, taken from a review paper
  that appeared in Die Naturwissenschaften 60, Pages 399-406,
  in 1973. New sections and some revisions have been made,
  updating the data.

# I.  INTRODUCTION

The application of platinum coordination complexes to the treatment of tumors in animals and man arose from the discovery that *cis*-dichlorodiammineplatinum(II), and some analog structures were potent anti-tumor agents against sarcoma 180 and leukemia L1210 in mice.(*1*)  This was an unexpected finding.  The history leading to the testing of its activity against tumors (a classic case of serendipity) has been described in earlier pages (*2*,*3*) and does not bear repeating here.  It is surprising and somewhat disconcerting that an entire sophisticated branch of chemistry, that of metal coordination complexes, had been largely ignored in the search for new drugs for cancer chemotherapy.  Since 1970, however, the National Cancer Institute of the United States, the Chester Beatty Institute in England, and numerous other laboratories and institutes have been making extensive efforts to redress the balance.  The literature is now large, and rapidly increasing.  While the major motivations for these studies are the applications to cancer chemotherapy, some laboratories have shown a broader scope of biological activities of these complexes including bacteriocidal, viricidal, immunosuppressive, and anti-arthritic activities.  Thus, we have a new, large class of chemical structures with a wide variety of potential biological and medical applications, the exploration of which has only just begun.  I shall restrict this review only to some recent developments in the field of cancer chemotherapy with platinum coordination complexes.

Large numbers of square planar platinum(II) complexes now have been screened for anti-tumor activity and, from these results, some simple "rules of thumb" have emerged relating structure and *in vivo* activity.  A variety of tumor systems in animals are used in such screening tests, and the number and types of tumor systems showing positive results suggest that these complexes are broad spectrum, anti-tumor agents.  The retention times and distribution patterns of these complexes in animals and man are now becoming known.  The sites of the primary lesions in the cells, leading to tumor destruction, are believed to be on the nuclear DNA.  However, *in vitro* tests indicate a large number of possible modes of reaction of the complexes with the nucleic acid and its constituents.  Events subsequent to the primary attack that lead to anti-tumor activity are largely unknown, but some evidence has been found suggesting the involvement of the hosts' immune response in the anti-tumor activity.  The toxic side effects in animals and man primarily are damage to renal tubules, the gastrointestinal epithelium, and bone marrow; with the kidney damage being the dose-limiting effect in man.  Recently, it has been found that hydration, with or without osmotic diuretics such as D-mannitol, decrease the renal toxicity without substantially depleting the drug from the body.  Thus, at allowed higher doses, other side effects are enhanced, as is the

anti-cancer activity.  Experimental clinical studies on a variety
of tumor types, both in the high-dose therapy and in combination
therapy, indicate that significant responses can be obtained.  In
testicular cancer, nearly 100% of the patients with metastatic
tumors responded, and in almost all of them the response was complete and of long duration.  The clinicians have called these therapies "probably curative".  Other cancers are beginning to show an
approach to these response levels.  These include ovarian carcinoma,
head and neck carcinomas, and bladder carcinomas.  Studies of other
cancers are as yet incomplete.  These results suggest that this first
platinum drug will be a valuable addition to cancer chemotherapy.

## Structure-Activity Relations for Platinum Complexes

The broad area of metal coordination chemistry has now been
broached in the search for new anti-tumor drugs.  It is of some
value to identify avenues and pockets of high potential success in
this search.

With our present state of ignorance, it is necessary to screen
as wide a variety of complexes as possible, particularly those for
which no logical connection to cancer chemotherapy has yet been established.  This massive, nonselective screening is most properly
the job of large institutions such as the Drug Research and Development Branch of the National Cancer Institute, which, indeed, has en-
thusiastically embraced this function.  They welcome the submission
of any such chemicals for their screening program.

For smaller groups, the area of research must by some means be
delineated.  Two groups, Thomson, Williams, and Reslova(4) and Cleare
and Hoeschele(5,6) have attempted to develop some guidelines.  Both
start with the observations that the presently established active
drugs, a few of whose structures are shown in Figure 1, exhibit some
common features.  These are:  (1) the complexes exchange only some
of their ligands quickly; (2) the complexes are neutral (although
the biologically active form may be charged after ligand exchange
*in vivo*); (3) the geometry of the complexes are either square planar
or octahedral; (4) two *cis* monodentate (or one bidentate) leaving
groups are required, the corresponding *trans* isomers of the monodentate leaving groups are generally inactive; (5) the rate of exchange of the leaving groups should fall in a restricted "window of
lability" roughly centered on that of the chlorides in 1 (the
palladium analog of 3, with a reaction rate some $10^5$ faster, has no
anti-tumor activity); (6) the leaving groups are spaced approximately
3.3 angstroms apart; (7) the ligands *trans* to the leaving groups
appear preferentially to be strongly bonded, relatively inert amine
type systems, probably due to a low thermodynamic probability of
substitution (although reactions with carbonyl groups on the pyri-
midines may be possible as discussed below).

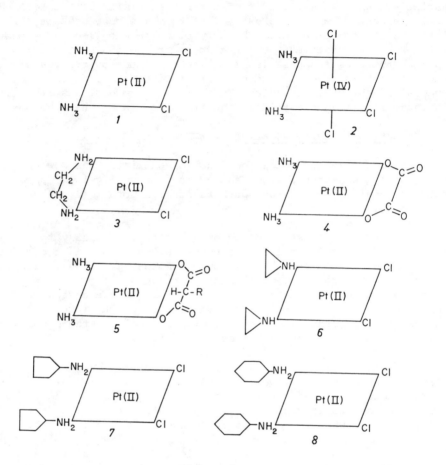

Figure 1

1. Structural Formulae of Some Representative Active Anti-tumor
   Complexes of Platinum: *1   cis*-dichlorodiammineplatinum(II);
   *2 cis*-tetrachlorodiammineplatinum(IV); *3* dichloroethylene-
   diamineplatinum(II); *4* oxalatodiammineplatinum(II); *5* substituted (R) malonatodiammineplatinum(II); *6 cis*-dichloro-
   bis-(ethyleneimine)-platinum(II); *7 cis*-dichloro-bis-
   (cyclopentylamine)-platinum(II); *8 cis*-dichloro-bis-
   (cyclohexylamine)-platinum(II)

Some modifications of the above features are necessary to explain the *in vivo* activity of the bidentate ligands. For example, while all of the monodentate *cis* leaving groups such as $Cl^-$, $Br^-$, $NO_3^-$, etc., are rapidly exchanged in solution, the bidentate groups are quite stable. This requires, if we wish to retain rules 1 and 5, a biochemical "deus ex machina" to activate these groups. Two possible processes are nonspecific oxidative cleavage of the C-C bonds, or enzymatic cleavage of the Pt-0 or C-C bonds. Additional studies are necessary here.

A second modification is required to explain the enormous decrease of the toxicity of the complexes when the ammines are substituted by cyclic amine ligands without a concomitant marked change in the anti-tumor activity, as found by Connors et al.(7)

The appearance of potent anti-tumor activity is a relatively rare occurrence in metal coordination complexes. While over 1,000 complexes have been screened so far, only 80 or so are highly active. We have, however, noted some other surprising biological activities of some of these complexes. For example, a number of complexes are extremely low in toxicity, the $LD_{50}$ (the single injected dose that kills 50% of the animals) for the tetraammineplatinum(II) ion, which is very soluble, is about 60 mg/kg. A similar low toxicity for all 10 soluble complexes of *cis*-dichlorodiammineplatinum(II) with methionine has been found. The most nontoxic complex reported so far, the *cis*-dichloro-bis (cyclohexylamine)-platinum(II) reported by Connors et al.(7) has an $LD_{50}$ of 3200 mg/kg. This complex is very insoluble, but is highly active against the ADJ/PC6 myeloma at a dose level of 12 mg/kg.

Other complexes are extremely toxic neuromuscular poisons, causing death within 20 minutes after injection. Two examples are oxalatoethylenediamine platinum(II) and the tris(ethylenediamine)-platinum(II) ion.

These preliminary results show a wide range of biological activities and toxicities for both soluble and insoluble complexes of this group, and precious few guidelines to allow predictions to be made.

In seeking the second-generation drugs to enter into clinical trials, the clinicians are faced with having to choose among the approximately 80 other active complexes. Criteria have now been established for the rational choice of a limited number of these for entering such trials. These criteria are: (1) high solubility (for potential oral administration); (2) less kidney toxicity; (3) less nausea and vomiting (although this appears to be modifiable by tetrahydrocannabinol given either orally or parenterally or marijuana by smoking); (4) a better penetration of the blood-brain barrier so as to allow treatment of central nervous system cancers;

(5) an improved therapeutic index; (6) potentially different mechanisms of action; (7) drugs that can exhibit synergism when used in
combination therapy with other anti-cancer drugs.

## Anti-Tumor Effects in Animal Systems

The first drug of this class to undergo extensive screening
against a wide variety of different tumor-host systems in animals
is *cis*-dichlorodiammineplatinum(II). While this is by no means the
most active complex against certain tumor systems, it was the first
chosen by the National Cancer Institute for clinical trials on human
patients, which fact has invested this drug with the elements of
primacy and immediacy. I shall restrict the discussion of screening test results to this drug only.

The tumor-screening systems fall into three major categories:
(1) transplantable tumors; (2) virally induced tumors; and (3)
chemically induced tumors (a fourth category, autochthonous tumors
have so far played only a minor role in drug-screening tests). The
*cis*-dichlorodiammineplatinum(II) complex has been tested against
examples in all three major categories, with the preponderance of
work reported on transplantable systems; however, virally induced
and chemically induced tumors are probably more relevant to human
cancers. The drug has shown activity against tumors in all three
categories. I have listed in Table 1 examples of the results of
such tests from a number of laboratories. I emphasize that I have
chosen, for the sake of simplicity, to list only the best results
for each test system, rather than average results, since animal
perversity and limited test results make either best or average results of dubious numerical value, and I merely want to convey a
qualitative impression here.

A number of points can be made from these results; these are:
(1) the drug exhibits marked, rather than marginal anti-tumor activity; (2) it is a broad-spectrum drug that is active against drug-
resistant as well as drug-sensitive tumors; (3) it is active against
slow-growing as well as fast-growing tumors; (4) it has some activity
against a tumor insensitive to "S" phase inhibitors; (5) it regres-
sess transplantable, virally induced and chemically induced tumors;
(6) there is no evidence of animal specificity, since it is active
against tumors in mice and rats, both of inbred and random-bred
strains, and in chickens; (7) it is useful against disseminated as
well as against solid tumors; (8) it is potent in rescuing animals
near death from advanced tumors of certain types.

In most of the tests, a solution of the drug in physiologic
saline was injected intraperitoneally. The drug is somewhat less e
effective when given intramuscularly or subcutaneously. It is ineffective against L1210, but it is still very effective against the
Walker 256 carcinosarcoma when given orally, but a much higher dose
level is required in the latter case.

TABLE 1

BEST RESULTS OF THE ANTI-TUMOR ACTIVITY
OF *CIS*-DICHLORODIAMMINEPLATINUM(II) IN ANIMAL SYSTEMS

| Tumor | Host | Best Results |
|-------|------|--------------|
| Sarcoma-180 solid | Swiss white mice | T/C=2-10% |
| Sarcoma-180 solid (advanced) | Swiss white mice | 100% cures |
| Sarcoma-180 ascites | Swiss white mice | 100% cures |
| Leukemia L1210 | $BDF_1$ mice | % ILS=379%; 4/10 cures |
| Primary Lewis lung carcinoma | $BDF_1$ mice | 100% inhibition |
| Ehrlich ascites | BALB/c mice | % ILS=300% |
| Walker 256 carcino-sarcoma (advanced) | Fisher 344 rats | 100% cures;T.I.>50 |
| Dunning leukemia (advanced) | Fisher 344 rats | 100% cures |
| P388 lymphocytic leukemia | $BDF_1$ mice | % ILS=533%; 6/10 cures |
| Reticulum cell sarcoma | C+ mice | % ILS=141% |
| B-16 melano-carcinoma | $BDF_1$ mice | % ILS=279%; 8/10 cures |
| ADJ/PC6 | BALB/c mice | 100% cures;T.I.=8 |
| AK leukemia (lymphoma) | AKR/LW mice | % ILS=225%; 3/10 cures |
| Ependymoblastoma | C57BL/6 mice | % ILS=141%; 1/6 cures |
| Rous sarcoma (advanced) | 15-I chickens | 65% cures |
| DMBA-induced mammary carcinoma | Sprague Dawley rats | 77% total regressions 3/9 free of all tumors |
| ICI 42, 464-induced myeloid and lymphatic leukemias | Alderly Park rats | %ILS=400% |

T/C= $\frac{\text{Tumor mass in treated animals}}{\text{Tumor mass in control animals}}$ x 100.

% ILS=% increase in lifespan of treated over control animals.

T.I.=Therapeutic index $(LD_{50}/E.D._{90})$, $E.D._{90}$=effective dose to inhibit tumors by 90%.

The drug failed to produce a marked response in the rabbit $VX_2$, in a Walker 256 strain with acquired resistance to alkylating agents(8) and in the syngeneic system of sarcoma 180 in the BALB/c mouse.(9) The cross-resistance of the alkylating agent-resistant strain is a significant result in that it suggests that the platinum drug may have a similar mechanism of transport, or action, to the bifunctional alkylating agents, as Drobnik has hypothesized. Fortunately, as discussed below, a number of responses in human patients have been reported against tumors that were already shown to be resistant to alkylating agents; thus, the situation of cross-resistance is by no means settled.

Retention Times and Organ Distributions of Platinum Drugs
in Animals

As a first step toward understanding the mechanism of action
of the drugs, it is necessary to determine the fate and the kinetics
of passage of injected pulse doses of the platinum drugs.  The first
such study was performed by Toth-Allen,(10) using Swiss white mice
(female), half with sarcoma 180 tumors and half that were normal.
The cis-Pt(II) (NH$_3$)$_2$Cl$_2$ at 8 mg/kg (the therapeutic dose) in saline solution was injected intraperitoneally.  At various times
afterward, the animals were sacrificed and the organs were separated and pooled.  The method of analysis used was neutron activation
and gamma spectrometry, which had the requisite sensitivity for low-
level platinum detection.  Other techniques now available include
the use of radioisotopes ($^{195m}$Pt, a gamma emitter suitable for whole
body counting or $^{14}$C-labeled non-exchanging ligands) and atomic
absorption spectrophotometry with graphite ovens.  Both latter techniques have confirmed the earlier results.

The drug is rapidly excreted, with a half time of about 1.6
hours, initially, to the extent of about 60% of the injected dose.
A much slower loss rate, with a half-time on the order of a week,
then occurs for the remaining drug.  The fast excretion is mainly
via urine, with a small portion found in the feces.  The drug appearing early in the urine has been found by Hoeschele (personal communication) to be unmodified, both for cis-dichlorodiammineplatinum(II)
and for malonatodiammineplatinum(II).  Tumored animals tend to retain
a slightly higher percentage of the drug, as compared with non-
tumored animals.  This may reflect a tumor-mediated influence on
the kidney function.  The loss kinetics of trans-dichlorodiammine-
platinum(II) follows a roughly similar time course as does the
isomer.  Thus, the lack of anti-tumor activity of the trans isomer
cannot be attributed to a shorter body retention time.

The distribution in the various organs of the body, 108 hours
after injection reported by Hoeschele and Van Camp(11) is shown in
Table 2.  The largest depots found are the excretory organs, the
liver, and the kidney.  Despite the high load in the liver, no animal
or man has ever exhibited any hepatic damage, either functionally or
histologically apparent.  It would be of value to know the form in
which the platinum drug is bound in the liver.  The kidney does
suffer damage, as described below, most probably from the bound
platinum complex and not from the unmodified form of the drug in
transit.  The spleen and thymus also exhibit damage due to the high
concentration found in these organs.  Most important from the point
of understanding the mechanism of action, there is no selective uptake of the platinum in the tumor tissue.  I conclude that the tumor
cells are more sensitive than normal tissue cells to the intracellular effects of the platinum drug, causing increased cell death
and/or an enhanced host response that leads to the selective destruction of the tumor.

TABLE 2

DISTRIBUTION OF $^{195m}$PLATINUM IN MAJOR ORGANS OF SWISS WHITE MICE
108 HOURS AFTER PULSE INTRAPERITONEAL INJECTION, 8 mg/kg cis-Pt(II)
(NH$_3$)$_2$Cl$_2$

| Organ | µgm Pt/gm of wet tissue | |
| --- | --- | --- |
| | cis-Pt(II)(NH$_3$)$_2$Cl$_2$ | trans-Pt(II)(NH$_3$)$_2$Cl$_2$ |
| Gastro-Intestinal Tract | | |
|   Tumored | 0.55 | 0.51 |
|   Non-Tumored | 1.1 | 0.75 |
| Liver | | |
|   Tumored | 10 | 2.2 |
|   Non-Tumored | 8.4 | 2.7 |
| Kidney | | |
|   Tumored | 12 | 1.3 |
|   Non-Tumored | 4.1 | 2.2 |
| Spleen | | |
|   Tumored | 8.5 | 4.3 |
|   Non-Tumored | 6.0 | 5.9 |
| Thymus | | |
|   Tumored | 9.1 | --- |
|   Non-Tumored | 3.4 | 1.5 |
| Tumor (Solid Sarcoma 180) | | |
|   Tumored | 2.5 | 2.1 |
|   Non-Tumored | --- | --- |
| Lungs | | |
|   Tumored | 2.1 | 1.4 |
|   Non-Tumored | 3.1 | 1.4 |
| Brain | | |
|   Tumored | 0.19 | 0.50(?) |
|   Non-Tumored | 0.15 | 0.04 |
| Stomach and Esophagus | | |
|   Tumored | not detected* | --- |
|   Non-Tumored | not detected* | --- |
| Heart | | |
|   Tumored | 0.65* | --- |
|   Non-Tumored | 0.54* | --- |

*Results of Toth-Allen (10)

A final point of interest is the very low concentration found
in the brain. This correlates well with the fact that the drug produces no detectable neural toxicity in any animal or man. This,
however, leads to a paradox: since the drugs are excreted unchanged
for hours after injection, and since the drugs are neutral molecules,
with low dipole moments, one would have expected penetration to some

degree of the so-called "blood-brain barrier." More recently, Ridgway and her associates have reported(*12*) that 1,2-diaminocyclohex-
anemalanatoplatinum(II) was found in the brain tissue of dogs as the
fourth major repository, at a level comparable to that in the kidney,
liver, and spleen. This is the first platinum complex that appears
to penetrate the blood-brain barrier readily to allow treatment of
central nervous system tumors.

## Biochemistry and Molecular Biology of the Platinum(II) Complexes

*Cis*-Dichlorodiammineplatinum(II) is injected as a neutral molecule in physiologic saline solution. It probably remains as the unchanged neutral structure in the extracellular fluid of the body as
this has a high enough chloride concentration (0.112M) to prevent
the hydrolysis reaction. Once within the cell, however, the lower
intracellular chloride concentration (0.004M) allows hydrolysis to
proceed via the sequential reactions:

$$[Pt(II)(NH_3)_2Cl_2]^0 + H_2O$$
$$\rightleftharpoons [Pt(II)(NH_3)_2Cl(H_2O)]^+ + Cl^-, \quad (1)$$

$$[Pt(II)(NH_3)_2Cl(H_2O)]^+ + H_2O$$
$$\rightleftharpoons [Pt(II)(NH_3)_2(H_2O)_2]^{2+} + Cl^-. \quad (2)$$

Depending upon the pH, the diaquo species may also lose protons
to form the monohydroxy and the dihydroxy species. At present, it
is believed that the active species are the aquo or hydroxy-substi-
tuted hydrolysis products, and it is these that react with the various cell receivers.

Lippert and his coworkers(*13,14,15*) have found that under varying conditions of pH and concentration, the reactions described
above are not the only ones possible. In addition to the monomeric
diaquo species of equation 2, they discovered a centrosymmetric
hydroxo-bridged dimer, a hydroxo-bridged cyclic trimer, and a dimer
of hydroxo-bridged dimers (a tetramer). The chemistry and biologic
actions of these different species have yet to be analyzed.

The effects of the drug on cellular biosyntheses were investigated simultaneously and independently by Howle and Gale(*16*) and by
Harder and Rosenberg(*17*) using tissue culture techniques. The first
study used Ehrlich ascites tumor cells, while the second used human
embryonic AV$_3$ cells. Tritiated thymidine, uridine, and leucine were
incorporated in the growth media to monitor the synthesis of DNA,
RNA, and protein, respectively. This was done after pulse dosing
with *cis*-dichlorodiammineplatinum(II), either the established cells
in the tissue culture flasks, or in one case, BALB/c mice who were
sacrificed and the cells then plated. There is general agreement in
the results of these two studies. The major results were: (1) at

low drug-dose levels (equivalent to the amount found in the tumor tissue, ~5μM after a therapeutic dose), the synthesis of DNA is selectively and persistently inhibited; (2) RNA and protein syntheses are not markedly effected; (3) the level of inhibition is dose dependent; (4) the onset of inhibition is slow, reaching a nadir about four to six hours after the drug pulse dose was removed. There is not a high cell kill under these conditions and many grow into giant cells, which, after three to four days, begin to show multi-nucleated structures, finally dividing into apparently normal cells. The syntheses of precursors for the DNA and the transport of such precursors through the cell membranes are not inhibited. Most platinum complexes with anti-tumor activity displayed similar effects, whereas the inactive complexes showed no effects until very high dose levels were reached that were frankly toxic to the cells. In these dose levels, all syntheses were inhibited. The inhibition of DNA syntheses could not be reversed by extensive washing or dialysis of the cells, indicating a very tight binding of the reacted platinum complexes to the cell receivers.

These results are consistent with the suggestion that the primary lesion in the cell caused by the active species of the *cis*-dichlorodiammineplatinum(II) is an attack upon the DNA of the cell. This attack prevents new DNA syntheses, but not transcription and translation. The attack is slowly reversed due either to further chemical reactions removing the attached platinum species, or by cellular DNA repair mechanisms, most probably the latter. While DNA polymerase and DNase activity is inhibited by the *cis*-dichlorodiammineplatinum(II) in *in vivo* tests, the DNA polymerase activity in treated cells is enhanced over the controls by a factor of about four times. This may reflect an enhanced repair activity in the drug-treated cells.

Nicolau(*18*) has shown that the *cis*-dichlorodiammineplatinum(II) interacts with erythrocyte ghost membranes by observing a fluorescence-quenching effect. This has been verified by Pant (personal communication) in this laboratory. This is the only evidence so far of a membrane interaction of the platinum drug. Its significance has yet to be determined.

Interactions of the platinum complexes with RNA, proteins, polysaccharides, and lipids are in very preliminary stages. Some enzyme proteins are inactivated by incubation with the drug, as mentioned above; others are not. Stone and Sinex(*19*) report "minimal" binding to commercially available histone preparations, and that chromatin appears to bind less of the drug than comparable amounts of pure DNA.

It thus appears that while the platinum drug reacts with many biochemicals other than DNA, evidence for these reactions being in the direct path leading to anti-tumor activity is lacking. The most

probable pathways are the creation of direct lesions on the DNA
structure.

Drobnik (personal communication) was the first to suggest that
a parallelism should be found between the platinum drug and the
classic bifunctional alkylating agents such as the nitrogen mustards.
Indeed, some parallelism does exist as shown in Table 3; therefore,
since it is believed that crosslinking of double-stranded DNA by the
bifunctional alkylating agents is the primary lesion leading to anti-
tumor activity, it suggests that this should also be true for the
platinum drugs. However, recent evidence by Roberts[20] of the
amount of crosslinking at toxic doses in tissue cultures indicates
that, while crosslinking does occur, it may not be relevant for the
further biologic actions of the drug.


TABLE 3

PARALLEL PROPERTIES AND EFFECTS OF BIFUNCTIONAL ALKYLATING AGENTS
AND $CIS$-Pt(II)(NH$_3$)$_2$Cl$_2$

1. Two chloride leaving groups

2. Giant cell formation

3. Persistent inhibition of cell division

4. Selective inhibition of DNA synthesis at therapeutic dose levels

5. Filamentation in bacteria

6. Enhanced DNA polymerase and DNase activities in treated cells·

7. Induction of lysogenic bacteria

8. Crosslink double-stranded DNA


It is obvious, however, that a geometric problem exists. The
classic bifunctional alkylating agents require that the two chloride-
leaving groups be about 5-7 Angstroms apart in order to show marked
anti-tumor activity. This is presumed to be due to the similar
spacing between N-7 groups of the guanine bases on opposite strands
of the Watson-Crick structure, which are the bridging sites. The
two chloride-leaving groups of $cis$-Pt(II)(NH$_3$)$_2$Cl$_2$ are only 3.3
Angstroms apart; thus, other crosslinking sites must be involved.
Thomson (personal communication) and Roberts and Pascoe[21] have
suggested the involvement of 6-NH$_2$ groups of adenine in an ApT sequence; 2-NH$_2$ groups of guanine in the narrow groove; and 6-NH$_2$ groups
of cytosine in a CpG sequence in a deep groove.

Other modes of attack on DNA also must be considered. Here, from *in vitro* studies, we have an embarrassment of riches. Mansy, Rosenberg, and Thomson(22) have used U.V. difference spectroscopy to investigate modes of interaction of the platinum drugs with nucleic acid components. The *cis*-isomer forms a bidentate chelate with either 6-NH and N-7, or 6-NH and N-1 of adenosine, and 4-NH and N-3 of cytidine. The *trans*-isomer interacts monofunctionally at N-7 and N-1 of adenosine and N-3 of cytidine. Both isomers bind monofunctionally to N-7 of guanosine and inosine. No evidence was found of binding of either isomer to uridine or thymidine.

Thomson and Mansy(23) have measured the interactions of the *cis* and *trans* isomers with dinucleotides, using circular dichroism and found that one molecule of the *cis*-isomer reacts with ApA to stabilize the stacked arrangement, consistent with a bifunctional attack in which the two chlorides are replaced by the 6-$NH_2$ groups of the adenines; whereas two *trans*-isomer molecules react with one ApA, and destabilize the structure, consistent with each *trans* molecule reacting monofunctionally with the 6-NH group. These results, which require additional testing, taken in conjunction with the facts that the *cis*-isomer inhibits single-stranded as well as double-stranded bacteriophage, and that the base-stacking distance of the Watson-Crick structure is 3.4 Angstroms, suggests that intrastrand dimers may also occur in DNA. More recently, Mansy and Rosenberg(24) have used Laser-Raman scattering to investigate the interactions of the platinum complexes with polynucleotides. The results indicate no evidence of any interactions of the platinum complexes with the phosphate or sugar moieties of the polynucleotides or DNA.

Theophanides and his coworkers(25) have attempted to study the stereospecificity of the platinum drug actions; viz., *cis* configurations are active while *trans* configurations are not, by examining the possible interactions of the platinum complexes with bases of the DNA. Logically, it is difficult to believe that the complex structure of DNA with its varieties of dislocations and its necessary plasticity could account for the severe stereoselectivity. Since the molecular structure of the individual bases are retained intact, it appears more likely to be the site for such stereoselectivity. Previous studies had indicated that guanine was the most likely base for this interaction. Theophanides and Macquet presented some evidence that the *trans* complex could attack the N-1 and N-7 sites of guanine in a monodentate attack, as could the configuration; however, the latter could form a crosslink chelate between the N7-06 of guanine, which the *trans* cannot. The involvement of the 06 of guanine in the interaction is interesting in that recent evidence on the mutagenicity and carcinogenicity of alkylating agents suggests that a minority component of the reaction ($\sim$ 10%), alkylation of the 06 site, may be largely responsible for the biologic action. While there are certainly differences between platination and alkylation, it could be reasonably expected that such chelation with platinum would increase the positive charge on the oxygen, and therefore, decrease its ability to hydrogen bond in the usual Watson-Crick pairing with the 4-$NH_2$ site of cytosine. This would lead on replication to a mispairing with adenine or thymine, which, on further cell replication, would lead to a base substitution mutation. The Ames bacterial test results showed that the configuration is indeed a base substitution mutagen (but not a frame shift mutagen), consistent with the hypothesis of chelation. The *trans* complex recently has been reported by Beck (personal communication) not to produce mutations, even at much higher dose levels than those used for the *cis* configuration. It now requires harder chemical evidence to justify this chelation reaction. In any case, while it could possibly explain the mechanism for mutagenicity of the platinum complexes, it will still require additional hypotheses to make it relevant to the anti-cancer activity.

Horacek and Drobnik(26) have studied the interaction of *cis* Pt(II)($NH_3$)$_2Cl_2$ with DNA using U.V. difference spectrophotometry. They found a shift in the U.V. absorption maximum of the DNA from 259 to 264 nm, and a hyperchromicity upon reaction with the hydrolyzed platinum drug at a Pt/P ratio of 1.0. The reacted DNA at much lower Pt/P ratios also showed marked renaturation after a heating and cooling cycle, suggesting crosslinking. Compounds added to the reaction mixture that affect DNA stability, such as putrescine, spermidine, histones, $Mg^{2+}$, $SO_4^-$, and $NO_3^-$ ions, had little effect upon either the reaction rates or the final equilibrium. Chlorides, however, greatly retarded the reaction rates (presumably by affecting the hydrolysis process of the platinum drug, which may be the rate-limiting step). The activation energy for the rate constant (experimental) for the platinum complex - DNA interaction was 18,000 ± 630 cal/mole, quite close to the value of 17,100 cal/mole found for the activation energy for inactivation of bacteriophages by the platinum drug. Interestingly, we have found that the hydrolysis rate of *cis*-dichlorodiammineplatinum(II) in pure water occurs with an activation enthalpy of 18,000 cal/mole. This confirms that the aquation reaction may be the rate-limiting step for the DNA interaction and the inactivation of bacteriophages.

Robins(27) has also measured the rate of reaction of DNA with dichloroethylenediamineplatinum(II) using a [14]C label on the ethylenediamine. He found slow rates of reactions with the purines, adenine, and guanine, and the nucleoside, deoxycytidine, and no reaction with thymidine (as also reported by Mansy et al.(22)) Guanosine and deoxyguanosine reacted an order of magnitude faster than the purine base alone, while the corresponding nucleotides and nucleosides of adenosine showed no change in reaction rate. He hypothesized that guanine residues were an important site of attack on DNA for the platinum drugs, particularly at N-7, as is the case for alkylating agents. More recently(28), he has concluded, in agreement with Drobnik, that neither polymerization nor the state of the helical structure affect the reaction rates of guanosine. He also found that the reaction rates with adenosine were greatly increased in the sequence:

poly d(AT)<ApA<AMP<PolyA,

and suggested that the presence of a phosphate group increased the reaction rate in some as yet unknown way. Since Mansy et al. showed no evidence for a phosphate interaction with Laser-Raman scattering, it is likely that only a short-lived, intermediate reactant between the platinum drug and phosphate may exist, which accelerates the binding of the hydrolyzed platinum drug to the bases. This is an area requiring much further study.

## Toxicology of Platinum Drugs in Animals and Man

Studies from many laboratories have established the dose of $cis$-dichlorodiammineplatinum(II) which, given as a single injection intraperitoneally, will kill 50% of the animals ($LD_{50}$dose). For mice, it is between 12-14 mg/kg; for rats, 11-13 mg/kg; for young chickens, 5-6 mg/kg; for dogs (beagles), about 2.5 mg/kg; for rhesus monkeys, no single dose toxicities were determined, but five daily injections of 1.25 mg/kg is considered a high toxic dose.(29) From Phase I clinical trials on man (terminal cancer patients) it is estimated that single intravenous doses above 2 mg/kg would lead to unacceptable toxicities.

The earliest study of toxicology in mice was reported by Toth-Allen.(10) She found at the therapeutic dose of 8 mg/kg used for treating sarcoma 180 in Swiss white mice, the following toxic side effects: (1) temporary cellular inhibition of the gastrointestinal mucosa; (2) lymphocyte depletion of the thymus and spleen; (3) inhibition of splenic hematopoietic elements; (4) pycnosis and vacuolization of the renal tubular epithelium; (5) leukopenia; (6) no evidence of liver damage. She concluded that the drug appears to attack rapidly proliferating cells almost exclusively, with little if any damage to other major body organs. All pathological effects were reversible.

A more detailed study of the pathology of the rat, given $LD_{50}$ doses of $cis$-dichlorodiammineplatinum(II), was described by Kociba and Sleight.(30) Major organs affected were the gastrointestinal tract, lymphoid organs, and bone marrow. While the erythrocyte number, packed cell volume, and hemoglobin concentration remained within normal limits, there was a detectable panleukocytopenia, reticulocytopenia, depressed platelet number, and decreases in serum proteins, such as alkaline phosphatase, lactic dehydrogenase, and serum glutamic oxalotransaminase activities. These effects have been verified by others.(*31, 32*)  In particular, the kinetics of blood element changes were studied by Zak et al.(*32*)

The major histological changes evident in mice and rats are: (1) denudation of intestinal epithelium (the major dose-limiting effect); (2) bone marrow depression; (3) thymic and splenic atrophy; and (4) acute nephrosis.  These pathologic changes were all reversible in recovered animals.

In dogs and monkeys, the toxic effects are similar:  (1) damage to the gastrointestinal tract (evidenced by emesis, anorexia, abdominal tenderness, and diarrhea); (2) renal tubular necrosis in dogs and nephrosis in monkeys; (3) lymphoid atrophy and hypoplasia of the bone marrow.  In these latter animals, the kidney damage has become the major dose-limiting effect.  But again, no irreversible side effects were noted in animals recovering from high toxic doses.

In clinical trials on human cancer patients, many of the predicted side effects have been noted.  Table 4 compiles the results of many clinicians' observations.  As with dogs and monkeys, the major dose-limiting pathologic effect is renal tubular damage.  Surprisingly, it does not occur with uniform severity.  It may, however, reflect some uniform damage that manifests itself more severely in patients whose kidney reserve capacity has been compromised.(*33*) The platinum drug is one of the few active anti-tumor agents where renal toxicity is dose limiting, and in its early stages of experience, it was a cause of some anxiety among clinicians.  The reports of high-frequency hearing loss have been variously attributed to eighth nerve damage or to cochlear damage.  Some evidence for the latter has now been reported by Stadnicki et al. in guinea pigs,(*34*) and in monkeys.(*35*)

TABLE 4

MAJOR PATHOLOGICAL EFFECTS IN HUMANS
FROM PHASE I CLINICAL TRIALS OF *CIS*-DICHLORODIAMMINEPLATINUM(II)

1.  Renal toxicity at higher dose levels (> 1 mg/kg) not invariable

2.  Hematopoietic toxicity - occasional

3.  Hypoplastic bone marrow

4.  Nausea and vomiting

5.  Transient decrease in hemoglobin - rare so far

6.  Tinnitus - occasional

7.  High frequency hearing loss - occasional

Krakoff, Cvitkovic, and their coworkers(36) at the Sloan-Kettering Institute reasoned that heavy metal kidney toxicity could be amerliorated by administration of an osmotic diuretic such as D-mannitol with hydration of the patient.  While it has not been shown that the platinum drug damage to the kidney is the same as that produced by heavy metal poisoning, their experimental results were significant.  This simple pharmacologic trick somehow protected the kidney against the drug without excessive removal of the drug from the animal.  This was confirmed by the enhancement of the other toxic manifestations of the drug.  The technique was then tested in humans, and it was found that the dose could be safely increased by 300% to a value of approximately three mg/kg.

Venditti and his coworkers(37) at the National Cancer Institute provided the first evidence in animal-tumor systems that the platinum drug exhibited additivity or synergism when given in combination with a number of other anti-tumor drugs.  Other laboratories have corroborated this with every other anti-tumor drug tested (with the possible exception of methotrexate).  The reasons for the additivity or synergism of the platinum drug in these combinations are not known, but these results provide a rationale for its use in combination chemotherapy in humans, as described below.

*Cis*-dichlorodiammineplatinum(II) entered human clinical trials in 1972 under the auspices of the National Cancer Institute (and a few months earlier at the Wadley Institute of Molecular Medicine in Dallas, Texas).  The preclinical studies of toxicology and pharmacology at different dose levels and schedules in dogs and monkeys established a safe, low, starting dose and predicted certain toxicities that would occur when the dose level was escalated.  The most severe toxicity was, as mentioned earlier, damage to the proximal convoluted tubules of the kidney, with less stringent toxicities in the blood-forming elements of the bone marrow, and intense nausea and vomiting (since the nausea and vomiting are ameliorated by oral or parenteral administration of tetrahydrocannabinol, or smoking marijuana, it is possible that this toxicity is a central nervous system reaction, rather than an indication of gastrointestinal damage).  An additional toxicity that emerged in the human testing was damage to the hair cells of the organ of Corti in the inner ear, leading to transient high-frequency hearing loss, and in a few cases, total deafness.

The drug was administered to patients terminally ill with cancer and no longer responsive to other treatments, and who signed informed consent agreements.  These patients, whose physical vitality has already been extremely sapped, both by the cancer and by subsequent therapies, could not be reasonably expected to show marked responses to the drug; however, from these studies, invaluable information on appropriate dose levels and schedules were obtained.

Nevertheless, some patients did indeed benefit from the drug, with partial or complete remissions in about 20% of the cases, for various durations. The drug seemed to produce more responses in patients with genitourinary cancers ($\sim$ 80% for testicular cancers and $\sim$90% for ovarian carcinomas); head and neck cancers ($\sim$ 40%); and some lymphomas ($\sim$ 40%). It proved a total failure in colon carcinoma.

In 1973, the clinicians felt that this was too dangerous a drug for general use (due to the kidney toxicity) but too good a drug to drop; but the testicular cancer work of Wallace, Holland, and coworkers(38) at Roswell Park, and the ovarian carcinoma work of Wiltshaw(39) at the Royal Marsden Hospital gave sufficient impetus to prevent the early demise of the drug.

Cvitkovic, Krakoff and coworkers at the Sloan-Kettering Institute, in developing their hydration technique and testing the drug at higher dose levels (up to 3.5 mg/kg) found markedly enhanced responses in their patients, particularly in testicular cancers. They incorporated the platinum therapy into a previously developed combination therapy to form the new VAB III combination with vinblastine and bleomycin and began to achieve close to 100% responses in testicular cancer patients, approaching completeness in most cases, and of long duration. They are now extending this combination therapy treatment to other cancers as well. Wittes et al.(40) showed excellent activity against head and neck cancers, and recently Yagoda(41) has reported effective responses in bladder carcinomas with the platinum drug alone or in various combination therapies.

Holland, Bruckner, and coworkers(42) at Mt. Sinai Hospital in New York, extended the initial work of Wiltshaw on ovarian carcinoma to include a combination therapy that now consists of the platinum drug, adriamycin and cytoxan. They now report greater than 70% response; most of these responses are complete, and some have been verified by second-look surgery. These responses are of longer duration than have been previously reported.

Einhorn(43) at Indiana University has evolved a combination therapy using platinum at low dosage with vinblastine and bleomycin. He reports that, even in patients with far-advanced disease, they could achieve complete remission rates of 72%, and overall disease-free status of 85% in nearly 40 patients. The duration of the remissions extends to over 27 months, and it is obvious that this regimen is producing long-term survivors better than the best previous regimen, wherein the average duration of remission was about six months. Similar results have been reported by Merrin(44) at Roswell Park. Some of the more recent clinical results are compiled in Table 5.

TABLE 5

PRELIMINARY CLINICAL TRIALS OF *CIS*-DICHLORODIAMMINEPLATINUM(II)

| Tumor Type | Drug Therapy | # Evaluable Patients | Complete Remissions (Durations) | Partial Remissions (>50%) | Total Responses (%) |
|---|---|---|---|---|---|
| 1) Testicular Cancers (metastatic)[1] | cis-Dichlorodiammine-platinum(II) + Vin-blastine + Bleomycin | 39 | 85% (3+ to 24+ mo.) | 15% (3+ to 24+ mo.) | 100% |
| 2) Epidermoid Carcinoma of head and neck (for advanced disease)[2] | High Dose cis-Dichloro-diammineplatinum(II) | 26 | 7% (2+, 6+ mo.) | 23% (1,2,3,4,5+,6+ mo.) 38% (measurable responses) | 69% |
| 3) Ovarian carcinoma (advanced, failed prior therapy)[3] | cis-Dichlorodiammine-platinum(II) + Adria-mycin | 18 | 33% | 33% | 66% (89% survival in remission) |
| 4) Bladder cancer[4] | cis-Dichlorodiammine-platinum(II) | 24 | 0% | 33% 16% (measurable responses) | 49% |

[1] L. H. Einhorn and B. Furnas, Proc. of III Int. Sym.; Journal of Clinical Hematology and Oncology 7, No. 2, April (1977) in press.

[2] R. E. Wittes et al. Ibid.

[3] H. W. Bruckner et al. Ibid.

[4] A. Yagoda et al. Cancer Treat. Rep. 60, 917-923, (1976)

At this time, the high-dose therapy with the platinum drug, and combination therapy, both at low and high dose levels, are being extended to the treatment of other classes of cancers.

## REFERENCES

1.  Rosenberg, B., et al., Nature 222, Page 385, 1969.

2.  Rosenberg, B., Platinum Metals Review 15, Page 3, 1971

3.  Gale, G. R., Handbuch der Experimentellen Pharmakologie, Springer Verlag, Berlin, Page 829, 1975.

4.  Thomson, A. J., Williams, R. J. P., Reslova, S., Structure and Bonding 11, Page 1, 1972.

5.  Cleare, M. J., Hoeschele, J. D., Bioinorganic Chemistry 2, Page 187, 1973.

6.  Cleare, M. J., Hoeschele, J. D., Platinum Metals Review 17, Page 1, 1973.

7.  Connors, T. A., et al., Chemico-Biol. Interactions 5, Page 415, 1972.

8.  Connors, T. A., Advances in Antimicrobial and Antineoplastic Chemotherapy 2, Page 237, University Park Press, Baltimore, 1972.

9.  Conran, P. B., Rosenberg, B., ibid, Page 235.

10. Toth-Allen, J., Ph.D., Thesis, Michigan State University, 1970.

11. Hoeschele, J. D., VanCamp, L., Advances in Antimicrobial and Antineoplastic Chemotherapy 2, Page 241, University Park Press, Baltimore, 1972.

12. Ridgway, H. J., et al., Journal of Clinical Hematology and Oncology 7, No. 1, Page 220, 1977.

13. Lippert, B., et al., Journal of the American Chemical Society 99, Page 777, 1977.

14. Lippert, B., et al., Journal of Inorganic Chemistry, in press, 1977.

15. Lippert, B., et al., ibid.

16.  Howle, J. A., Gale, G. R., Biochem. Pharmacol. 19, 2757, 1970.

17.  Harder, H. C., Rosenberg, B., Int. J. Cancer 6, Page 207, 1970.

18.  Hörer, O. L., Nicolau, C., F.E.B.S. Letters 14, Page 262, 1971.

19.  Stone, P. J., Sinex, F. M., Platinum Coordination Complexes in Cancer Chemotherapy (edited by T. A. Connors and J. J. Roberts) Page 68, Springer-Verlag, Berlin, 1974.

20.  Van Den Berg, H. W., Fraval, H. N. A., and Roberts, J. J., Journal of Clinical Hematology and Oncology 7, No. 1, 349, 1977.

21.  Roberts, J. J., Pascoe, J. M., Advances in Antimicrobial and Antineoplastic Chemotherapy 2, Page 249, University Park Press, Baltimore, 1972.

22.  Mansy, S., Rosenberg, B., Thomson, A. J., Journal of the American Chemical Society 95, No. 5, 1973.

23.  Thomson, A. J., Mansy, S., Advances in Antimicrobial and Antineoplastic Chemotherapy 2, Page 199, University Park Press, Baltimore, 1972.

24.  Mansy, S., Rosenberg, B., unpublished results.

25.  Theophanides, T., Macquet, J. P., Bioinorganic Chemistry 5,1 Page 59, 1975.

26.  Horacek, P., Drobnik, J., Biochim. Biophys. Acta. 254, 341, 1971.

27.  Robins, A. B., Chem.-Biol. Interactions 6, Page 35, 1973.

28.  Robins, A. B., Chem.-Biol. Interactions 7, Page 11, 1973.

29.  Dixon, R. L. et al., Advances in Antimicrobial and Antineoplastic Chemocherapy 2, Page 243, University Park Press, Baltimore, 1972.

30.  Kociba, R., Sleight, S. D., Cancer Chemother. Rep. 55, 1, 1971.

31.  Thompson, H. S., Gale, G. R., Toxicol. Appl. Pharmacol. 19, Page 602, 1971.

32.  Zak, M., Drobnik, J., Rezny, Z., Cancer Research 32, 595, 1972.

33.  Rossof, A. H., Slayton, R. E., Perlia, C. P., Cancer 30, Page 1451, 1972.

34.  Stadnicki, S. W., et al., F.A.S.E.B. Meeting Abstract, 1973.

35. Stadnicki, S. W., et al., Cancer Chemother. Rep., Part 1 59, No. 3, Page 467, 1975.

36. Hayes, D., et al., Proceedings AACR 17, Page 169, 1976.

37. Woodman, R. J., et al., Proceedings American Association Cancer Research 12, Page 24, 1971.

38. Higby, D. J., et al., Cancer 33, Page 1219, 1974.

39. Wiltshaw, E., Kroner, T., Cancer Treatment Rep. 60, 55, 1976.

40. Wittes, R. E., et al., Journal of Clinical Hematology and Oncology 7, No. 2, April 1977.

41. Yagoda, A., et al., Cancer Treatment Reports 60, No. 7, Page 917, 1976.

42. Bruckner, H. W., et al., Journal of Clinical Hematology and Oncology 7, No. 2, April 1977.

43. Einhorn, L. H., Furnas, B., Journal of Clinical Hematology and Oncology 7, No. 2, April 1977.

44. Merrin, C., AACR Abstracts, No. C-26, Page 243, May 1976.

*CHAPTER 11*

POTENTIAL CARCINOSTATIC ACTIVITY OF METAL COMPLEXES

Stanley Kirschner, Stanley H. Kravitz,

Department of Chemistry, Wayne State University
Detroit, Michigan  48202, U.S.A.

and

Ana Maurer, Coriolan Dragulescu

Centrul de Chimie, Timisoara, Romania

## I.   INTRODUCTION

For several years, there has been considerable controversy about the question of whether certain forms of cancer in humans are caused by viruses.  Luria(*1*) indicated in 1960 that there was already considerable evidence that many tumors have viruses associated with them.  In 1966, Kirschner et al.(*2*) proposed that certain complexes of the heavy transition metals should be active against tumor systems and viruses; namely, those that contain metals that have an affinity for the donor atoms on DNA and proteins (e.g., S, N, O) and which are of "moderate" stability; not so stable as to resist attack by these potential donor groups, but not so labile as to be attacked effectively by the many types of normal proteins and DNA in living systems.  They also reported the synthesis of several metal complexes that are active against various tumor systems.

## II.   DISCUSSION

It is proposed herein that at least seven approaches may be used whereby metal complexes can potentially exhibit activity in tumor systems.

A.   Effect of the Metal as a Donor Atom Acceptor

It has been proposed(*2*) that donor atoms from DNA and/or viruses can coordinate to metals in complexes by displacement of one or more ligands that are not tightly bound, as shown in Equation [1]:

$$m(Vi) + [M^{x+} (L^{y-})_n (L')_p]^{x-ny} = [M^{x+} (Vi)_m (L')_p]^{x+} + nL^{y-} \quad [1]$$

where
    L' is a neutral ligand, L is a negative ligand, and Vi is a
virus or DNA donor.  In the case of a virus, Equation [1] represents an alteration of the virus, which is expected to eliminate
or considerably reduce its disease-causing properties.  In the
case of DNA coordination, it is expected that this reaction would
significantly affect (perhaps eliminate) the ability of that DNA
to undergo replication.  Rosenberg and others(3) have postulated
that the powerful anti-tumor agent cis-[Pt(Cl)$_2$(NH$_3$)$_2$] acts to
inhibit the replication of DNA by either inter- or intra-strand
coordination of the DNA to the complex after the chlorides have
been displaced.

B.  The Effects of the Ligands

    Kirschner et al.(2) have proposed the use of complexes con-
taining ligands that are anti-tumor and/or anti-viral agents in
their own right, in an effort to enhance the activities of these
substances.  For example, it can be noted in Equation [1] that
when the ligand L$^{y-}$ is released, it is presumably available at the
site of the important biological activity of the complex.  Therefore, if the ligand has anti-tumor activity itself (e.g., 6-
mercaptopurine), the complex will have acted as a carrier for the
biologically significant ligand to the site where it can most
effectively exert its activity.

    However, it must be stressed that the bond strength between
such ligands and the metal must not be so strong that the ligand
cannot be separated from the metal.  These authors have reported
significant anti-tumor activity of the trans-[Pt(Cl)$_4$(6-mp)$_2$]$^=$
complex against sarcoma 180 and carcinoma 755, but it can be reported here that this complex is inactive against leukemia 1210,
even though the ligand itself possesses considerable activity against
this type cancer.

C.  The Use of Radioactive Metal Ions

    It is proposed by the authors that the use of metal complexes
containing radioactive metal ions should enhance the effectiveness
of these complexes as anti-tumor agents.  Not only might such metal
ions serve to find locations of relatively high concentration (and
activity) of the complex in living systems, but the radioactive
metals should be effective in helping to destroy tumor systems.
Since the radioactive sources will be very close to the significant
regions of biological activity, the inverse square law should permit strong radiation effects with low-level emitters, even those

having fairly short half-lives.    Wolf et al.(4) have synthesized complexes containing radioactive platinum and are studying the activity of such complexes as anti-tumor agents.

D.   The Use of Radioactive Ligands

It is also proposed that the use of radioactive ligands in these complexes should enhance their anti-tumor activity.  If such ligands are displaced from the complex according to Equation [1], then presumably they will be located in the region of significant biological activity, and, because they are close to active sites, low-energy (even short-lived) isotopes should be usable with considerable effectiveness.  If these ligands remain with the metal as part of the complex, their radiation still could be effective in preferential destruction of viruses or tumors.  For example, when 6-mp is used as a ligand, it is proposed that some $^{35}S$ might be incorporated into the ligand before the complex is synthesized. If the complex binds to DNA (or viruses) of tumor systems, the radiation could help to destroy such systems.

E.   The Use of Optically Active Complexes

There are many examples in the literature of biologically significant compounds that are also optically active.  Further, it is often found that one enantiomer of these compounds possesses significantly greater biological activity than the other.  Examples are to be found in *levo*-epinephrine and *dextro*-penicillamine.  It is proposed that those metal complexes that are potentially anti-tumor active, and that possess sufficient dissymmetry to be optically active, be resolved into their optical enantiomers and that these be screened separately.  It is likely that the individual enantiomers will not exhibit the same biological activity.

F.   The Use of Optically Active Ligands

Using reasoning analogous to that in Section E, when potentially physiologically active metal complexes possess ligands that are optically active (whether or not they possess anti-tumor activity in their own right), it is proposed that metal complexes be synthesized utilizing individual enantiomers of these dissymmetric ligands.  Not only will this significantly affect the optical activity of the complex, but it is expected to affect its physiological activity as well.  Examples of complexes and ligands possessing such optical activity are reported herein.

G.   The Internal Synergistic Effect

Since most metal complexes contain more than one molecule of ligand, it is proposed to synthesize metal complexes that contain

two or more different ligands ("mixed ligand" complexes), each of
which possesses anti-tumor activity alone.  Equation [2] illustrates
this proposal which is expected to result in a three-way "internal
synergistic effect"; an effect whereby one drug enhances the effectiveness of another(s).  In this case, the two ligands would be expected to each exhibit anti-tumor activity (and presumably, the
action of one could enhance the physiological activity of the
other).  Further, the physiological activity of both would be affected by the activity of the metal complex on the tumor system.  The
effect is referred to as "internal" since all three sources of
physiological activity are contained within the same molecule, and
all three are presumably released and become physiologically active
at about the same time.  Equation [2] is as follows:

$$m(Vi) + [M^X(L^{Y-})_n(L')_p(L'')_q]^{x-ny} = [M^{x+}(Vi)_m(L')_p]^{x+} + nL^{y-} + qL''$$

In Equation [2], both L and L'' are ligands that possess anti-
tumor activity in their own right.

## H.  Synthesis of Complexes

In this research group, complexes have been synthesized to test
several of the hypotheses listed above, but this group has not yet
synthesized complexes to test the radioactivity proposals.  These
complexes are described in Section 3, and results are described in
Section 4.

## III.  COMPLEXES AND LIGANDS

Table 1 lists some of the complexes that have been synthesized
during this study, along with their ligands.

TABLE 1

| Number | Complex | Ligand |
|---|---|---|
| I | $[Ni(cyl)_2].2H_2O$ | cyl = cyloleucine = |
| | | 1-aminocyclopentane- |
| II | $[Zn(cyl)_2].1/2H_2O$ | carboxylate anion |
| III | $[Pb(cyl)_2].H_2O$ | |
| IV | $[Mn(cyl)_2].H_2O$ | |
| V | $[Pd(cyl)_2].H_2O$ | |
| VI | $[Cu(cyl)_2].NaCl$ | |

TABLE 1 (Continued)

| Number | Complex | Ligand |
|--------|---------|--------|
| VII | $[Au(cyl)_2]Cl.3HCl$ | |
| VIII | $[Au(cyl)_2][AuCl_2]$ | |
| IX | $[Au(dzu)_2Cl_2].HCl$ | dzu = 5-diazouracil |
| X | $[Pt(dzu)_2Cl_4].2HCl$ | |
| XI | $[Co(N-ipyN'-hyu)_2Cl_2]$ | N-ipyN'-hyu = N-isopropyl-idine-N'-hydroxyurea |
| XII | $[Ni(N-ipyN'-hyu)_2Cl_2]$ | |
| XIII | $[Mn(N-ipyN'-hyu)_2]Cl_2$ | |
| XIV | $[Zn(N-ipyN'-hyu)_2]Cl_2$ | |
| XV | $[Mn(N-ipyN'-hyu)_2]\underline{D,L}-[Mn(\underline{d,l}-pdta)].4.5H_2O$ | $\underline{d,l}$-pdta = racemic-propylenediaminetetra-acetate anion |
| XVI | $[Mn(N-ipyN'-hyu)_2]\underline{D}-[Mn(\underline{l}-pdta)].4.5H_2O$ | |
| XVII | $\underline{D,L}-K_2[Mn(\underline{d,l}-pdta)].2.5H_2O$ | |
| XVIII | $\underline{D}-K_2[Mn(\underline{l}-pdta)].2.5H_2O$ | |
| XIX | $cis-[Pd(Cl)_2(N_2H_4)]$ | $N_2H_4$ = hydrazine |
| XX | $cis-[Pd(Cl)_2(pip)_2]$ | pip = piperdine |
| XXI | $cis-[Pt(Cl)_2(pip)_2].H_2O$ | |
| XXII | $cis-[Pt(Cl)_2(TSCZ)_2]$ | TSCZ = thiosemicarbazide |
| XXIII | $cis-[Pt(Cl)_2(N_2H_5)_2]Cl_2$ | $N_2H_5$ = hydrazinium cation |
| XXIV | $cis-[Pt(Cl)_2(morph)_2]$ | morph = morpholine |
| XXV | $cis-[Pt(Cl)_2(me-pipz)_2]$ | me-pipz = N-methylpiper-azine |

cont.

TABLE 1 (Continued)

| Number | Complex | Ligand |
|--------|---------|--------|
| XXVI | [Pd(HFPTSCZO)Cl | HFPTSCZO = 5-hydroxy-2-formylpyridine-thiosemicarbazone |
| XXVII | [Pt(HFPTSCZO)Cl] | |
| XXVIII | $trans$-Na$_2$[Pt(mp)$_2$Cl$_4$] | mp = 6-mercaptopurine |
| XXIX | Na$_2$[Bi(O)(mp)$_3$] | |

## IV.   TEST PROCEDURES AND RESULTS

### A.   Inhibition of DNA Synthesis(5)

This procedure involves incubation of murine leukemia L1210 tumor cells in culture with the test compound in DMF solution at a concentration of 1 mg/ml for 10 minutes at 37°.  Labeled thymidine (5 ml of a 100 mM solution) is added, and the solution is allowed to stand for another 10 minutes at 37°.  The DNA formed from un-destroyed tumor cells that incorporate labeled thymidine is deter-mined quantitatively with a liquid scintillation spectrometer. Table 2 lists the concentration of complex required to inhibit DNA synthesis by 50% (ID$_{50}$).

TABLE 2

| Complex | ID$_{50}$ Concentration ($\mu$g/ml) |
|---------|-------------------------------------|
| XIX | inactive |
| XX | 5 |
| XXI | 100 |
| XXIII | 350 |
| XXV | inactive |

B.    Filamentation Tests (6)

This test measures the percentage of filamentation in
in comparison to the effect on filamentation of the complex *cis-*
$[Pt(Cl)_2NH_3)_2]$ taken to be 100%.  The results are given in Table 3.

TABLE 3

| Complex | Test Result |
|---------|-------------|
| XIX | Weak Positive |
| XX | Positive (80%) |
| XXI | Positive (80%) |
| XXII | Positive |
| XXIII | No filamentation; "giant" cells formed |
| XXIV | Positive (80%) |
| XXV | Positive |

C.  *In Vivo* Tests; Swiss Female White Mice; Ascites S-180 (7)

Only compound V was tested by this procedure.  Six animals were
in each test group and each control group.  There were two test
groups and two control groups.  The best result in each group indicated an increased life span (%ILS) as indicated in Table 4.

TABLE 4

| Complex | Dosage | Percentage ILS |
|---------|--------|----------------|
| XXIII | 7 mg/kg | 55.6% |
| XXIII | 40 " | 52.1% |

Table 5 lists the activities of some complexes against two types of tumor systems (S 180 and Ca 755) in Swiss mice[a] or BDF$_1$ mice[b].

TABLE 5

| Compound | Test System | Tumor Wt (T/C) (mg) | % |
|----------|-------------|---------------------|---|
| XXVIII | S 180[a] | 92/1176 | 7 |
|  | Ca 755[b] | 0/984 | 0 |
| XXIX | S 180[a] | 170/1028 | 16 |
|  | Ca 755[b] | 0/485 | 0 |

It should be noted that the dosages were in the region of 25 mg/kg, and it also should be stressed again that for compound XXVIII, although the complex is active against S 180 and Ca 755 (as is the ligand itself), the complex is inactive against L 1210, even though the ligand is active against this tumor system. This indicates that the stability of the complex is too great for re-action [1] to occur, or perhaps, for the complex even to dissociate to an extent that would allow for DNA complexation to the metal. In addition, preliminary results indicate that compounds II and IV are active against Walker carcinosarcoma 256.

V.   CONCLUSIONS

The activity demonstrated by the above complexes is supportive of the proposals concerning the potential anti-tumor activity of coordination compounds, and certainly other related complexes should be synthesized and screened for such activity.  The work of Rosenberg et al. (8,9), Hill, Speer, Kahn, et al. (10), Thomson, Williams  et al. (11), Cleare and Hoeschele (12,13), and Connors, Tobe et al. (14,15) also implies that platinum complexes, even those that contain relatively simple ligands that do not possess anti-tumor activity, show significant anti-cancer activity when they possess the appropriate stability and stereochemistry to interact with DNA and/or viruses.

*ACKNOWLEDGEMENTS*

The authors wish to express their appreciation to the U. S. National Science Foundation and to the Romanian Council for Science and Technology for research grants that contributed significantly to the progress of this investigation.

*REFERENCES*

1.  Luria, S. E., Cancer Research 20, Page 669, 1960.

2.  Kirschner, Stanley, Wei, Young-Kang, Francis, Dawn and Bergman, John G., J. Med. Chem. 9, Page 369, 1966.

3.  Proceedings of Second International Symposium on Platinum Coordination Complexes in Cancer Chemotherapy, Oxford, 1973.

4.  Wolf, W., Manaka, R. C. and Leh, F. K. V., J. Clinical Hematology and Oncology, in press.

5.  Acknowledgement and thanks for these tests are accorded to Dr. David Kessel of the Milton Darling Memorial Center, Detroit, Michigan  48201.

6.  Tests performed at the Institute of Medicine, Timisoara, Romania, with thanks to Professor V. Topciu.

7.  Acknowledgement and thanks for these tests is accorded to Professor B. Rosenberg, Department of Biophysics, Michigan State University, East Lansing, Michigan.

8.  Rosenberg, B., Van Camp, L. and Krigas, T., Nature 205, Page 698, 1965; Rosenberg, B., Van Camp, L., Grimley, E. and Thomson, A. J., J. British Chemistry 242, Page 1347, 1967. Rosenberg, B., Renshaw, E., Van Camp, L., Hartwick, J. and Drobnik, J. Bacteriology 93, Page 716, 1967; Rosenberg, B., Van Camp, L., Trosko, J. E., Mansour, V. H., Nature (London) 222, Page 385, 1969.

9.  Rosenberg, B., Naturwissenschaften 60, Page 390, 1973, Plat. Met. Review 15, Page 3, 1971; Van Camp, L., Cancer Research 30, Page 1799, 1970.

10. Hill, J. M., Speer, R. J., Loeb, E., MacLellan, A., Hill, N.O. and Khan, A., Wadley Medical Bulletin 1, Page 121, 1971; Cardona, F. A., Hill, J. M., Loeb, E., MacLellan, A., Hill, N. O. and Khan, A., Wadley Medical Bulletin 2, Page 45, 1972; Astaldi, C. G. and Yalcin, B., Wadley Medical Bulletin 3, Page 7, 1973.

11. Thomson, A. J., Williams, R. J. P. and Reslova, S., Struct. and Bond. 11, Page 1, 1972; Strivastava, R. C., Froehlich, J. and Eichhorn, G. L., The Effect of Platinum Complexes on the Structure and Function of DNA, in press; Horer, O. L., Nicolau, C., FEBS Letters IN, Page 262, 1971; Drobnik, J. and Horacek, P., Chem-Biol Interactions F, Page 223, 1973; Munchausen, L.L., Proceedings National Academy Science, U. S. A., in press.

12. Cleare, M. J. and Hoeschele, J. D. H., Proceedings of the VIIth International Congress of Chemotherapy, Prague, 1970, Avicenum, Prague, in press.

13. Cleare, M. J. and Hoeschele, J. D., Bioinorganic Chemistry 2, Page 187, 1973; Cleare, M. J., Chem. Reviews 12, Page 349,1974.

14. Connors, T. A., Platinum Met. Review 17, Page 3, 1973; Connors, T. A., R. R. C. R 48, (19), in press; Higby, D. J., Wallace, H. J., Jr., Drs Albert and J. Holland, J. Urology 112, Page 100, 1973; Higby, D., Wallace, H. J. Jr. and Holland, J., Cancer Chemotherapy Reports, Part I, pp. 57, 459, 1973.

15. Connors, T. A., Jones, M., Ross, W. C. J., Braddock, P. D., Khokhar, A. R. and Tobe, M. L., Chem.-Biol. Interactions 5, Page 415, 1972.

CHAPTER 12

ANTI-TUMOR VIRUS ACTIVITY OF COPPER-BINDING DRUGS

Warren Levinson,* Peter Mikelens, Jean Jackson
Department of Microbiology, University of California, San Francisco,
San Francisco, California 94143

and

William Kaska

Department of Chemistry, University of California, Santa Barbara,
Santa Barbara, California 93106

ABSTRACT

Several, structurally different, copper-binding ligands can inhibit the RNA-dependent DNA polymerase of Rous sarcoma virus (RSV)
and can inactivate the ability of the virus to malignantly transform
chick embryo cells. These ligands include the anti-microbial agents,
thiosemicarbazones, 8-hydroxyquinolines, isonicotinic acid hydrazide,
and others. Many of these compounds bind to DNA and RNA in the presence of copper, which may play a role in their anti-viral activity.
However, not all agents active against RSV bind to nucleic acids and
not all ligands that bind to nucleic acids are active against RSV.
Some copper-binding ligands are neither active against RSV, nor bind
nucleic acids. It appears that there is no simple relationship between the anti-viral activity of copper-binding ligands and their
nucleic acid-binding ability. The biological importance of thio-
semicarbazone-copper complex binding to nucleic acids is supported
by the observation that treatment of intact RSV virions with the
complex causes the genome 70S RNA to sediment abnormally in velocity
sucrose gradient analysis.

---

* Person to whom correspondence should be addressed.

## I.  INTRODUCTION

Some organic ligands that bind metals of the first transition series, such as ortho-phenanthroline(1,2,3,4,5) and N-methyl isatin β-thiosemicarbazone (M-IBT),(6,7) inhibit DNA and RNA polymerases. It was hypothesized that inhibition was due to the binding of the ligand to zinc ions in the active site of the enzyme.(1,2,3,4,5) Inhibition of polymerases and other enzymes by metal-binding compounds has been used as indirect evidence that the enzyme is a metalloprotein and recent studies have directly demonstrated the presence of zinc in *E. coli* DNA polymerase I,(3) *E. coli* RNA polymerase,(1) and in the RNA-dependent DNA polymerase of avian myeloblastosis virus.(4,5)

We have presented evidence that one of these ligands, M-IBT, complexes with cupric ion and binds to nucleic acids.(8)  In view of this finding, we proposed that the inhibition of polymerases by some metal complexing agents may be due to interaction with the template rather than with the enzyme.  In this paper, we report that a variety of compounds inhibit the RNA-dependent DNA polymerase and the transforming ability of Rous sarcoma virus (RSV) and that some of these compounds bind to DNA and RNA in the presence of copper. However, not all copper-chelating compounds that affect RSV were found to bind to nucleic acids, which indicates that another mechanism may be involved.

Many of the compounds tested have well-documented anti-viral, anti-bacterial, or anti-tumor activity.  For example, M-IBT interferes with the replication of smallpox and vaccinia viruses(9), and is useful clinically in the treatment of some vaccination complications(10) and in the prevention of smallpox.(11)  In addition to the inhibition of poxviruses, M-IBT inactivates the RNA-dependent DNA polymerase activity and transforming ability of Rous sarcoma virus (RSV) upon *in vitro* exposure to the compound.(6)  Other RNA tumor viruses,(7) herpes simplex viruses,(12) and arenaviruses(13) are also inactivated upon *in vitro* exposure.  The inactivation of these viruses by M-IBT is prevented and reversed by competing chelating agents such as EDTA, 2-mercaptoethanol, and histidine.(2,12,13) In addition, M-IBT inhibits the RNA-dependent RNA polymerase activity of influenzavirus.(14)  Another thiosemicarbazone, thiacetazone, is used in combined therapy with isonicotinic acid hydrazide against tuberculosis.(15)  Some of the α-N-heterocyclic thiosemicarbazones (TSC), such as 2-formylpyridine TSC (PY-TSC) and 1-formylisoquinoline TSC (IQ-TSC), which complex with first transition series metals, exhibit antineoplastic activity.(16,17,18)  The inhibition of ribonucleoside diphosphate reductase has been proposed for their antitumor activity.(19)  In addition, kethoxal bis (thiosemicarbazone) (KTS) has been shown to possess anti-tumor activity(20), and the copper chelate complex appears to be the active form.(20,21,22) The radioprotective agents, cysteamine (2-mercaptoethylamine) and

3-mercaptopropylamine, which bind copper, have anti-tumor activity also.(23)

Two other types of metal-binding ligands, selenocystamine and the ortho-phenanthroline derivative, bathocuprein, inhibit the RNA-dependent RNA polymerase activity of influenza virus.(14,24)   D-Penicillamine, which is used clinically to remove excess copper from patients with Wilson's disease, inhibits the replication of poliovirus.(25)   Bis-benzimidazole inhibits the growth of some arenaviruses, for example, lymphocytic choriomeningitis virus,(26) and some picornaviruses, for example, poliovirus and rhinovirus.(27)

8-hydroxyquinoline (8-HQ) inhibits the growth of *Staphylococcus aureus* in the presence of copper,(28) is active as an anti-fungal agent,(29) and inhibits the RNA-dependent DNA polymerase of avian myeloblastosis virus(4) and of RSV.(30)   The derivative of 8-HQ (enteroviofform) is used clinically to treat skin infections and inhibits the RNA-dependent DNA polymerase of RSV.(30)   Isonicotinic acid hydrazide (isoniazid) (INH), a copper chelator, is well known as the drug of choice in the treatment of tuberculosis.(31)   Tetracycline is a copper-chelating, broad-spectrum antibiotic.(32)   Weak binding of tetracycline to DNA in the presence of zinc has been reported.(33)   Aurin tricarboxylic acid (ATA) inhibits protein synthesis *in vitro*,(34) DNA-dependent RNA polymerase of *E. coli* and coli phage T4,(35) RNA-dependent RNA synthesis of phage Qβ(35) and of vesicular stomatitis virus,(36) and RNA-dependent DNA polymerase of avian myeloblastosis virus(37) and murine leukemia virus.(38) ATA also prevents the binding of *lac* repressor to *lac* operator DNA.(33)   ATA froms brilliantly colored "lakes" in the presence of heavy metals, especially aluminum and iron.(39)   Although *cis* platinum (NH$_3$)$_2$Cl$_2$ is not a copper-chelating agent, its anti-tumor activity(40) and its DNA-binding ability(41) have been reported.  We, therefore, tested its activity against Rous sarcoma virus and its binding to DNA and RNA in our system.

## II.   RESULTS

The inhibition of the RNA-dependent DNA polymerase and the inactivation of the transforming ability of RSV by several thiosemicarbazones and their copper complexes is shown in Table 1.  M-IBT and PY-TSC are active, both as the free ligand and as the preformed copper complex.  IQ-TSC is also active as the free ligand; the copper complex was not available.  In contrast, KTS, the side-chain TSC, and dithizone (a thiocarbazone, not a thiosemicarbazone) are much less active as the free ligand than as the preformed complex. It is possible that those compounds that are active as the free ligand can complex with copper or other metal present in the virion or in the solutions.  This possibility is supported by our finding that EDTA can prevent the inhibitory activity of the free ligand, M-IBT.(6)

TABLE 1

EFFECT OF THIOSEMICARBAZONES ON RSV POLYMERASE AND TRANSFORMATION

| Compound | μMolar[b] | % Inhibition Polymerase Activity | Transforming Ability |
|---|---|---|---|
| M-IBT | 40 | 95 | 99 |
| M-IBT-copper[a] | 40 | 95 | 99 |
| PY-TSC | 10 | 98 | 99 |
| PY-TSC-copper[a] | 10 | 99 | 99 |
| IQ-TSC | 10 | 99 | 99 |
| KTS | 70 | 40 | 40 |
| KTS-copper[a] | 7 | 95 | 99 |
| TSC | 50 | 88 | 63 |
| TSC-copper[a] | 10 | 99 | 99 |
| Dithizone | 8 | 40 | 80 |
| Dithizone-copper[a] | 0.5 | 96 | 99 |
| Thiacetazone | 40 | 0 | 0 |

[a] Preformed, purified copper complex used.

[b] Molarity calculated on the basis of a 1:1 ligand metal complex.

The data in Table 2 demonstrates that 8-HQ and its 5-chloro, 7-iodo derivative are active both as the free ligand and as the preformed copper complex, but INH is active only as the copper complex. In contrast to the compounds previously described, O-phenanthroline and ATA have an unusual pattern of activity, since they inhibit the polymerase, but fail to inactivate the transforming ability except at much higher concentration. We suspect that this finding is due to the reversal of the polymerase inhibition inside the infected cell, since we found that proviral DNA is made normally within the cell infected with O-phenanthroline-treated RSV, despite inhibition of the polymerase activity *in vitro*.

TABLE 2

EFFECT OF 8-HYDROXYQUINOLINES,  ISONICOTINIC ACID HYDRAZIDE, O-PHENANTHROLINE, AND AURIN TRICARBOXYLIC ACID ON RSV

| | | % Inhibition | |
| | | Polymerase | Transforming |
| Compound | $\mu$Molar[b] | Activity | Ability |
| --- | --- | --- | --- |
| 8-HQ | 0.5 | 95 | 99 |
| 8-HQ copper[a] | 0.5 | 95 | 99 |
| 5-Cl, 7-I 8-HQ | 1 | 95 | 99 |
| 5-Cl, 7-I 8-HQ copper[a] | 1 | 95 | 99 |
| INH | 100 | 0 | 0 |
| INH copper[a] | 30 | 90 | 99 |
| O-Phenanthroline | 80 | 97 | 0 |
| ATA | 10 | 95 | 0 |
| ATA | 100 | 99 | 99 |

[a] Preformed, purified copper complex used.

[b] Molarity calculated on the basis of a 1:1 ligand metal complex.

The compounds in Table 3; selenocystamine, cysteamine, tetra-cycline, bis-benzimidazole, D-penicillamine and cis-platinum dia-mine chloride have little if any activity against the RSV functions tested. In order to detect latent activity with these compounds, 2 μM CuSO$_4$ was added; however, no increase in activity was observed.

In view of the correlation between the anti-RSV activity of M-IBT and its ability to bind to DNA and RNA in the presence of copper,[8] we tested the ability of the other compounds to bind to DNA and RNA. Our working hypothesis was that compounds with anti-viral activity would bind to the nucleic acids and compounds with-out anti-viral activity would bind less or not at all. The data in Table 4 uses the binding by 50 μM M-IBT, and 50 μM CuSO$_4$ as a 100% reference point. By comparison, as much as 200 μM M-IBT alone binds a maximum of 10%. The preformed M-IBT copper complex is approximately as effective as the components added separately.

TABLE 3

EFFECT OF SEVERAL CHELATING AGENTS ON RSV

| | | % Inhibition | |
| | | Polymerase | Transforming |
| Compound | μMolar | Activity | Ability |
| --- | --- | --- | --- |
| Selenocystamine | 50 | 33 | 0 |
| Cysteamine[a] | 100 | 0 | 0 |
| Tetracycline[a] | 400 | 0 | 0 |
| Bis-benzimidazole[a] | 100 | 0 | 0 |
| D-penicillamine[a] | 400 | 0 | 0 |
| Cis-Platinum (NH$_3$)$_2$Cl$_2$ | 75 | 0 | 0 |

[a] Ligand used with and without 2 μM copper sulfate. This con-centration of copper sulfate was maximum which, by itself, had no effect on either function.

PY-TSC is similar to M-IBT in that the free ligand has anti-RSV activity but does not bind to nucleic acid; however, it is different from M-IBT in that the addition of copper does not cause binding. In this case, it is cobalt that is effective. This supports the previous observation that PY-TSC forms complexes with cobalt more avidly than with copper.(42)  IQ-TSC follows the same pattern as M-IBT; that is, the free ligand does not bind, but the addition of copper sulfate causes binding. The preformed copper complex was unavailable.

KTS is unusual since it is poorly active against the virus as the free ligand. It doesn't bind DNA or RNA itself, but does when copper is added; however, the preformed copper complex that is strongly anti-viral does not bind DNA or RNA. This indicates that our hypothesis that anti-RSV activity is due to nucleic acid binding may not be correct. It also suggests that KTS-copper complexes may form more than one type structure with different properties.

TSC, the side chain containing the chelation sites, follows the pattern of its derivative, M-IBT; that is, the free ligand does not bind, but the addition of copper or the use of the preformed copper complex causes binding. The interaction of TSC-copper complexes with DNA has been confirmed using a variety of spectrophotometric techniques.(43)

Dithizone is unusual since it does not bind nucleic acids, even in the presence of copper, despite a distinct color change upon the addition of $CuSO_4$. The dithizone-copper complex, although quite active against RSV, does not bind nucleic acids, which is similar to the results with the KTS-copper complex.

Thiacetazone, despite its inability to inhibit RSV functions, binds to DNA and RNA effectively in the presence, but not in the absence, of copper.

It can be seen in Table 5 that 8HQ, which inhibits RSV activity, does not bind to nucleic acids as the free ligand, but does so when approximately equimolar copper is added; however, in contrast to M-IBT, the preformed copper complex does not bind to nucleic acids. The 5-chloro, 7-iodo derivative, which is also active against RSV, does not bind to DNA or RNA as the free ligand. When 10 µM $CuSO_4$ was added to 60 µM ligand, perhaps encouraging the 2:1 complex rather than the 1:1 complex, significant binding to DNA but not to RNA was observed. The loss of inhibitory activity of 8-HQ against *Staphylococcus aureus* by altering the ratio of ligand to copper, a phenomenon termed "concentration quenching" has been reported.(44)  The preformed 5 Cl, 7I, 8-HQ copper complex also binds to DNA, but not RNA, at 6 µM.

TABLE 4

BINDING OF THIOSEMICARBAZONES TO DNA AND RNA*

| Compound | RSV Inhibition[a] | μMolar | CuSO$_4$ μMolar[b] | % Binding DNA | RNA |
|---|---|---|---|---|---|
| M-IBT | + | 50 | - | 10 | 1 |
| M-IBT | + | 200 | - | 10 | 5 |
| M-IBT | + | 50 | 50 | 100[c] | 100 |
| M-IBT-copper | + | 40 | - | 100 | 140 |
| PY-TSC | + | 200 | - | 0 | 1 |
| PY-TSC | N.D. | 200 | 1000 | 10 | 60 |
| PY-TSC | N.D. | 200 | 500[d] | 115 | 50 |
| IQ-TSC | + | 40 | - | 0 | 0 |
| IQ-TSC | + | 600 | - | 0 | 0 |
| IQ-TSC | N.D. | 40 | 50 | 85 | 130 |
| KTS | - | 500 | - | 0 | 0 |
| KTS | N.D. | 500 | 500 | 50 | 115 |
| KTS-copper | + | 500 | - | 0 | 0 |
| TSC | + | 200 | - | 0 | 0 |
| TSC | N.D. | 40 | 50 | 100 | 140 |
| TSC-copper | + | 40 | - | 140 | 95 |
| Dithizone | - | 500 | - | 0 | 0 |
| Dithizone | N.D. | 500 | 500 | 0 | 0 |
| Dithizone-copper | + | 500 | - | 0 | 0 |
| Thiacetazone | - | 200 | - | 0 | 0 |
| Thiacetazone | N.D. | 50 | 50 | 100 | 120 |

*Footnotes for Tables 4 and 5 are on pages 169 and 170.

TABLE 5

BINDING OF VARIOUS COMPOUNDS TO DNA AND RNA

| Compound | RSV Inhibition[a] | μMolar | CuSO$_4$ μMolar[b] | % Binding DNA | % Binding RNA |
|----------|:-----------------:|:------:|:------------------:|:-------------:|:-------------:|
| 8-HQ | + | 600 | – | 0 | 0 |
| 8-HQ | N.D. | 600 | 500 | 50 | 50 |
| 8-HQ-copper | + | 200 | – | 0 | 0 |
| 5Cl, 7I-8HQ | + | 60 | – | 30 | 5 |
| 5Cl, 7I-8HQ | N.D. | 60 | 10 | 100 | 25 |
| 5Cl, 7I-8HQ-copper | + | 6 | – | 100 | 10 |
| INH | – | 1400 | – | 0 | 5 |
| INH | N.D. | 1400 | 1500 | 0 | 40 |
| INH-copper | + | 50 | – | 70 | 80 |
| O-Phenanthroline | ± | 200 | – | 65 | 15 |
| O-Phenanthroline | N.D. | 200 | 200 | 75 | 60 |
| ATA | ± | 500 | – | 0 | 0 |
| ATA | N.D. | 500 | 500 | 0 | 0 |

Footnotes FOR TABLES 4 and 5

[a] This column refers to the data presented in Tables 1, 2 and 3.

+ Indicates a compound that inhibited RSV greater than 75% at 50 μM or less. The concentration at which RSV inhibition was tested does not necessarily correspond to that used in the binding assay.

– Indicates a compound that did not inhibit RSV greater than 75% at more than 50 μM.

Cont.

Footnotes for Tables 4 and 5 (Continued)

± Means polymerase activity inhibited but not transformation when
low concentrations were used.

N.D. Indicates not done.

[b] Concentration of $CuSO_4$ added to the sample. The amount of $CuSO_4$
in buffer and compound is unknown.

-- Indicates no $CuSO_4$ added.
     No binding by $5000 \mu M$ $CuSO_4$ itself was observed.

[c] Defined as 100% binding. This represents [3]H Hela DNA (550 ng/ml)
containing approximately 4000 cpm and [32]P Rous sarcoma virus RNA (460
ng/ml) containing approximately 3000 cpm. This represents approximately
75% and 70% of acid-precipitable cpm of DNA and RNA, respectively.

[d] Cobalt chloride not copper sulfate.

---

INH binds to neither DNA nor RNA but does bind selectively to
RNA when equimolar copper is added. The preformed INH-copper complex loses this specificity, again indicating that different structures may arise under different conditions of formation.

O-Phenanthroline binds to DNA to a greater extent than to RNA as
the free ligand, but both nucleic acids are bound to approximately
the same extent when equimolar copper is added.

ATA, although effective in inhibiting the polymerase activity of
RSV at low concentration, does not bind to either DNA nor RNA in the
presence or absence of copper; however, some interaction of ATA with
DNA may occur, since 6 μM ATA can block the binding of 50 μm-IBT-
copper complex when added to the DNA before but not after the M-IBT-
copper complex (P.M., unpublished results).

Selenocystamine, which does not inhibit RSV functions, does not
bind to DNA nor RNA (Table 6). Cysteamine, which also does not inhibit RSV, does not bind to nucleic acids as the free ligand, but
does when copper is added. Tetracycline and bis-benzimidazole

manifest a similar pattern as cysteamine, since they show no anti-RSV activity, but bind nucleic acids in the presence of copper. Bis-benzimidazole at low concentration shows some selective binding of DNA rather than RNA.  D-Penicillamine has no effect on RSV, and does not bind DNA nor RNA with or without copper.  Lastly, cis-platinum $(NH_3)_2Cl_2$ binds neither DNA nor RNA in this assay.

TABLE 6

BINDING OF VARIOUS COMPOUNDS TO DNA AND RNA

| Compound | RSV Inhibition[a] | μMolar | CuSO4 μMolar[b] | % Binding DNA | RNA |
|---|---|---|---|---|---|
| Selenocystamine | − | 100 | − | 0 | 0 |
| Selenocystamine | − | 100 | 50 | 0 | 0 |
| Cysteamine | − | 500 | − | 0 | 0 |
| Cysteamine | − | 50 | 50 | 100 | 135 |
| Tetracycline | − | 600 | − | 0 | 0 |
| Tetracycline | − | 80 | 100 | 100 | 125 |
| Bis-benzimidazole | − | 200 | − | 0 | 0 |
| Bis-benzimidazole | − | 5 | 50 | 150 | 125 |
| Bis-benzimidazole | − | 5 | 10 | 100 | 28 |
| D-Penicillamine | − | 500 | − | 0 | 0 |
| D-Penicillamine | − | 500 | 1000 | 0 | 0 |
| Cis-platinum$(NH_3)_2Cl_2$ | − | 500 | − | 0 | 0 |

Since nucleic acids bind to M-IBT copper complexes *in vitro*, it was of interest to determine whether the interaction observed in the test tube with purified nucleic acids was biologically pertinent. Some information regarding this question is available since we found that M-IBT-copper complexes inhibit transfection of lambda phage DNA in *E. coli*.(45)  We report here our efforts to determine whether a nucleic acid, M-IBT-copper complex, was formed within RSV virions

when they were exposed under conditions similar to those used to inactivate the biological activities of the virus.

Purified RSV was exposed to either 50 μM M-IBT, 50 μM CuSO$_4$, or
a combination of the two in a buffer approximating that used in the
polymerase reaction.  After incubation at 37° for 15 minutes, 2%
deoxycholate, to disrupt the virion, and excess calf thymus DNA, to
react with unreacted M-IBT-copper complexes, were added.  After further incubation at 37° for 5 minutes to ensure release of the RSV-
RNA, the samples were centrifuged and processed as described in the
legend to Figure 1.  It can be seen that exposure to 50 μM CuSO$_4$
has little effect on the sedimentation of the RSV RNA, whereas exposure to 50 μM M-IBT results in the loss of approximately 50% of
the RNA.  Treatment with both M-IBT and  CuSO$_4$ results in the complete loss of RNA.  Presumably, the RNA was pelleted rather than degraded, since there are no counts at the top of the gradient.

Two control experiments to determine the reliability of these
observations were performed.  One experiment tested whether the
loss of RNA could be due to nonspecific trapping in aggregates of
DNA that had interacted with M-IBT copper complexes.  It was found
that when RSV was added after the DNA, the M-IBT, and the CuSO$_4$
then treated with deoxycholate, the RNA sedimented in the position
of Sample A in Figure 1.  This indicates that trapping is unlikely
to be the explanation.  Another experiment tested whether EDTA, which
we reported prevents inhibition of the RSV polymerase by M-IBT,(6)
could prevent the loss of RNA in the gradient.  We found that the
addition of 500 μM EDTA directly after exposure to the 50 μM M-IBT
and the 50 μM CuSO$_4$ completely prevented the loss of RNA in the
gradient.  This supports the hypothesis that copper is important in
the binding of M-IBT to the RNA in the virion.

We conclude that several, structurally different copper-binding
ligands can inhibit the RNA-dependent DNA polymerases of RSV, perhaps by binding to DNA or RNA.  However, not all metal-binding ligands, which inhibit polymerase activity, bind efficiently to DNA or
RNA in the presence of copper; for example, KTS, dithizone, and ATA.
It is possible that binding to nucleic acids may involve a different
metal.  On the other hand, there are some compounds such as thiacetazone, cysteamine, tetracycline, and cis-benzimidazole, which bind
to DNA and RNA in the presence of copper, but do not inhibit polymerase activity.  There are two metal-binding ligands, selenocystamine and D-penicillamine, which neither inhibit polymerase activity
nor bind to DNA.  It appears that there is no simple relationship
between the antiviral effect of metal-binding ligands and their ability to bind to nucleic acids.  This suggests that a second mechanism
may be involved, namely, that the virion polymerase may be the site
of action rather than the nucleic acid for some of these compounds.

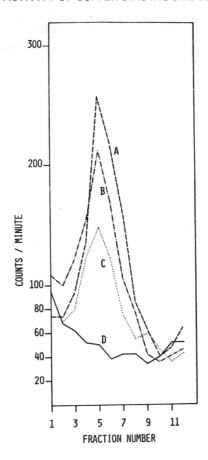

Figure 1

Effect of M-IBT and $CuSO_4$ on RSV 70S RNA

Purified [3]H-uridine labeled RSV (SR strain) was incubated in 0.2 ml of a buffer containing 0.1 M phosphate pH 7.5 and 0.05 M NaCl at 37° for 15 minutes in the presence of (a) no additions; (b) 50 µM $CuSO_4$; (c) 50 µM M-IBT; (d) 50 µM M-IBT and 50 µM $CuSO_4$. 1.8 ml of buffer containing 2% sodium deoxycholate and 20 µg/ml calf thymus DNA were added, incubated 37° for five minutes and then centrifuged in a 15% to 30% sucrose gradient for three hours at 40,000 rpm in an SW 41 rotor. Sucrose solutions were prepared in a buffer containing 0.02 M phosphate pH 7.5 and 0.1 M NaCl. Fractions were collected, acid precipitated, trapped on filters, and counted in a liquid scintillation spectrometer.

III.  METHODS

## RNA-Dependent DNA Polymerase Assay

Purified RSV, suspended in 200λ of 0.05 M phosphate-buffered
saline pH 7.4, was exposed to different concentrations of the various compounds by addition of a 2λ aliquot after 30 minutes at 37°,
20λ of a solution containing 2 μc $^3$H-TTP (sp. act. 13 Cu/millimole),
0.5% NP40 (final concentration 0.05%).  The reaction mixture was
incubated at 37° for two hours and acid-precipitable counts obtained.(6)   Since many of these compounds were dissolved in 100%
dimethylsulfoxide, we tested its effect on enzyme activity.  No
inhibition by 1% DMSO was observed.

## Transformation Assay

Before adding the $^3$H-TTP in the polymerase assay, a 5λ aliquot
was diluted into 0.5 ml 199 + 4% calf serum and assayed for focus
formation on chick embryo cells as described.(46)

## Nucleic Acid-Binding Assay

The binding assay(8) contained $^3$H-thymidine-labeled HeLa cell
double-stranded DNA or $^{32}$P labeled RSV 70S RNA in 0.05M phosphate
buffer pH 8.0 to which aliquots of drug and copper sulfate were
added.  The mixture was incubated at 0° for 10 minutes and then
passed through a 0.45μ pore nitrocellulose filter.  After washing,
the filters were dried and counted in a liquid scintillation spectrometer.  Appropriate aliquots of 100% DMSO retained no DNA on the
filter.

*ACKNOWLEDGEMENTS*

This investigation was supported by U. S. Public Health Service
Grants CA 12705-05, AI 08293, AI 00299; Contract No. NO1 CP 33293,
within the Special Virus Cancer Program of the National Cancer
Institute and the American Cancer Society Grant VC-70.

## ABBREVIATIONS

| | |
|---|---|
| M–IBT | N-methyl isatin beta-thiosemicarbazone |
| RSV | Rous sarcoma virus |
| EDTA | ethylene diamine tetra acetic acid |
| TSC | thiosemicarbazide or thiosemicarbazone |
| KTS | kethoxal bis-(thiosemicarbazone) |
| Py-TSC | 2-pyridine thiosemicarbazone |
| IQ-TSC | isoquinoline 1-formyl thiosemicarbazone |
| 8-HQ | 8-hydroxyquinoline |
| 5 Cl,7I-8HQ | 5-chloro, 7-iodo, 8-hydroxyquinoline |
| INH | isonicotinic acid hydrazide |
| ATA | aurin tricarboxylic acid |
| dithizone | diphenylthiocarbazone |
| thiacetazone | para-aceto amino benzaldehyde thiosemcarbazone |
| bis-benzimidazole, 1,2-Bis | (5-methoxy-1 H-benzimidazole-2-yl)-1,2-ethanediol |

## REFERENCES

1. Scrutton, M., Wu, C. and Goldthwait, D., Proceedings National Academy Science U.S.A. 68, Page 2497, 1971.

2. Valenzuela, P., Morris, R., Faras, A., Levinson, W. and Rutter, W., Biochem. Biophys. Res. Commun. 53, Page 1036, 1973.

3. Springate, C., Mildvan, A., Abramson, R., Engle, J. and Loeb, L., J. Biol. Chem. 248, Page 5987, 1973.

4. Auld, D., Kawaguchi, H., Livingston, D. and Vallee, B., Proc. National Academy Science U.S.A. 71, Page 2091, 1974.

5. Poiesz, B., Seal, G. and Loeb, L., Ibid. Ref. 4, Page 4982.

6. Levinson, W., Faras, A., Woodson, B., Jackson, J., and Bishop, J. M., Ibid. Ref. 4, 70, Page 164, 1973.

7.  Levinson, W., Faras, A., Morris, R., Mikelens, P., Ringold, G.,
    Kass, S., Levinson, B. and Jackson, J., <u>Virus Research</u> (ICN-
    UCLA Symposium), F. Fox and W. Robinson, Editors, Academic
    Press, New York, Page 403, 1973.

8.  Mikelens, P., Woodson, B., Levinson, W., Biochem. Pharmacology
    <u>25</u>, Page 821, 1976.

9.  Easterbrook, K., Virology <u>17</u>, Page 245, 1962.

10. Douglas, R., Lynch, E. and Spira, M., Arch. Internal Medicine
    <u>129</u>, Page 980, 1972.

11. Bauer, D., St. Vincent, L., Kempe, C., Young, P. and Downie, A.,
    American J. Epidemiology <u>90</u>, Page 130, 1969.

12. Levinson, W., Coleman, V., Woodson, B., Rabson, A., Lanier, J.,
    Witcher, J. J. and Dawson, C., Antimicrob. Agents Chemother <u>5</u>,
    Page 398, 1974.

13. Logan, J., Fox, M., Morgan, J., Makohon, A. and Pfau, C., J.
    Gen. Virol. <u>28</u>, Page 271, 1975.

14. Oxford, J., J. Gen. Virol. <u>23</u>, Page 59, 1974.

15. Citron, K., British Medical J. <u>1</u>, Page 426, 1972.

16. French, F., Blanz, E., Jr., Doamaral, J. and French, D., J.
    Med. Chem. <u>13</u>, Page 1117, 1970.

17. Blanz, E., Jr., French, F., Doamaral, J. and French, D., Ibid.
    Ref. 16, Page 1124.

18. Agrawal, K. and Sartorelli, A., Ibid. Ref. 16, Page 431.

19. Sartorelli, A., Agrawal, K. and Moore, E., Biochem. Pharmacol.
    <u>20</u>, Page 3119, 1971.

20. Petering, H., Buskirk, H. and Underwood, G., Cancer Research
    <u>24</u>, Page 367, 1964.

21. Crim, J. and Petering, H., Cancer Research <u>27</u>, Page 1278, 1967.

22. Bhuyan, B. and Betz, T., Cancer Research <u>28</u>, Page 758, 1968.

23. Apffel, C., Walker, J. and Issarescu, Cancer Research <u>35</u>,
    Page 429, 1975.

24. Oxford, J., J. Gen. Virol. <u>18</u>, Page 11, 1973.

25. Merryman, P., Jaffe, I. and Ehrenfield, E., J. Virol. 13, Page 881, 1974.

26. Stella, J., Yankaskas, K., Morgan, J., Fox, M. and Pfau, C., Antimicrob. Agents Chemother. 6, Page 754, 1974.

27. Schleicher, J., Aquino, F., Rueter, A., Roderick, W. and Appel, R., Applied Microbiology 23, Page 113, 1972.

28. Rubbo, S., Albert, A. and Gibson, M., Br. J. Exp. Pathology 31, Page 425, 1950.

29. Gershon, H., Parmeciani, R. and Nickerson, W., Applied Micro- biology 10, Page 556, 1962.

30. Rohde, W., Mikelens, P., Jackson, J., Blackman, J., Whitcher, J. and Levinson, W., Antimicrob. Agents Chemother. 10, Page 234, 1976.

31. Cymmerman-Craig, J., Nature 177, Page 480, 1956. Reiber, M. and Bemski, G., Arch. Biochem. Biophys. 131, Page 655, 1967.

32. Doluisio, J. and Martin, A., J. Med. Chem. 6, Page 16, 1963.

33. Kohn, K., Nature 191, Page 1156, 1961.

34. Stewart, M., Grollman, A. and Huang, M., Proc. Natl. Acad. Sci. USA, 97, 1971.

35. Blumenthal, T. and Landers, T., Biochem. Biophys. Res. Commun. 55, Page 680, 1973.

36. Hunt, D. and Wagner, R., J. Virol. 16, Page 1146, 1975.

37. Leis, J. and Hurwitz, J., J. Virol. 9, Page 130, 1972.

38. Liao, L., Horowitz, S., Huang, M., Grollman, A., Steward, D. and Martin, J., J. Med. Chem. 18, Page 117, 1975.

39. Smith, W., Sager, E. and Siewers, I., Anal. Chem. 21, 1134, 1949.

40. Rosenberg, B. and Van Camp, L., Cancer Research 30, 1799, 1970.

41. Macquet, P. and Theophanides, T., Bioinorganic Chemistry 5, Page 59, 1975.

42. Agrawal, K., Booth, B., Michaud, R., Moore, E. and Sartorelli, A., Biochem. Pharmacology 23, Page 2421, 1974.

43.  Pillai, C., Nandi, V. and Levinson, W., Bioinorganic Chem.
     (in press).

44.  Albert, A., Selective Toxicity, Chapman and Hall, London,
     Page 371, 1973.

45.  Levinson, W. and Helling, R., Antimicrob. Agents Chemother. 9,
     Page 160, 1976.

46.  Levinson, W., Virology 32, Page 74, 1967.

CHAPTER 13


REACTION OF COPPER COMPLEXES WITH EHRLICH CELLS

David H. Petering

Department of Chemistry
University of Wisconsin-Milwaukee
Milwaukee, Wisconsin  53201

For many years, medicinal chemistry has been largely the province of organic and natural products chemists, with the great majority of all chemotherapeutic agents being metal-free organic or biochemicals.  Yet where metal complexes have been used, or the involvement of metals in the mechanism of action of organic compounds recognized, there is ample evidence of the enormous potential that metal
complexes have in drug design.  Considering cancer chemotherapy,
there are several major examples in which metal complexes have been
shown to have substantial anti-tumor activity or to be cytotoxic to
tumor cells.  As shown in Figure 1, bis(thiosemicarbazonato)
copper(II) complexes, copper-bleomycin, *cis*-dichlorodiammine plat-
inum(II) complexes, some rhodium(II) carboxylates, and recently,
iron and copper complexes of α-N-heterocyclic formyl thiosemicarbazones fall into this category.(1-5)

That transition or other heavy metals can perturb biochemical
processes has been known for years.  Metal ions have been used as
reagents to modify or denature isolated enzymes, deoxyribonucleic
acids, mitochondria, and other membranous structures.(6-8)  The
widespread interaction of metal ions with cellular components is
due to the fact that all of these structures contain a variety of
functional groups that can act as metal-binding ligands.  Not only
can such effects be elicited by so-called toxic metals, but they can
be observed with transition metal ions that are normally considered
essential to cells. Members of the latter group can certainly function in uncontrolled ways in cells as long as they escape their normal metabolic pathways.  The problem is how to obtain these inter-

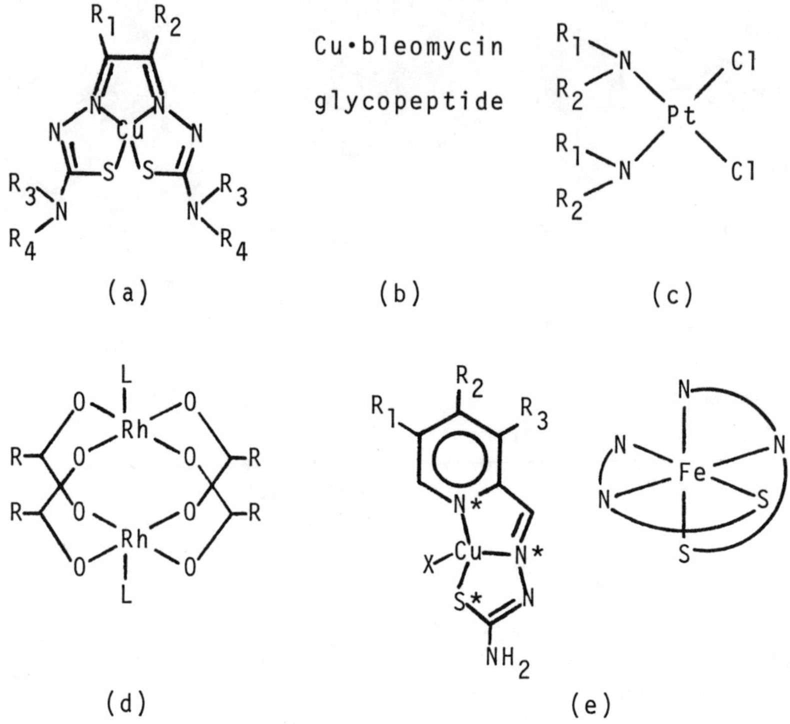

Figure 1

Structures of Complexes
a.  bis(thiosemicarbazonato) Cu(II);  c.   cis-dichlorodiammine Pt(II);
d.  rhodium carboxylate; e.   α-N-Heterocyclic formyl thiosemi-
    carbazonato copper(II) and iron(II,III).

actions in cells and organisms where non-polar membranes exist to
hinder the movement of charged metal ions into the cell, where a
myriad of metal-binding sites exist to compete for the metal ion,
and where specificity of cellular interaction must occur in order
to obtain therapeutic value.  Some possible answers to this question can be set forth here using existing experimental results.

In general, metal-ligand complexes must be used (1) which have
sufficient lipid solubility to permit transport of the metal across
membranes; (2) which have high enough thermodynamic stability to
allow the complex to reach the site without being dissociated; and
(3) which then react as metal complexes with cells to produce a

selective effect.  These points can be illustrated with thiosemicarbazonato metal complexes.

In the early 1960's, French and Freelander, and H. G. Petering
and coworkers showed that 3-ethoxy-2-oxobutyraldehyde bis(thiosemicarbazone), $H_2KTS$, was a highly active anti-tumor agent in rats
against several established, solid tumors.(9-11)  Mihich and Nichol
also found the compound to have wide-spectrum activity against
transplanted and spontaneous tumors.(12)  In the early mechanistic
investigation of the compound, it was concluded that in animals or
in a metal-controlled *in vitro* system, the compound itself is not
active.  In fact, it is the copper complex, CuKTS, that constitutes
the cytotoxic entity.(1,13,14)  At the outset of a more detailed
analysis of the mode of interaction of CuKTS with cells, it was
recognized that several different classes of reactions might be
involved as listed in reactions 1-4, and that a knowledge of the
chemical properties of this complex would be useful in directing
the investigation of its reaction with tumor cells.

$$ML_n + mL' \underset{k_{-1}}{\overset{\overset{\textstyle K_{eq}}{k_1}}{\rightleftharpoons}} ML'_m + nL \qquad \text{Ligand Substitution} \qquad (1)$$

$$M_{ox}L + L'_{red} \rightleftharpoons M_{red}L + L'_{ox} \qquad \text{Redox Reaction} \qquad (2)$$

$$ML_n + L' \rightleftharpoons ML_n - L' \qquad \text{Adduct Formation} \qquad (3)$$

$$ML_n + X \rightleftharpoons ML''_n \qquad \begin{array}{l}\text{Modification of} \\ \text{Coordinated Ligand}\end{array} \qquad (4)$$

CuKTS has large thermodynamic stability, having a conditional
formation constant at pH 7.4 of $10^{18.8}$ which is much larger than
those for copper complexes involving simple biological ligands.(15,16)
On this basis, it was not expected to be dissociated by competing
ligands, and indeed, in a model biological fluid, human blood plasma,
no dissociation is observed.(17)  In addition, this is a lipid soluble complex and so has substantial mobility in biological systems.
Its pattern of movement, of course, differs quantitatively and qualitatively from $CuCl_2$ as judged in experiments utilizing [64]Cu-labeled
materials in mice.(18)

In contrast to this case are the bis(thiosemicarbazonato)

zinc(II) complexes.  At one time, ZnKTS was thought to be an independent cytotoxic agent in animals, for ZnKTS is an active compound.(19,20)  However, *in vitro* under metal-free conditions, this
chelate is not effective.(14)  Here it could be shown that the formation constant is not large enough to prevent complete dissociation
of ZnKTS in plasma to release free ligand.(17)  What must occur in
animals, therefore, is that ZnKTS serves a donor of ligand which
then complexes available copper to generate the active species
CuKTS.  Nevertheless, 3-ethoxy-2-oxobutyraldehyde bis(N$^4$-dimethyl-
thiosemicarbazone) does form a biologically stable complex with
zinc to produce a chelate that is cytotoxic to tumor cells *in vitro*,
depresses incorporation of thymidine into DNA, and inhibits oxidative
phosphorylation.(14,17,21,22)

Returning to the chemistry of CuKTS, it does not form adducts
of any stability with Lewis bases and does not appear to be readily
alkylated (reactions 2, 4).  However, the complex can be stoichio-
metrically reduced and dissociated with dithiothreitol according to
the reaction.(23)

$$Cu(II)KTS + 2RSH \longrightarrow Cu(I)SR + H_2KTS + 1/2RSSR \qquad (5)$$

The half-wave reduction potential of CuKTS (-120 mv, pH 6.6; -178
mv, pH 9.1) and the stability of copper(I) mercaptides favor this
reaction.(23)  This redox process was used as a starting point for
the examination of the reaction of CuKTS with Ehrlich tumor cells
and, in fact, now appears to represent the general type of reaction
that does occur.(24)

Figure 2 shows the dissociation of CuKTS by cells as monitored
spectrophotometrically at 469 nm.(24)  This is a pseudo first-order
process, which also can be shown to depend on the concentration of
cells.  A variety of techniques including epr spectroscopy, atomic
absorption spectrophotometry, the use of reagents to measure cop-
per(I) and thiols support the conclusion that this is a redox reaction in which thiols are the reducing agents as described in
Equation (5).  Interestingly, this is a nonspecific reaction in
which copper is deposited throughout the cell and causes lesions in
several different biochemical processes including DNA, RNA, and
protein synthesis, oxidative phosphorylation; and thymidine uptake,
of which the first is most sensitive to CuKTS.(24-26)

A test of this mechanism comes from the variation in activity
of bis(thiosemicarbazonato) copper(II) complexes substituted in
$R_1$-$R_4$ positions (Figure 1a).  Table 1 summarizes the comparative
properties of these complexes.(26-27)  It is evident in this set of
chelates that chemical, biochemical, and cellular properties do
parallel one another.  In particular, pseudo first-order rate constants for thiol oxidation of bis(thiosemicarbazonato) copper(II)

complexes and similar constants for the cellular reaction with these materials are both linearly correlated with reduction potentials for these complexes as illustrated in Figure 3.

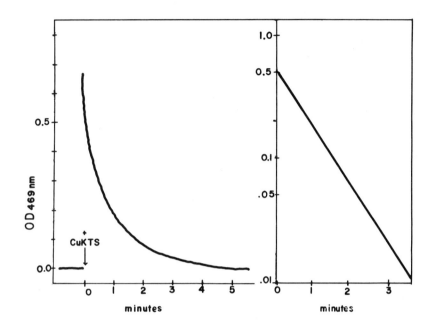

Figure 2

Reaction of CuKTS with Ehrlich Cells
45 mg/ml Cells in Eagle's Medium and Earle's Salts

An instructive comparison in mechanism involves 2-formyl-pyridine thiosemicarbazonato copper(II), $CuL^+$. This complex has been shown to be cytotoxic to Ehrlich ascites cells.(5) It is highly stable, $\log K^{Cu}_{CuL}$ = 13.3 at pH 7.4, and not dissociated by plasma.(16,28) It has a high half-wave potential, +2 mv, and reacts rapidly with thiols.(16,29) In addition, it forms adducts with Lewis bases, utilizing its availability in plane coordination site.(16) Since Ehrlich cells have a large sulfhydryl content, it was surprising to find that $CuL^+$ is not reduced upon uptake into these cells (Table 1, Figure 3). In fact, it is irreversibly taken up into the Ehrlich cell and remains a part of it.(30) However, $CuL^+$ may be forming adducts that are important in its mechanism of cytotoxicity. Evidence for adduct species come from low-temperature epr spectra of the complex in cells as exemplified in Figure 4.(30)

Table 1

Comparative Properties of Copper Complexes

| Complex | $R_1$ | $R_2$ | $R_3$ | $R_4$ | Relative in vitro Cytotoxicity[a] | $E_{1/2}$ (V) | $k/k_0$[b] (dtt) | $k/k_0$[c] (cells) |
|---|---|---|---|---|---|---|---|---|
| 1. CuKTS | CH(OEt)CH$_3$ | H | H | H | (+) | -0.178 | 1.0 | 1.0 |
| 2. CuKTSM | CH(OEt)CH$_3$ | H | CH$_3$ | H | (+) | -0.188 | 0.84 | 0.43 |
| 3. CuKTSM$_2$ | CH(OEt)CH$_3$ | H | CH$_3$ | CH$_3$ | (-) | -0.283 | 0.007 | 0.004 |
| 4. CuPTS | CH$_3$ | H | H | H | (+) | -0.188 | 3.7 | 0.47 |
| 5. CuPTSM | CH$_3$ | H | CH$_3$ | H | (+) | -0.208 | 3.7 | 0.52 |
| 6. CuPTSM$_2$ | CH$_3$ | H | CH$_3$ | CH$_3$ | (-) | -0.278 | 0.015 | 0.001 |
| 7. CuGTS | H | H | H | H | (-) | -0.098 | 165 | 0.013 |
| 8. CuL$^+$ |  |  |  |  | (+)[d] | +0.002 | 110 | 0.004 |

[a]Ref 14.   [b]Ref 27.   [c]Ref 26.   [d]Ref 5.

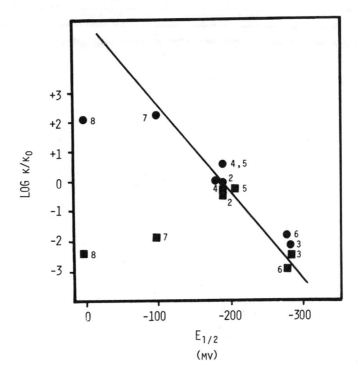

Figure 3

Linear Free-Energy Correlation of Reaction of bis
(thiosemicarbazonato) Copper Complexes with Ehrlich Cells.
Numbers refer to complexes in Table 1.

Reaction with dithiothreitol (●).   Reaction with cells (■).

The appearance of a new set of hyperfine lines in the $g_{||}$ region
of the spectrum is an indication that an adduct species may exist
in the cell. As with CuKTS, this copper chelate inhibits DNA synthesis at low concentration. Yet this effect and the overall cytotoxicity to Ehrlich cells must occur by a distinctly different mode
of reaction.

These examples, along with other compounds shown in Figure 1,
support the contention that metal complexes, even different complexes of a given metal, may show wide array of chemical inter-

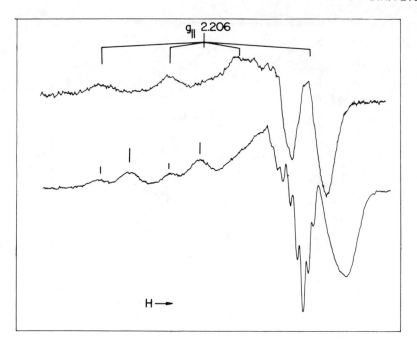

Figure 4

Electron Paramagnetic Spectra

a.  CuL$^+$; b.  CuL$^+$ in Ehrlich cells.  Modulation frequency, 100 kHz; modulation amplitude, 8 g; microwave frequency, 9.108; temperature, 77°K.

actions with cells that may be finely tuned by structural modifications of the ligands.  In addition, it should be emphasized that if the metal complex is dissociated during its reaction with cells, both the metal and the ligand may cause cytotoxic effects.  Such an example may involve the natural product, bleomycin.(31)

Although bleomycin is isolated from *Streptomyces verticillis* as a copper complex, which is an active anti-tumor agent in animal systems, it is now used and studied exclusively as the free ligand. Recently, studies have shown that Cu·bleomycin is significantly more cytotoxic to tumor cells than bleomycin itself (Figure 5).(32) This difference may be due to the intrinsic effects of Cu·bleomycin or may result if Cu·bleomycin breaks down in the tumor cell to yield copper ion and free bleomycin, both of which have independent activity.

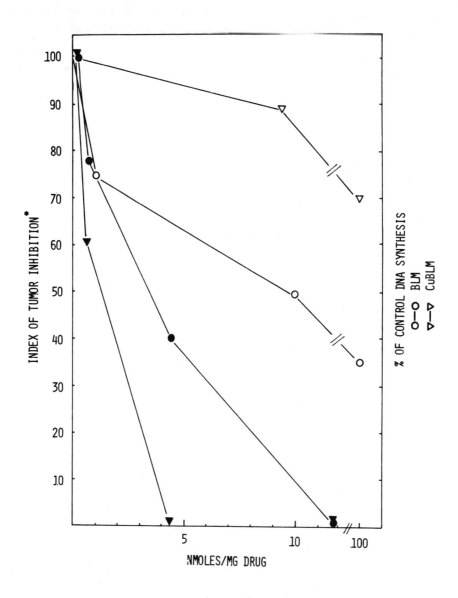

Figure 5

Cytotoxicity of Bleomycin and Copper Bleomycin

Experimental conditions:  reference 5; Blm  (●); Cu Blm  (▼)

Index = (time in days to develop 10 g tumor in controls)/(time in days to develop 10 g tumor in drug-treated animals) x 100.

How is selective cytotoxicity achieved by metal complexes? Considering the thiosemicarbazones, it is interesting to observe in Table 2 that CuKTS, $CuL_2^+$, $FeL_2^+$, and $CdKTSM_2$ are all potent inhibitors of thymidine incorporation into DNA and generally seem to affect DNA synthesis at lower concentration than, for example, oxidative phosphorylation.(22)  With CuKTS and $CdKTSM_2$, inhibition of DNA synthesis correlates with cytotoxicity; hence, as with a number of organic anti-tumor agents, specificity or therapeutic value may depend upon the differential rates of growth of normal and neoplastic cells.  While many tissues may be exposed to the drug, those with a requirement for rapid growth are more sensitive; however, in other cases, concentration of drugs that completely inhibit DNA synthesis are not directly related to cytotoxic effects.  This is strikingly evident with $FeL_2^+$ and its unbound ligand, HL.  On a more specific level, since CuKTS interacts with cellular thiols, it may be argued that the complex will react preferentially with tissues having a relatively high concentration of thiols.  Hence, it may be possible to design complexes that react selectively with cells containing an abundance of a given type of molecule.

Table 2

Inhibition of Ehrlich Tumor Cell Properties

| Complex | Zero[b] Growth | DNA Synthesis[c] 90% Inhibition (nmoles/mg) | Cell Respiration[d] 90% Inhibition (nmoles/mg) |
|---|---|---|---|
| CuKTS (26,33)[a] | 5 | 1.1 | 20 |
| $CuL^+$ (5,30) | >30 | 0.8 | >42[e] |
| $FeL_2^+$ (22,30) | >80[e] | 0.5 | -- |
| HL (22,30) | >325[e] | 8.5 | -- |
| $CdKTSM_2$ (34) | >20 | 4 | 49 |

[a]Reference numbers in parentheses.  [b]Thirty-minute incubation of drug with cells (nmole/mg) in metal-free medium followed by injection into host.  [c]Measured by $^3$H-thymidine incorporation in DNA.  Incubation time 15-30 minutes.  [d]Incubations, CuKTS—240 min, $CuL^+$ and $CdKTSM_2$—60 min.  [e]No measurable effect.

Finally, one can ask which metals should be examined, given the variety that have been shown to have activity in some metal complexes. In the past, there has been an emphasis on biologically nonessential or toxic heavy metal complexes. Such studies have proved fruitful. At the same time, the use of complexes involving biologically essential metals such as Mn, Fe, Cu, and Zn, also seems attractive for the reason that organisms have homeostatic mechanisms for metabolizing these metals. If complexes of these metals are broken down during the course of their reactions with components of the biological system, the liberated metal ion may then be incorporated naturally into the organism to prevent some of the extraneous heavy metal toxicity that results when nonessential metal ions are introduced into the system.

## ACKNOWLEDGEMENT

The author's research is currently supported by NIH Grant CA 16156-03, and by a grant from the American Cancer Society, Milwaukee Section.

## REFERENCES

1. Crim, J. A. and Petering, H. G., Cancer Research 27, Page 1278, 1967.

2. Ishiznka, M., Takayama, H., Takeuchi, T. and Umezawa, H., J. Antibiotics, Ser. A, 20, Page 15, 1967.

3. Rosenberg, B., and Van Camp, L., Cancer Research 30, Page 1799, 1970.

4. Erck, A., Rainer, L., Whileyman, J., Chang, I. M., Kimball, A. P. and Bear, J., Proceedings Soc. Exp. Biol. Med. 145, Page 1278, 1974.

5. Antholine, W., Knight, J. and Petering, J. Med. Chem. 19, Page 339, 1976.

6. Vallee, B. L. and Ulmer, D. D., Annual Review Biochemistry 41, Page 91, 1972.

7. Eichhorn, G. L., Inorganic Biochemistry, Vol. 2, G. L. Eichhorn, Editor, Elsevier, New York, Page 1210, 1973.

8. Chvapil, M., "Effect of Zinc on Cells and Biomembranes," in The Medical Clinics of North America--Trace Elements, Vol. 60, No. 4, W. B. Saunders Co., Philadelphia, Pennsylvania, Page 799, 1976.

9.  French, F. A. and Freelander, B. L., Cancer Research 21,
    Page 505, 1960.

10. Petering, H. G. and Buskirk, H. H., Federal Proceedings 21,
    Page 163, 1962.

11. Petering, H. G., Buskirk, H. H. and Underwood, G. E., Cancer
    Research 24, Page 367, 1964.

12. Mihich, E. and Nichol, C. A., Cancer Research 25, Page 1410, 1965.

13. Petering, H. G., Buskirk, H. H. and Crim, J. A., Cancer
    Research 27, Page 1115, 1967.

14. Van Giessen, G. J., Crim, J. A., Petering, D. H. and
    Petering, H. G., J. National Cancer Institute 51, Page 139,
    1973.

15. Petering, D. H., Bioinorganic Chemistry 1, Page 273, 1972.

16. Antholine, W., Knight, J. M. and Petering, D. H., Inorganic
    Chemistry, in press.

17. Petering, D. H., Biochem. Pharmacology 23, Page 567, 1974.

18. Lieberman, L. M., Young, D., Petering, D. H. and Minkel, D.,
    Society Nuclear Medicine, presented at 23rd meeting, June,
    1976.

19. Booth, B. A., Donnelly, T. E., Jr., Zettner, A. and Sartorelli,
    A. C., Biochem. Pharmacology 20, Page 3109, 1971.

20. Petering, D. H. and Petering, H. G., "Metal Chelates of 3-
    Ethoxy-2-oxobutyraldehyde Bis(thiosemicarbazone), $H_2HTS$,"
    A. C. Sartorelli and D. G. Johns, Editors, Antineoplastic and
    Immunosuppressive Agents II, Springer-Verlag, New York,
    Page 841, 1975.

21. Minkel, D. T., Chan-Stier, C. and Petering, D. H., Mol.
    Pharmacology, in press.

22. Saryan, L. A. and Petering, D. H., unpublished information.

23. Petering, D. H., Bioinorganic Chemistry 1, Page 273, 1972.

24. Minkel, D. T. and Petering, D. H., submitted for publication.

25. Booth, B. A. and Sartorelli, A. C., Mol. Pharmacology 3,
    Page 290, 1967.

26.  Minkel, D. T., Saryan, L. A. and Petering, D. H., submitted
     for publication.

27.  Winkelmann, D. A., Bermke, Y. and Petering, D. H., Bioinorganic
     Chemistry 3, Page 261, 1974.

28.  Antholine, W. E., Knight, J. M., Whelan, H. and Petering,
     D. H., Mol. Pharmacology, in press.

29.  Minkel, D. T. and Petering, D. H., unpublished information.

30.  Saryan, L. A., Mailer, K., Antholine, W. and Petering, D. H.,
     to be published.

31.  Pietsch, P., "Phleomycin and Bleomycin," in Antineoplastic
     and Immunosuppressive Agents II, A. C. Sartorelli and D. G.
     Johns, Editors, Springer-Verlag, New York, Page 859, 1975.

32.  Solaimon, D., Antholine, W., Saryan, L. A. and Petering, D. H.,
     presented at the 17th Annual Meeting of the American Society
     of Pharmacognosy, Cable, Wisconsin, July, 1976.

33.  Chan-Stier, C., Minkel, D. T. and Petering, D. H., Bioinorganic
     Chemistry 6, Page 203, 1976.

34.  Solaimon, D., Saryan, L. A. and Petering, D. H., unpublished
     information.

*CHAPTER 14*


THE INHIBITORY EFFECT OF COPPER ON ETHIONINE CARCINOGENESIS*

Zbynek Brada and Norman H. Altman

Papanicolaou Cancer Research Institute at Miami
and Department of Pathology
University of Miami, Miami, Florida   33123

## I.   INTRODUCTION

The application of metabolic inhibitors in biological systems plays a vital role in biomedical research.  By the use of different inhibitors, we may gain new insight into the mechanisms of carcinogenesis.

## II.   COPPER AS AN INHIBITOR OF HEPATOCARCINOGENESIS IN RATS

There are many reports concerning the protective effect of copper salts on hepatic toxicity and tumorigenesis produced by a variety of chemical substances (Table 1).   Sharples[4] first observed that increased amounts of copper in the diet of rats fed 4-dimethylaminoazobenzene resulted in an extended induction time of hepatic tumors.  These results were confirmed by many authors.[5,6,7,8]

In a system where the carcinogenic substance produced tumors in the liver and at the other sites, the simultaneous administration of cupric acetate prevented only the formation of liver tumors, while the incidence of extrahepatic tumors remained unchanged.[9]

---

*   This study was supported by USPHS Grant CA-11071 from the
    National Cancer Institute, NIH.  A part of this work was published previously.[1,2,3]

TABLE 1

EFFECT OF COPPER ON LIVER DAMAGE AND CARCINOGENESIS

| Toxic substance | Effect of copper | Author |
|---|---|---|
| 4-Dimethylaminoazobenzene | Increased induction time for liver tumor formation | G.R. Sharples (4) |
| 3'-Methyl-4-dimethylamino-azobenzene | Inhibition of tumor formation | E. Pedrero and F.L. Kozelka (5) |
| Thioacetamide | Minimal damage of liver restricted to some portal areas | G. Fare (10) |
| Fluorenylacetamide | Cholangiofibrosis, cholangio-carcinoma and hepatoma were all absent | G. Fare (11) |
| Dimethylnitrosamine | Protected from ductular cell proliferation and cholangio-fibrosis; tumorigenesis not studied | G. Fare (11) |
| α-Naphthylisothiocyanate | Copper delayed but did not pre-vent ductular cell prolifera-tion | G. Fare (11) |
| Ethionine | Decreased ductular cell prolifera-tion and cholangiofibrosis; tumorigenesis not studied | G. Fare (11) |
| Ethionine | Inhibition of tumor formation | Kamamoto et al. (12) |

In all cases the copper was administered in salt form in the diet together with the
particular toxic substance.

Reports on the mechanism of the protective effect of copper on
hepatic carcinogenesis are rather conflicting. A comparative study
revealed that the anionic part of the molecule of copper salts is
not essential for the protective action. King et al.(8) suggested
that the protective effect could be attributed to the destruction
of azo dye in the diet catalyzed by copper, resulting in a decreased
amount of ingested azo dye. They observed a lower hepatic level of
total and bound azo dye during five weeks of the carcinogenic regimen in rats fed a diet with a high content of copper salts. Contrary to this suggestion, Fare(10,11) demonstrated that the investigated hepatotoxins were not inactivated by copper salts *in vitro*

during diet storage. Howell(7) attempted to investigate whether a
chemical alteration of dimethylaminazobenzene occurs under the influence of CuAc in the gastrointestinal tract during digestion.
He administered CuAc and the carcinogen alternately. Unfortunately,
the experiments were inconclusive. As is evident from Table 1, the
copper salts are effective in decreasing the toxicity of hepatotoxins of unrelated chemical structure. The majority of them,
except for ethionine, require activation by a nonspecific microsomal system.

Y. Yamane and K. Sakai(13) studied the role of the cation in
metal salts in 3'-methyl-4-dimethyl-aminoazobenzene carcinogenesis
and they determined that copper can be replaced by manganese or
nickel. Zinc was found to have no such protective effect. The
effect of these metal salts in inhibiting the carcinogenesis of azo
dye was observed to go parallel with their capacity to decrease the
concentration of protein-bound dye and to enhance the hepatic activity of azo dye reductase in liver.

### III.  THE METABOLISM OF ETHIONINE IN RATS

Dyer(15) carried out the first *in vivo* investigation with
ethionine, a methionine antimetabolite. In these experiments,
ethionine, a synthetic ethyl homolog of methionine, could not substitute for methionine in supporting the growth of rats. This important discovery was followed by many other studies of its pathological and biochemical effects (see reviews *16*,*17*). These studies
culminated when Popper and coworkers reported that feeding rats a
diet containing DL-ethionine induced tumor-like nodules in the
liver.(*18*) These findings were confirmed by Farber,(*19*) who also
demonstrated that ethionine in rats induced hepatocellular carcinoma. The similarities in chemical structure and metabolism between
ethionine and methionine provide some unique experimental oppor-
tunities not available with other hepatic carcinogens.

Metabolism of DL-ethionine proceeds in rats in four basic pathways (see Figure 1):

a.  the inversion of D-ethionine into L-ethionine via α-keto-
    γ-ethiolbutyric acid;(*20*,*21*)

b.  the oxidation of both ethionine isomers to ethionine sulf-
    oxides and the subsequent acetylation to N-acetylethionine
    sulfoxide (this pathway represents about 50% of metabolized
    ethionine after a single ethionine injection); (*20*,*22*)

c.  the activation of ethionine to S-adenosylethionine with
    the help of the enzyme ATP-S-adenosyl transferase (this
    pathway represents about 30% of the metabolized ethionine
    after a single ethionine injection);(*17*)

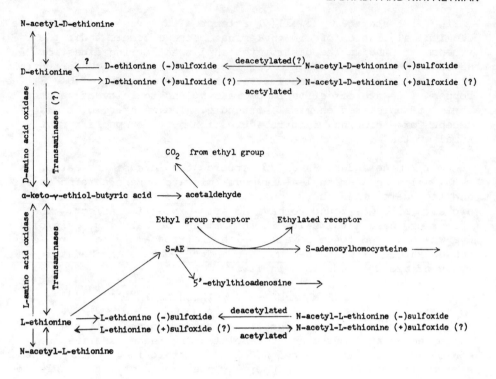

Figure 1

Metabolic Pathway of DL-ethionine in Rat *In Vivo*

d.    the oxidative pathway of the ethyl group of ethionine via α-
      keto-γ-ethiolbutyric acid

     The currently accepted view in chemical carcinogenesis is that
a carcinogenic chemical must react irreversibly with cellular macromolecules to initiate the transformation of somatic cells.  All
macromolecules that are present in target cells can be considered
as possible and biologically plausible candidates for interaction
with different carcinogens.  Evidently, the most attractive and
most studied candidates are proteins, RNA's and DNA.  At this time,
it is difficult to make any judgment concerning the relative importance of any of these interactions.  The modification of DNA is the
simplest possible mechanism, specifically because such an explanation provides a direct analogy to mutagenesis.  On the other hand,
the genetic mechanism may include the modification of RNA, which
could be subsequently transcribed into DNA.  Also open for discussion

is an interaction with proteins involved in the fidelity of copying the DNA.

From the analogy of the function of S-AE, which is a donor of the methyl group in biological systems, it is likely that the S-AE may also donate its ethyl group. The hypothesis that the ethyl donor S-AE plays a decisive role in the ethionine carcinogenesis is based on logical molecular-biological speculations, but it is supported only by circumstantial evidence.

## IV. THE INHIBITORY EFFECT OF CUPRIC ACETATE ON THE INDUCTION OF HEPATOCELLULAR CARCINOMA BY DL-ETHIONINE

As shown in Table 1, the addition of CuAc to a diet containing ethionine inhibits the induction of hepatocellular carcinoma. In our experiments, we have found hepatocellular carcinoma in 100% of the rats sacrificed after nine months of ethionine treatment. The addition of the same amount of CuAc completely abolished the carcinogenic effect of ethionine (Figure 6).

A. Chemical Interaction Between Ethionine and Cupric Acetate

Ethionine and CuAc form an insoluble complex. The molar ratio of copper to ethionine in this complex was determined by the titration of ethionine solution with CuAc. The end point of the interaction was determined by the measurement of the remaining soluble ethionine in the reaction mixture and was found at the ratio 1:2. The nonprecipitable portion of ethionine in the solution was small and was probably caused by the presence of small amounts of ethionine sulfoxide and ethionine sulfone in the available commercial preparations of $C^{14}$-ethionine. Both those compounds do not form insoluble complexes.(2)

B. The Effect of Cupric Acetate on Ethionine Metabolism in Acute Experiments

The absorption of free ethionine from the gastrointestinal tract is rapid and is completed within two hours after administration. When a suspension of an insoluble complex (L-ethionine-CuAc 1:1) was administered by gavage, the absorption process took considerably more time and was finished within 16 hours after administration (Figure 2). The absorption of free ethionine from the gastrointestinal tract proceeded very uniformly; in the mixture with CuAc, the absorption rate was variable.

When larger amounts of the ethionine-CuAc mixture were administered in bigger rats, a part of the complex remained in an undissolved state in the small intestine and in the caecum and the ethionine radioactivity was not extractible by water, but by tri-

chloroacetic acid solution. The liquid portions obtained from the
lumen of rats treated with free ethionine and, with the CuAc complex,
were analyzed chromatographically. The chromatographic pattern of
the ethionine label changed characteristically as a function of
time after ethionine administration. More extensive changes were
observed, when the rats were kept on an exclusive carbohydrate diet
for a few days before the experiments. Such a diet apparently increased the bacterial flora in the small intestine. The chromatographic changes were probably caused by the formation of new metabolites that appeared partially as new peaks and partially increased
the background label across the chromatogram. These effects were
almost totally absent in the presence of CuAc. The alteration in
the absorption rate of ethionine from the gastrointestinal tract
was accompanied by expected corresponding differences in the concen-

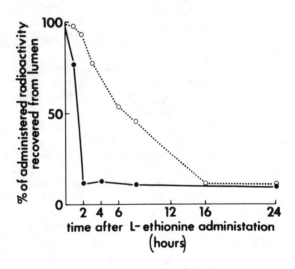

Figure 2

The effect of CuAc on the absorption of L-ethionine from gastrointestinal tract after p.o. administration. L-ethyl-1-$^{14}$C-ethionine
(12.5 mg/100 g body weight) or a mixture of L-ethyl-1-$^{14}$C-ethionine
and CuAc (12.5 mg ethionine + 12.5 mg CuAc) in solution were administered by stomach tube to rats that were made to fast for 16 hours.
The volumes of ethionine solutions were kept at 2.0 ml/100 g body
weight. The rats were sacrificed at the indicated time, the gastrointestinal tract was removed and rinsed out with cold 0.9% NaCl
solution. The washings were combined, acidified by diluted HCl
and an aliquot was used for determination of radioactivity after
the solids were dissolved in Hyamin. L-ethionine (●), L-
ethionine + CuAc (O)

tration of total ethionine metabolites and of S-AE in liver as a
function of time after p.o. administration of ethionine or ethionine
+ CuAc. The highest S-AE concentration in liver was observed five
hours after the administration of free ethionine and 24 hours after
administration of the ethionine-CuAc mixture. The radioactivity of
the total substances soluble in trichloroacetic acid showed the
same pattern as did S-AE.

These results were corroborated by the measurement of the
excretion pattern of ethionine metabolites into urine. Fifty percent of the p.o. administered radioactivity of labeled free ethionine was excreted into urine within 48 hours. This was not dependent on the weight of the rats. When ethionine was administered in
the form of its mixture with CuAc, small rats excreted significantly
less metabolites within the first 24 hours; however, this deficit
was compensated for in the second 24 hour-period (Figure 3). In
rats weighing over 200 g, the total amount excreted within 48 hours
was significantly decreased. The amount of the labeled ethionine
in both cases was 12.5 mg ethionine per 100 g body weight.

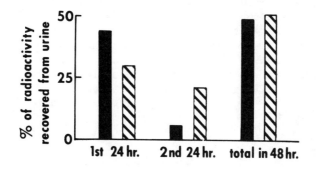

Figure 3

The excretion of L-ethyl-1-$^{14}$C-ethionine metabolites into urine
after p.o. administration of ethionine and its copper complex.
See Figure 2 for the description of the ethionine administration.
The rats were kept in metabolic cages for 48 hours. Water and
food were given *ad libitum*. Dark columns: L-ethionine; dashed
columns: L-ethionine + CuAc.

The quantitative analysis of excreted ethionine metabolites in
urine after p.o. administration of ethionine and of the mixture of
ethionine with CuAc revealed significant differences. As a result
of the simultaneous administration of labeled ethionine and cupric
acetate, the excretion of ethionine sulfoxide was increased at the
expense of its acetylated form. The change in the ratio of ethio-

nine sulfoxide : N-acetylethionine sulfoxide is a function of the
route of administration, since this ratio was not significantly
altered when ethionine was administered one hour after pretreatment of rats with an i.p. injection of the highest tolerated amount
of CuAc.  This result suggests that the decrease in the acetylated
form of ethionine sulfoxide is not a direct effect of cupric ions
on the transacetylation as could be expected, based on the observation that copper can inhibit the acetylation *in vitro.*(23)

C.   The Effect of Cupric Acetate on Ethionine Metabolism in
     Chronic Experiments

A complete pathological examination was performed on rats in
chronic experiments where ethionine, CuAc, or ethionine + CuAc were
fed for 28 and 55 days.  Characteristic changes as previously described were observed in the ethionine-fed groups.  The rats fed
ethionine and CuAc had mild changes consisting mainly of neutro-
philic infiltration and scattered hepatocellular necrosis.  The
livers of rats fed only CuAc were essentially normal.

A striking increase in the hepatic concentration of S-AE in
rats ingesting ethionine + CuAc was observed (Table 2).  The difference between S-AE concentrations in rats fed only ethionine and
those fed ethionine + CuAc can be attributed to the timing of the
sacrifice of the rats.  Furthermore, CuAc changes the time pattern
of ethionine absorption from the intestinal lumen and can modify
the concentration curve of S-AE plotted against time.  The data
collected during the entire 24-hour cycle demonstrated (Figure 4)
that whatever causes the increase in the concentration, the in-
crement was observed at any time of the cycle.  This is the first
recorded observation of the inhibition of ethionine carcinogenesis
accompanied by a distinct rise of the S-AE level in liver.  The
cause can be in an increased synthesis of this compound or in a
considerably decreased catabolism.  The results are in good agreement with recent findings of Yamane et al.(14) who observed that
the activity of the enzyme synthetizing S-AE increased in rats fed
a diet containing different amounts of copper before the experiment.

In order to determine the changes in ethionine metabolism in
chronic experiments, two groups of female rats were investigated.
One group was fed 0.25% ethionine; the second group was fed 0.25%
ethionine + 0.25% CuAc.  At different periods of ethionine treatment, the cold ethionine was removed, and radioactive L-ethionine
was administered p.o. in a single dose (12.5 mg/100 g body weight).
The urine collected within 48 hours was analyzed for the presence
of radioactive ethionine metabolites.  In the first group, a short
time exposure to DL-ethionine increased the excretion of free ethionine and of S-AE at the expense of total ethionine sulfoxide.  With
the extended feeding period, the excretion of total ethionine sulfoxide became normalized while free ethionine and S-AE decreased.

Table 2

THE EFFECT OF CuAc ON THE CONCENTRATION OF S-AE
IN THE LIVER OF ETHIONINE-FED RATS

| Treatment[a] | Duration of experiment (days) | S-adenosyl ethionine $\mu$ moles/g dry fat-free substances |
|---|---|---|
| 0.3% ethionine | 28 | 1.23±0.23[b] |
| 0.3% ethionine + 0.3% CuAc | 28 | 3.46±0.51[c] |
| 0.3% ethionine | 56 | 2.20±0.58 |
| 0.3% ethionine + 0.3% CuAc | 56 | 4.20±0.27[c] |

[a]   The rats were sacrificed after a 16-hr period of fasting

[b]   Mean ± S.D.

[c]   Statistically significant

During the entire period of observation, the acetylated fraction of ethionine sulfoxide was slightly reduced. The fraction of free ethionine sulfoxide increased gradually and was five to seven times higher than in normal rats. In the second group, the excretion of total ethionine sulfoxide was decreased and that of S-AE was increased during the entire feeding period. The excretion of acetylated ethionine sulfoxide was decreasing up to 150 days of feeding and was accompanied by an increase in free ethionine sulfoxide, which represented more than 50% of the excreted radioactivity (Figure 5). These results enable us to suggest an explanation of the mechanism for the increased concentration of S-AE in liver due to the addition of CuAc to the diet. In chronic experiments, where ethionine alone was administered in the diet, the ingested ethionine was quickly oxidized to ethionine sulfoxide, with the exception of a short period after the beginning of the experiment. Then ethionine sulfoxide was acetylated to N-acetylethionine sulfoxide and excreted. The constant concentration of S-AE in liver was maintained during the 24-hour cycle, primarily with the aid of the reduction of the available ethionine sulfoxide to ethionine. After the addition of CuAc, the increased concentration of S-AE in liver may be, at least partly, a result of the diminished capacity of rats

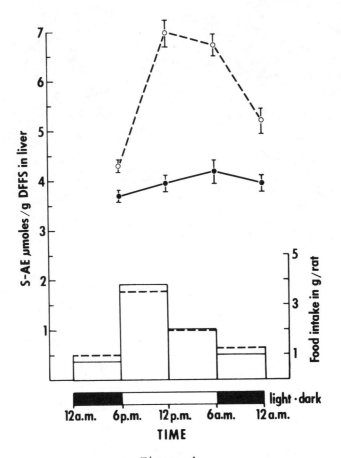

Figure 4

The effect of CuAc on the rhythm of hepatic S-adenosylethionine
concentration in rats fed DL-ethionine.  Two groups of rats were
fed for 28 days a diet containing 0.3% DL-ethionine (o) or 0.3%
DL-ethionine + 0.3% CuAc (●) ad libitum.  Four rats from each
group were sacrificed at the given time, and S-AE was determined
in the liver.  On the first day of the experiment, the food intake
was measured every six hours.


to acetylate ethionine sulfoxide.  As a consequence of this diminished acetylation, the concentration of ethionine sulfoxide and
free ethionine in liver is higher and the amount of free ethionine
in liver is rather a function of ethionine intake, than of the reduction of ethionine sulfoxide to ethionine.  The ultimate result
of the alteration of the regulation of the free ethionine level in
liver is the observed diurnal variation in the concentration of S-AE
in rats treated by CuAc (Figure 4).

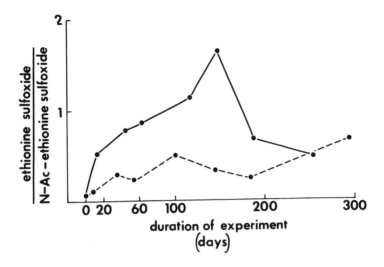

Figure 5

The effect of CuAc on the ratio between ethionine sulfoxide and
N-acetylethionine sulfoxide excreted into urine as a function of
the duration of ethionine feeding.  One group of rats was fed a
diet containing 0.25% DL-ethionine (---) and a second group, a
diet containing 0.25% DL-ethionine + 0.25% CuAc (___).  Before
the experiment, the diet containing ethionine was replaced for
48 hours by the basal diet without ethionine.  At 5 p.m. on the
day before the experiment, the diet was removed, and rats were
kept starving over night.  The next day at 9 a.m., L-ethyl-1-$^{14}$C-
ethionine was administered p.o. (12.5 mg/100 g body weight; spec.
activity, 5 μCi/12.5 mg).  The rats were then placed in metabolic
cages and the urine was collected within a period of 48 hours.
An aliquot of the urine was analyzed by chromatography on an
AG 50 W column.(20)


We have not studied in our laboratory the ethylation of cellular macromolecules in the presence of CuAc and the only available
recently published data are from Yamane et al. (14)  They observed
a decrease in the ethylation of t-RNA in rats chronically treated
with ethionine and CuAc.  These authors used minimal amounts of
labeled ethionine after 24 hours of food deprivation.  As we have
demonstrated, the level of ethionine metabolites in rats treated
with CuAc reached a maximum 24 hours after administration of ethionine.  The observed decrease in the ethylation (30%) may be a result of the dilution of radioactive ethionine by the cold ethionine
and, therefore, this problem needs further clarification.

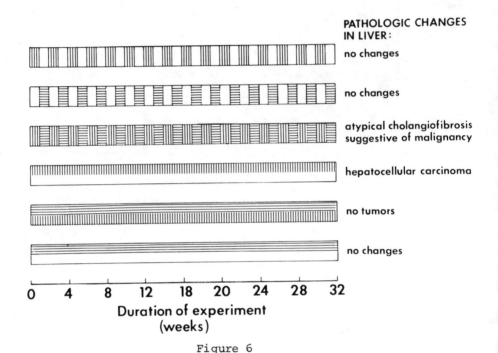

Figure 6

The Design of the Feeding Experiments

Legend for Figure 6:  The rats were fed ad libitum, the following diets:

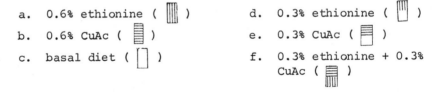

a.  0.6% ethionine (    )          d.  0.3% ethionine (    )

b.  0.6% CuAc (    )               e.  0.3% CuAc (    )

c.  basal diet (    )              f.  0.3% ethionine + 0.3%
                                       CuAc (    )

D.   The Effect of the Alternate Weekly Feeding of DL-ethionine, CuAc, and the Basal Diet on the Development of Pathologic Changes in Liver

An important basic question is whether the protective effect can be demonstrated when CuAc is not administered together with ethionine. Therefore, the following experiment was undertaken:

> In the first group, rats were alternately one week on a diet containing a double amount of DL-ethionine (0.6%) and one week on a basal diet. The second group was alternately fed a diet with a double amount of CuAc (Figure 6). Using these regimens, the total administered amounts of DL-ethionine or of CuAc remained the same as in the original experiment using the simultaneous feeding of both agents. After eight months of feeding, all rats were sacrificed and the livers were examined histologically. Pathologic changes were not found in the first and second groups. In the livers of the third group, extensive cholangio-fibrosis was observed with some areas suggestive of cholangiocarcinoma.

*ABBREVIATIONS*

S-AE:   S-adenosylethionine

CuAc:   cupric acetate [$Cu(C_2H_3O_2) \cdot H_2O$]

*REFERENCES*

1.   Brada, Z, Altman, N. H. and Bulba, S., Proceedings American Society Cancer Research 15, Page 145, 1974.

2.   Brada, Z, Altman, N. H. and Bulba, S., Cancer Research 35, Page 3172, 1975.

3.   Brada, Z and Bulba, S., Federal Proceedings 35, Page 557, 1976.

4.   Sharples, G. R., Federal Proceedings 5, Page 239, 1946.

5.   Pedrero, E. and Kozelka, F. L., A.M.A. Arch. Pathology 52, Page 455, 1951.

6.   Clayton, C. C., King, H. J. and Spain, J. D., Federal Proc. 12, Page 190, 1953.

7.   Howell, J. S., British J. Cancer 12, Page 594, 1958.

8.  King, H. J., Spain, J. D. and Clayton, C. C., J. Nutrition 63, Page 301, 1957.

9.  Fare, G. and Howell, J. S., Cancer Research 24, 1279, 1964.

10. Fare, G., American J. Pathology 46, Page 111, 1965.

11. Fare, G., British J. Cancer 30, Page 569, 1966.

12. Kamamoto, Y., Makiura, S., Sugihara, S., Hiasa, Y., Arai, M. and Ito, N., Cancer Research 33, Page 1129, 1973.

13. Yamane, Y. and Sakai, K., Gann 64, Page 563, 1973.

14. Yamane, Y., Sakai, K. and Kojima, S., Gann 67, Page 295, 1976.

15. Dyer, H. M., J. Biol. Chem. 124, Page 519, 1938.

16. Farber, E., Advanced Cancer Research 7, Page 380, 1963.

17. Stekol, J. A., Advanced Enzymol. 25, Page 369, 1963.

18. Popper, H., de la Huerga, J. and Yesinick, C., Science 118, Page 80, 1953.

19. Farber, E., Arch. Pathology 62, Page 445, 1956.

20. Brada, Z., Bulba, S. and Cohen, J., Cancer Research 35, Page 2674, 1975.

21. Brada, Z. and Bulba, S., Proceedings American Association Cancer Research 17, Page 60, 1976.

22. Smith, R. C. and Beeman, E. A., Biochem. Biophys. Acta 208, Page 267, 1970.

23. Weber, W. W., Metabolic Conjugation and Metabolic Hydrolysis, W. H. Fishman, Editor, Academic Press, New York, P.249, 1973.

# Part III

# Nutrition and Trace Elements in Cancer

## CHAPTER 15

DIET, NUTRITION, AND CANCER

Harold G. Petering

Department of Environmental Health
University of Cincinnati Medical Center
Kettering Laboratory, Cincinnati, Ohio

## I. INTRODUCTION

The roles we are beginning to assign to nutrition and diet as facotrs in the causation of cancer are only one aspect of the realization that these are of major importance to human health in many ways other than just in growth and development. Nutritional science is coming to have a special application in surgery, in the treatment and prevention of cardiovascular diseases, and it is even being recognized as important in studies of pharmacology and toxicology.

We have touched on the subject of Nutrition and Cancer in a number of ways earlier in this conference, but today we expect to treat this subject more intensively, albeit still in a manner too brief for its importance. We need, therefore, at the outset, to define a few terms and recognize something of the scope of the subject with which we are dealing.

Nutritional science deals with the study of the 50 or more essential elements or nutrients that go to furnish the body with the building blocks necessary for the sustenance of life and health in an optimal fashion. It deals with the quality and chemical characteristics of these materials as well as with the quantitative aspects of their intakes. It also deals with the balance with which these nutrients are optimally utilized, and furthermore, is concerned with how these building blocks are metabolized and how they function in the body. So we have a concern for amounts of nutrients and calories, as well as with the kinds of amino acids, vitamins, and minerals required.

We obtain our nutrients in the food and water (or drink) that constitutes our diet, but we get more than the basic nutrients in natural foods. For example, we get non-nutritive colors, flavors, and fiber, and some of these have been shown to be beneficial and some may be harmful to health. In addition, food now contains additives and residues from materials used in harvesting or processing the foodstuff. When we realize that 80% or more of cancer in man is caused by environmental factors, and most of these are chemical, we have reason to suspect that some active carcinogens may actually occur in foods and feed.(1)

The history of the study of the relationship of nutrition to cancer is much older than many realize, even though it is not ancient. It goes back in this country to Tannenbaum's classic studies beginning in 1940,(2,3,4) and includes the work of Kensler et al., Mider et al., and many others.(5,6) In 1966 in a review of the work that had been performed up to that time, Petering(1) indicated that we needed to become more concerned with the presence of potent carcinogens in foods and feeds, which had then just begun to be recognized as being in feeds as a result of the work of Lancaster et al.(7) on aflatoxins.

Since we cannot go into detail of all of the many interesting facets of our subject, this discussion will be limited to indicate some of the basic concepts that need to be considered, and to some specific illustrations of these.

Our diet, from which we gain our nutritional elements, as we all know, furnishes proteins, carbohydrates, and fats as the bulk energy components, each of these also supplying important building blocks of amino acids, carbohydrates, and fatty acids for organ and cell structures, for enzymes and the like. In addition, we must take in essential vitamins and minerals, and all of these as we are learning, should be in definite quantities and in a more or less definite balance for optimal utilization and for the healthful function of the organism.

In addition to recognizing some basic considerations about the scope of nutritional science, we also need to be aware of some of the complexities of the cancer problem in order to find meaningful applications of nutrition to cancer. Carcinogenesis (or tumorigenesis as it is also known) is a multifaceted process, and we need constantly to realize that something which affects the initiation phase may not affect the promotion phase, or vice versa, and that clinical expression of cancer is greatly dependent on host factors where nutrition may play an important role. Cancer incidence or morbidity undoubtedly depends upon genetic determinants, life styles, or cultural patterns, and on health status, as well as exposure to specific carcinogens. Cancer mortality depends on many unspecified and undefined factors involving detection, therapy, and related factors in which nutrition may play an important role. The steps involved in cancer formation are illustrated in Figure 1, which is adapted from a report by Vitale.(8)

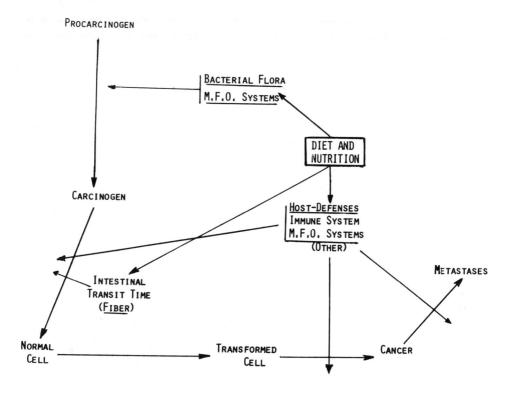

Figure 1

Schematic diagram showing the multistep process involved
in chemical carcinogenesis.  Arrows indicate the steps
that can be affected by diet and nutrition directly or
indirectly through influencing metabolic processes.
(Diagram is a modification of one presented by Vitale(8).)

As John Cairns pointed out recently in Nature(9), 90% of cancers in man are epithelial carcinomas that are closely related to
environmental causes of cancer, and involve sites related to the
portal of entry of or exposure to environmental agents.  He also
emphasized that in the human situation we are probably dealing with
weaker carcinogens or at lower levels of exposure than is often the
case in experimental situations.

In an issue of Cancer Research devoted entirely to the subject
of Nutrition and the Causation of Cancer, Hegsted(10) discussed
"The Relevance of Animal Studies to Human Diseases".  In his summary
he pointed out (a) that diet is an environmental factor in all bio-

logical studies and results based on tests without concern for diet
may be extremely erroneous and frightening to contemplate; (b) that
there are both unity and a diversity in metabolic patterns of animals
and that both can be explored to understand cancer processes; and
(c) commercial diets vary in exact composition of ingredients from
day to day as a result of the cost of raw materials; so at the very
least may deliver varying amounts of non-nutritive agents, some of
which may affect the cancer process.

About 37 years ago, Albert Tannenbaum(2) began publishing a
provocative series of articles in which he explored the effect of
restricting caloric intake or underfeeding on the incidence of tumors
and longevity of inbred mice genetically susceptible to cancer.  His
work showed that cancer incidence was reduced, the appearance of
cancer delayed, and longevity increased by caloric restriction or
by underfeeding.  Tannenbaum and Silverstone(3), furthermore showed
that their animal data were similar to actuarial information in the
United States, which indicated that cancer death rate can be directly related to obesity, and that underweight in man alone predisposes to lower cancer mortality.  A summary of some of their work
showing the effect of caloric restriction on spontaneous tumor incidence taken from a recent review by Clayson(11) is found in Figure 2.

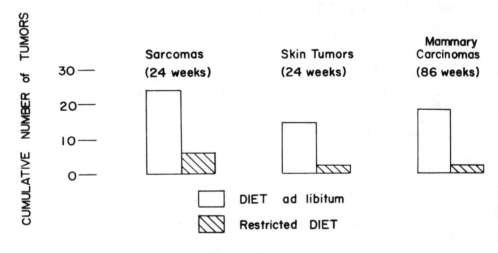

Figure 2

Data of A. Tannenbaum as presented by Clayson(11) in which
the effects of caloric restriction on incidence of carcinogen-induced (B(a)P) sarcomas and skin tumors and of spontaneous mammary carcinoma in DBA mice are depicted.

Related to this early work on spontaneous tumor incidence are the results showing that caloric restriction also influences the appearance of carcinogen-induced tumors, as shown in Figure 3, also based on Clayson's review.(11)

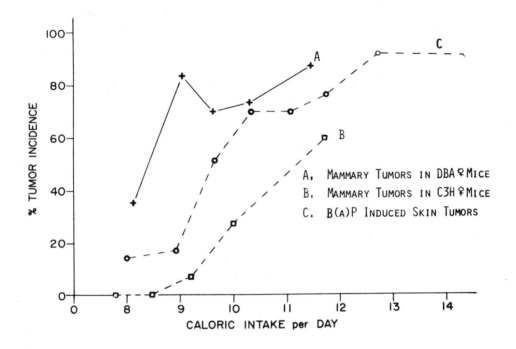

Figure 3

Data of A. Tannenbaum as presented by Clayson(11), in which the effects of caloric restriction on the incidence of spontaneous mammary tumors in two strains of mice and on the efficacy of B(a)P are depicted.

In this presentation, I would like to draw your attention to several areas not specifically and obviously addressed by other members of this conference.

## II.  CARCINOGENS IN FOODS AND FEEDS

As mentioned above(1), it has been shown that a variety of carcinogenic chemicals are present in foods and feeds, some occurring naturally and some occurring as contaminants due to processing or due to fungal growth during storage.  Wogan(12) has recently reviewed this subject, citing in addition to a variety of mycotoxins

also the presence of safrol, thiourea, and tannic acid in some
foodstuffs, which need further evaluation as carcinogens.  Sinnhuber, et al.(13) have also reported that sterculic and malvalic
acids present in cottonseed meal and cottonseed oil can potentiate
the carcinogenicity of aflatoxin B₁.  Compounds with cyclopropenylene
groups occur in many plants.  Shubik(14) has written an excellent
review of the problem of possible carcinogenicity of food additives
and contaminants, some of which are shown in Figure 4.  We also
know that diethylstilbestrol and other estrogens are carcinogenic
and that their use in animal husbandry could lead to their ingestion if proper precautions to reduce their carcass residues are not
followed before marketing occurs.  The presence of synthetic food
colors with carcinogenic potentialities is a constant concern to
many food scientists.

1. MYCOTOXINS

   AFLATOXINS

   LUTEOSKYRIN

2. CYCASIN (METHYLAZOXYMETHANOL)

3. NITROSAMINES

4. TANNINS

5. CONTAMINANTS AND RESIDUES - (ESTROGEN, PESTICIDES, METALS)

6. CO-CARCINOGENS

STERCULIC ACID $(CH_3 \cdot KH_2)_7 \cdot C = C -(CH_2)_7 \cdot COOH$ with $\overset{CH_2}{\diagup\diagdown}$

MALVALIC ACID $(CH_3 \cdot (CH_2)_7 \cdot C = C -(CH_2)_6 \cdot COOH$ with $\overset{CH_2}{\diagup\diagdown}$

7. POLYCYCLIC AROMATIC HYDROCARBONS

Figure 4

List of Carcinogens Found in Foods and Feeds

The presence of nitrosamines that are potent experimental carcinogens in foods or feeds and their formation in the intestinal
tract is a subject of great concern; this may depend on the presence, or formation of nitrite ion, which, in turn, is related to
the type of bacterial flora in the gut, and the nature of the dietary intake as well as the nutritional quality of the food.

## III.   NON-NUTRITIVE ELEMENTS IN FOOD

Diet is the vehicle by which we obtain our nutrients and we need to realize that foods contain non-nutritive elements that can and do affect our use of the nutrients as well as our metabolism. The list of natural materials and additives in foods is a long one; therefore, we must limit our consideration to several of these that seem to have very important roles in the disposition of cancerogenic agents.  The ones we shall discuss are fiber, and agents in food that can alter microsomal mixed functional oxidase activities.

A.   Fiber

Dietary fiber and the effects of intestinal bacterial flora on orally ingested carcinogens or procarcinogens has come to be an important area for prophylaxis and treatment of colon cancer.  Shils[15] has indicated that colon cancer in the United States and England is second only to lung cancer in males and breast cancer in females in respect to mortality, accounting for 12% to 14% of all deaths due to malignancy.  Therefore, the influence of dietary constituents on this form of cancer is of great importance.

In several very incisive and searching articles on the relation of diet to cancer, Ackerman[16] and Burkitt[17,18] have indicated that fiber in the diet probably is an important factor in preventing colon cancer because of its effect in decreasing transit time and in altering bacterial flora of the gut.  Increased fiber increases excretion of sterols and bile acids, and this reduces enterohepatic recycling of these compounds, and also decreases the concentrations of these for possible conversion to polycyclic aromatic hydrocarbon carcinogens by gut flora.[19]  Renwick and Drasor[20] offer another hypothesis, suggesting that retoxification of PAH metabolite conjugates by hydrolysis due to gut bacteria is an important process and that bile acids may act as cocarcinogens in the action of the free carcinogens.

The net result of increased fiber is the establishment of more rapid transit time of gut contents and lower concentration of carcinogen and cocarcinogen in a given area of the intestinal tract. The importance of the prophylactic action of dietary fiber becomes more obvious when viewed in the light of John Cairns' reminder that 90% of cancer in man is the result of low-grade processes in which constant removal or elimination of carcinogens or cocarcinogens is imperative.[9]

B.    Inducers of Microsomal Mixed-Function Oxidase (MFO) Activities

Other non-nutritive factors present in foods are the natural
and added chemicals that can induce the activity of microsomal
mixed-function oxidases in liver, lung, intestines and perhaps other
tissue.

In his review in Cancer Research(21), Wattenberg points out
that there are two types of dietary constituents that affect the
metabolism of chemical carcinogens by MFO systems; i.e., (a) naturally occurring inducers present in stock diets, derived particularly
from plants such as substituted indoles from cruciferous vegetables,
and flavonol compounds found in citrus fruits; and (b) phenolic antioxidants such as butylhydroxyanisole (BHA) now widely found in processed foods; and (c) pesticide contaminants, PCBs, and even carcinogens like B(a)P itself.

These inducers of MFO systems, which tend to metabolize some
carcinogens to inactive compounds but also may activate some procarcinogens, are found to act on enzymes in the intestinal tract,
the liver and the lungs; so we must ultimately understand this system in man, and use it to protect him from fortuitous exposure to
chemical carcinogens.

In his earlier review(22), Wattenberg also pointed out the way
in which other dietary factors affect the MFO system. In rats, the
activity is completely lost by 72 hours of starvation and is at a
very low level when purified diets are used. It can be stimulated
in rats on purified diets if inducer chemicals are given. These
inducers may be in bedding of rat cages or may be delivered by in-
sect sprays. We therefore must be concerned about these factors in
designing experiments.

The action of the dietary inducers is not well understood. In
rats, flavone inducers altered MFO in liver, small bowel, and lung
but in mice it did not affect the liver enzyme system. The inducers
have been found to have direct effect, as shown by the action of
flavone on skin carcinogenesis.

Mixed-function oxidases not only affect polycyclic aromatic
hydrocarbon carcinogens, but can also activate aromatic amines by
N-hydroxylation or inactivate these compounds by ring hydroxylation.
The balance between these two reactions is important, but the factors that influence the rates of these reactions are not well understood. It is still questionable as to whether the net result ever
is enhanced carcinogenesis.

Zannoni and Sato(23), in reviewing the effects of vitamin deficiencies on hepatic MFO, show that nutritional deficiencies of

ascorbic acid, riboflavin and α-tocopherol cause significant decreases in this system without an effect on apparent Km's with
Type I or Type II substrates.  There seems to be no alteration of
the effect of inducers such as phenobarbital in any case.

Campbell and Hayes(24) participating in the same symposium,
pointed out that severe protein deficiency causes a reduction in
MFO activity and in cytochrome P-450 content of hepatic cells, and
Wade and Norred(25) showed that increasing the level of corn oil
in the diet of rats led to increased MFO activities and to enhanced
response to inducing agents.  Finally, Becking(26) found that the
literature contains evidence suggesting that iron deficiency increases hepatic drug metabolism, while magnesium and potassium deficiency reduce hepatic MFO.

The literature then shows that nutritional elements as well as
non-nutritional constituents of the diet can markedly alter MFO of
liver or other tissues, which in turn, have important roles in the
disposition of ingested carcinogens.  When microsomal mixed-function
oxidases destroy carcinogens, the action is beneficial, but when
they lead to potent carcinogens by activating procarcinogens, the
activity is deterimental.  Their dietary induction or reduction of
MFO activity depends on the carcinogen or procarcinogen involved.

## IV.  ANTI-CARCINOGENESIS

A concept, the time for which seems to have arrived, is that
of anti-carcinogenesis, especially by nutritional elements.  This
concept was forcefully presented by H. Falk in 1969(27) who in turn
pointed out that it was then about 20 years old, having first been
proposed in 1947 by Crabtree.(28)  In a sense, we have been indirectly considering aspects of the subject in previous sections, but
in this one, particular emphasis on direct activity of specific
agents will be made.

In his discussion, Falk indicated the value from the experimental point of view and ultimately in control of human disease, of
putting much more effort on anti-carcinogenesis studies.  He showed
how the bioassay of a suspected carcinogen, using 100 animals, which
yields no tumors, still must assess the risk as about 4.5% at the
99% confidence level.  If 1,000 animals are used, and a 99% confidence level is assumed, the probable risk would still be 0.46% if
no tumors were found.  This extrapolated to 200,000,000 people (US
population) would mean that about 900,000 people might be at risk.
Thus, it is impossible to carry out studies with a large enough
animal population to really assess risk adequately.

The answer to this dilemma, he argues, is to be about the bus-
iness of finding anti-carcinogenic substances that can be given to

man.  His experimental design is to use a carcinogen at a dose that
would yield 25% to 50% tumors in reasonable time periods and then
determine the effects of agents that would reduce this incidence
figure to near the zero level.  Such a system would yield statistically significant results with animal populations of reasonable
numbers.  We might add that all animals in such experiments should
be under conditions of defined environmental protection; i.e., diet,
exposure to MFO-inducing agents, etc.

Viewed in this way, we see that the dietary or nutritional
effects on cancer incidence that we have been discussing, i.e.,
caloric restriction, fiber in the diet, or dietary substances and
nutrients that enhance the microsomal mixed-function oxidase systems, all may be considered anti-carcinogenic processes or agents.
OUr adaptation of the basic diagram of Vitale(8) as shown in Figure 1 illustrates the possible effects and points of action of
these dietary factors.

A.    Fatty Acids

Schramm(29), in 1962, reported that oral ingestion of ethyl
linolenate completely blocked the formation of liver tumors in rats
by 3'-methyl DAB, and that the carcinogenic activity of 4-dimethyl-
aminostilbene was greatly reduced.  Hepatic tumors and liver cirrhosis due to AAF were also reduced by ethyl linolenate, but carcinogenesis due to polycyclic hydrocarbons or urethane was not
affected.  Whether this effect was a specific one due to linolenic
acid, or more generally due to unsaturation was not clear.  In view
of the findings mentioned earlier that corn oil, an unsaturated fat
increased microsomal drug metabolizing activity, it would appear
that this observation of Schramm, which seems to have been forgotten,
may be understood as an expression of anti-carcinogenesis due to
enhancement of the host detoxification mechanism by a nutritional
element.

B.    Water-Soluble Vitamins

As noted above, riboflavin and ascorbic acid seem to enhance
MFO activity of the liver.  In 1941, Kensler et al.(5) found that
riboflavin had a definite anti-carcinogenic effect with respect to
azo dyes.  Miller(30) later showed that 3'-methyl DAB feeding to
rats reduced liver $B_2$ content.  All of this finally fell into place
when Fouts  et al. (31) found that the azo reductase of liver, which
splits azo dyes as well as azo chemicals such as prontosil, is a
flavoprotein.  The effects of dietary constituents on azo-dye carcinogenesis also involve the effects of copper and other B-complex
members.  It appears that the way to potentiate azo-dye carcinogenesis is to have a diet low in B-complex vitamins and in copper.

Again, we find that ascorbic acid not only affects MFO activity but has a definite inhibitory action *in vitro* and *in vivo* on the nitrosation of secondary amines, so that the formation of nitrosamine carcinogens is reduced or eliminated.(32,33,34) In addition, Edgar(35) found that carcinogens such as carbon tetrachloride and some alkylating agents including nitrosamines will deplete body stores of ascorbic acid.

## C.   Fat-Soluble Vitamins

Vitamin E or α-tocopherol deficinecy was found by Arrhenius(36) to cause a decrease of N-demethylase activity that would be expected to reduce the detoxification of certain carcinogenic aromatic amines and possibly increase ring-oxygenation such as occurs in the carcinogenic transformation of 2-aminofluorene. In an earlier paper, Haltuin and Arrhenius(37) had shown that vitamin E suppresses the carcinogenic effectiveness of 2-aminofluorene.

Vitamin E also has been indicated as a potent antioxidant or inhibitor of membrane lipid peroxidation.(38) Peroxidation of membrane lipids may lead to formation of peroxides and oxidant-free radicals that have been indicated as being carcinogenic. As was noted above, other antioxidants used in foods such as BHA have the property of inducing MFO, just as vitamin E does. Regardless of the mechanism of action, however, L. Haber and R. W. Wissler, in 1962,(39) reported that large excesses of dietary α-tocopherol given to C57 leaden female mice reduced the yield of sarcomas due to sc injection of 3-MC. In a second experiment in C57 black male mice, the same results were obtained.

One of the most exciting aspects of the role of vitamins in protecting against carcinogenesis is that of the action of vitamin A and some of its analogs. In this case, definitive early experiments had shown that vitamin A deficiency in animals led to epithelial changes, which may be considered precancerous; and Harris et al.(40) showed that topically applied vitamin A prevented the carcinogenic effect of concomitant application of DMBA to the cervix and vagina of animals. In 1965, Chu and Malmgren(41) showed that large dietary supplements of vitamin A to Syrian hamsters protected against cancer induction in the forestomach and small intestine by orally administered PAH, DMBA, and B(a)P. Following these reports, Salffiotti et al.(42) showed that cancer of the lungs in Syrian golden hamsters caused by intratracheal administration of B(a)P and hematite was almost completely eliminated when vitamin A palmitate in large doses was given beginning one week after B(a)P treatment was completed.

These observations have led to many studies to define the precise limitations and effectiveness of vitamin A as a preventive measure or prophylactic of carcinogenesis. I. Sanitzki and S. Goodman(*43*) found that retinol, retinoic acid, α-retinoic acid and a cyclopentyl analog of retinoic acid (R18-7699) were all active in preventing MC-induced hyperplasia, metaplasia, and parakeratosis in organ cultures of mouse prostatic tissue. The analogs of retinoic acid have no vitamin A activity. This indicated that the anti-carcinogenic activity was not dependent on vitamin A activity.

Bollag(*44*) describes a new aromatic analog of retinoic acid with as much or more anti-carcinogenic activity as the parent substance, retinol. This was confirmed by Sporn et al.(*45*) and extended to include three other analogs with definite activity, none of which had vitamin A activity. The structures of compounds having nti-carcinogenic activity are shown in Figure 5.

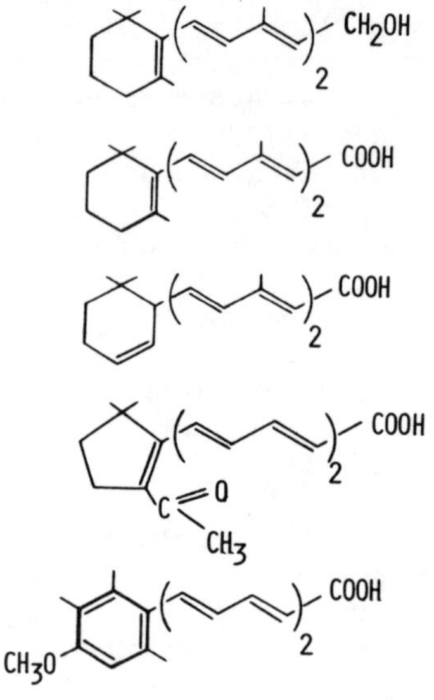


RETINOL - VITAMIN A

β-RETINOIC ACID

α-RETINOIC ACID

DIMETYLACETYLCYCLOPENTYL ANALOG

TRIMETHY-METHOXYPHENYL ANALOG

Figure 5

Structures of Retinol and Analogs Having Anti-carcinogenic Activity

The importance of the anti-carcinogenic action of retinol, β-retinoic acid, and analogs cannot be overemphasized because it indicates a new, direct approach to cancer control which, as we have seen, has other less dramatic facets. It also opens avenues for understanding carcinogenic processes and finding ways of controlling them. The question now rises as to what the mechanism of action is, and immediately, a very complex situation appears to be involved, which may be related to zinc and copper metabolism as well as with possible endocrine functions.

In 1969, Moore(46) pointed out the striking inverse relationship between serum levels of vitamin A and copper.  On the other
hand, we now know that there are similar inverse relationships between serum copper and zinc.  Furthermore, recent reports show a
very close relationship between vitamin A metabolism and zinc nutrition.  It is obvious that zinc and vitamin A metabolism may be
interrelated in many ways, but basically at the nutritional level.
It has been known for some time that zinc-deficient swine are low
in vitamin A;(47) and Saraswat and Arora(48) showed in lambs deficient in zinc and vitamin A that zinc supplementations were
necessary for effective vitamin A therapy.

Recently, Smith et al.(49) found that plasma levels of both
vitamin A and retinol-binding protein are low in zinc-deficient
rats, despite the fact that liver stores of vitamin A are adequate;
thus, zinc appears to be a trace metal necessary for vitamin A
metabolism.

D.   Trace Metals

Both essential and nonessential or toxic metals have been implicated as having a role in cancer.  M. K. Schwartz(50) who has
recently reviewed much of the literature on this subject, has indicated that there are many conflicting reports.  In examining these
reports, it becomes evident that many of them suffer seriously from
poor design in respect to nutritional control; and others fail to
distinguish between effects on initiation or promotion of the carcinogenic process or a separation of effects on growth of transplanted or spontaneous tumor and prevention of carcinogenesis.  A
good case in point is the effect of zinc.  In 1967, Petering et al.
(51) reported that restricting dietary zinc greatly inhibited the
growth of Walker 256 carcinosarcoma in rats and that increases in
tumor growth were related to the dietary level of zinc.  Furthermore, it was shown that the tumor growth response was sharper than
that of the carcass growth.  These findings have been confirmed by
DeWys et al.(52)   and McQuity et al.(53)   In other work, McGlashan
(54) and Stocks et al.(55) have implicated dietary intake of zinc
with the incidence of esophogeal and stomach cancer in man.  On the
other hand, Poswillo and Cohen(56) have shown that excess dietary
zinc suppresses DMBA carcinogenesis in the cheek pouch of the Syrian
golden hamster.  Following this work, Duncan et al.(57) and Duncan
and Dreosti(58) showed that azo-dye carcinogenesis in rats was reduced when dietary zinc was very low (0.4 ppm) or very high
($\leq$ 500 ppm), the toxic level being reported to be 2500 ppm.

These experimental reports are all compatible and not contradictory if one recognizes the differences in experimental design
that were used, and realizes that excessive dietary intake of zinc
(less than toxic level) upsets the balance of other trace elements.
This may have an effect mechanistically quite distinct from that

due to dietary zinc deficiency; although a very recent report by
Duncan and Dreosti(59) shows that both dietary zinc deficiency and
excess also result in reduction of DNA synthesis in grafted tumor
tissue.

As has been previously mentioned, copper has anti-carcinogenic
activity with respect to the action of azo dyes; and Yamane and
Sakai(60) found that manganese salts would also reduce azo dye
hepatic carcinogenesis, whereas zinc had no effect.  They suggested
that the activity of copper, manganese, nickel, and zinc in this regard paralleled their capacity to reduce hepatic protein-bound dye.
Kamamoto et al. (61) have also found that extra dietary copper reduces the carcinogenesis of ethionine.

There are many other aspects of trace element nutrition in relation to cancer, some of which have been touched upon in this conference already.  The role of selenium is of importance, but will
not be included here, since Schrauzer(62) has reviewed this subject.
It seems evident that the role of essential trace metals will be of
increasing interest in both cancer prevention and cancer therapy.

E.    Immunocompetence, Nutrition, and Cancer

As may have become evident by this time, the relationships of
nutrition to cancer seem to be an expanding web of interactions,
not all directly connected to the carcinogenic process.  We come
now to a most important and also a rather indirect way in which
nutrition and diet may affect cancer incidence and the treatment
of cancer; namely, the effect of nutrition on the immunity of an
organism or on the competence of an organism's immunologic mechanisms to deal with newly formed cancer cells.  This is of great importance, since immune processes seem to be involved in disposing
of transformed cells that may become cancerous, in disposing of
cancer cells, and obviously, in resisting concurrent infections
that are always a problem for a patient with cancer.

In 1961, Burnet(63) suggested that one of the important functions of the immune system was to eliminate mutant somatic cells
that otherwise would go on to form neoplasms.  In an excellent review of this subject, Berenblum(64) pointed out that evidence then
available showed that chemical carcinogenesis was facilitated by
using immunologically immature animals or by using thymectomized
animals.  Furthermore, he also pointed out that some carcinogens
themselves seemed to suppress immune responses.  In addition, he
suggested that some forms of cancer therapy actually could be harmful because of their immunosuppressive action.  This point has now
been recognized widely, and efforts are being made to find and use
therapeutic regimens that do not suppress immune response.

With these facts in mind, I believe it is worthwhile to dwell briefly on the subtle ways that nutrition and diet can affect immune responses and thus be a factor in the formation of cancerous cells, in their elimination, and in the treatment of malignancy. Some of these nutritional factors are suggested in Figure 6.

```
┌─────────────────────────────────────────────────────────┐
│                                                         │
│    RESTRICTION OF CALORIES                              │
│                                                         │
│    VITAMINS - PYRIDOXINE, PANTOTHENIC ACID,             │
│                                                         │
│              FOLIC ACID, RIBOFLAVIN, RETINOL,           │
│              ASCORBIC ACID                              │
│                                                         │
│    PROTEIN                    METALS - Zn, Fe           │
│                                                         │
└─────────────────────────────────────────────────────────┘
```

Figure 6

Nutrients that are Necessary for Immune Responses

Axelrod, in an excellent review, brings this subject of nutrition and immunity up to date as of about 1972.(65)  In this review, he shows that deficiencies of some B vitamins and essential amino acids lead to grossly impaired immune response.  The B vitamins most important in this regard are pyridoxine, pantothenic acid, folic acid, and possibly riboflavin.  In addition, data were discussed by Axelrod that indicated that deficiencies of vitamin A, vitamin C, and biotin might also impair secondary immune processes involving IgG antibodies.  Inanition did not affect antibody formation.

The early work of Scrimshaw and associates has also shown that nutrition plays an important role in the prevention of infectious diseases.(66)  In addition,  Law et al.(67) found that cell-mediated immunity in which T lymphocytes participate and which is vital to defense against foreign cells (transplants or cancer cells) is markedly depressed in severe adult human malnutrition.

Following this work, R. K. Chandra(68) also showed that thymus-dependent T-cell lymphocyte populations were decreased in malnourished children.  These depressions could be reversed by nutritional repletion.  The depression of immunocompetence by severe caloric and protein deficits could lead to increased susceptibility to the action of carcinogens.  This is in contrast to the reports that were discussed earlier that caloric restriction is beneficial in reducing tumor incidence or carcinogenic responses.  These, however, are not contradictory, but they rather show the subtlety of effects of diet

on immune responses and cancer.  This is evident in the recent report by Fernandes et al.(*69*) that moderate caloric and protein
restriction causes a potentiation of cell-mediated immunity and
permits the maintenance of a vigorous population of functional T
cells in mice susceptible to spontaneous tumors.  Thus, the beneficial effects of nutritional manipulation, so widely confirmed,
now seem to have a solid basis in probable mechanism of action.

This concept is further supported by the report of Mertin and
Hunt(*70*) that allograft survival as well as development of 3-MC-
induced tumors was decreased in mice fed a diet deficient in polyunsaturated fatty acids.  These findings must be ultimately related
to those mentioned earlier in which ethyl linolenate was found to
reduce the carcinogenic effect of 3'-methyl DAB(*29*) and the finding
that corn oil increased the resting levels of MFO enzymes.(*25*)

When we turn to the effects of minerals on immunocompetence, we
find that most work has been done on the relationships between iron
nutrition and metabolism.  Weinberg(*71*) has for many years written
about the needs of pathogenic microbes for readily available iron,
both in the intestinal tract and in the body as a whole.  Thus, he
has emphasized that reduction of available iron in plasma or the
gut by any means, i.e., nutritional deficit or presence of chelating
substances such as unsaturated transferrin and siderophones of all
kinds would be most unfavorable to microbial growth and infection.
Balanced against this viewpoint is that of Chandra(*72*) who argues
that we must consider the fact that immunity is lowered in iron deficiency, a fact that must be taken into account in evaluating the
effect of iron deficit on reduction of microbial growth.  This point
is particularly important in respect to virus infection and cancer.
He then cites many studies showing that microbial infections are
increased in patients with iron-deficiency states and that the situation is remedied by iron repletion.  There is evidence that a deficit of myeloperoxidase-containing cells occurs in iron-deficient
animals, who are also more susceptible to many infective agents.
There was a difference in the effect of parenteral ionic iron and
chelate iron, the latter being more efficacious.  Ionic iron increased infectivity and chelated iron gave protection.

In another study, Joynson et al.(*73*) found that delayed hypersensitivity and lymphocyte transformation in response to PPD were
impaired in adult anemia groups.  These defects were not found after
iron therapy and therefore could be interpreted to mean that cell-
mediated immunity, so important in preventing cancer cell establishment, was impaired.  The role of iron in this process is still controversial, but there seems to be good evidence that free or available iron is important in microbial growth, whereas, it also may be
important in developing immunocompetence.

It would seem that zinc would have an important role in immunity in general and specifically with respect to cancer, since it is a vital element in DNA and RNA synthesis and metabolism, and it is essential for protein synthesis in general. It is well known that in infections as well as some malignancies, serum iron and zinc are reduced, while serum copper is elevated during the active stages of the disease, but that this situation is reversed during the remission phases.

There is one other aspect of immunocompetence that should be mentioned because it not only relates to the subject of diet and cancer, but probably involves aspects of bioinorganic chemistry. The area to which I refer is the finding by a number of investigators(74,75,76) that both cadmium and lead, given in the diet of experimental animals severely reduce immune responses of animals to bacterial challenge or endotoxin administration, both leading to disease and death. The dietary or nutritional aspect of this situation is found in the facts(a) that most of our exposure to cadmium and lead is by oral ingestion; and (b) that the absorption of these toxic metals as well as their toxicity is greatly decreased if diets are high in calcium, iron, copper, zinc, selenium, and protein. It may well be that we need to consider the contradictory reports on the tumorigenic effects of cadmium and lead in the light of their immunosuppressive action.

## V.   SUMMARY

A review of the vast literature that exists with respect to the relationship of nutrition (or diet) to cancer leads one to conclude that a wealth of basic information has been available for useful clinical application, and has only recently been rediscovered for use in clinical studies. The main use of the basic information has been in the design of vitamin antagonists as cancer chemotherapeutic agents.

The recent activity in seeking to find ways of preventing carcinogenic responses with vitamin A and analogs represents a new and useful approach to a major part of the cancer problem. It would seem that anti-carcinogenesis research should be a major thrust of any crusade against cancer, and the role of nutrition and dietary manipulation in this aspect seems to be assured.

Our study has shown that specific nutrients or dietary constituents may have important effects of cancer incidence and development by virtue of their enhancement of or essentially for immune response to foreign cells, and because they enhance microsomal mixed function oxidase enzymes that can detoxify procarcinogens, carcinogens, and cocarcinogens.

Even though dietary Zn, Cu, Se, and Mn can be important factors in the role of nutrition as a preventive factor in cancer, this area has been given the least attention of any of the classes of nutrients. For this reason alone, much more research effort in bioinorganic chemical research in relation to cancer causes and prevention is urgently needed.

## TABLE OF ABBREVIATIONS

| | |
|---|---|
| PAH | polycyclic aromatic hydrocarbons |
| MFO | mixed-function oxidase |
| BHA | butylated hydroxyanisole or butylhydroxyanisole |
| PCB | polychlorinated biphenyl |
| B(a)P or BP | benzo(a)pyrene |
| Km | Michaelis constant |
| $P_{450}$ | cytochrome P450 of microsomes |
| DAB | 4-dimethylaminoazobenzene |
| AAF | 2-acetylaminofluorene |
| Vitamin $B_2$ $(B_2)$ | riboflavin |
| 3 MC or MC | 3-methylcholanthrene |
| DMBA | 7,12-dimethylbenz(a)anthrocene |
| Vitamin C | ascorbic acid |
| PPD | purified protein derivative (antigen from M. tuberculosis) |

This work was supported in part by USPHS Grant ES-00159 to the Center of the Study of the Human Environment, University of Cincinnati.

## REFERENCES

1.   Petering, H. G., Nutr. Review 24, Page 321, 1966.

2.   Tannenbaum, A., American J. Cancer 38, Page 335, 1940.

3.   Tannenbaum, A. and Silverstone, H., Advanced Cancer Research 1, Page 451, 1953.

4.  Tannenbaum, A. and Silverstone, H., Cancer, Vol. 1, R. W. Raven, Editor, Page 306, Butterworth and Co., Ltd, London, 1957.

5.  Kensler, C. J., Suguira, K., Young, N. F., Halter, C. R. and Rhoads, C. P., Science 93, Page 308, 1941.

6.  Mider, G. B., Tesluk, J. and Morton, J. J., Acta Univ. Intern. Contra. Cancrum 6, Page 409, 1948.

7.  Lancaster, M. C., Jenkins, F. P. and Philip, J. McL., Nature 192, Page 1095, 1961.

8.  Vitale, J. J., Cancer Research 35, Page 3320, 1975.

9.  Cairns, J., Nature 255, Page 197, 1975.

10. Hegsted, D. M., Ibid Ref. 8, Page 3537.

11. Clayson, D. B., Ibid Ref. 8, Page 3292.

12. Wogan, G. N., Prog. Expt. Tumor Res. 11, Page 134, 1969.

13. Sinnhuber, R. O., Wales, J. H. and Lee, D. J., Fed. Proc. 25, Page 555, 1966.

14. Shubik, Ibid Ref. 8, Page 3475.

15. Shils, M. E., Modern Nutrition in Health and Disease, M. E. Shils, Editor, Lea & Febiger, Philadelphia, Chapter 37, Page 493, 1973.

16. Ackerman, L. V., Nutrition Today, 2, 1972.

17. Burkitt, D. P., Nutrition Today 6, 1976.

18. Burkitt, D. P., Cancer 28, Page 3, 1971.

19. Hill, M. J., Cancer 34, No. 3 (Supplement), Page 815, 1974.

20. Renwick, A. G. and Drassar, B. S., Nature 263, Page 234, 1976.

21. Wattenberg, L. W., Ibid Ref. 8, Page 3326.

22. Wattenberg, L. W., Prog. Exp. Tumor Research 14, Page 89, 1969.

23. Zannoni, V. G. and Sato, P. H., Fed. Proceedings 35, Page 2464, 1976.

24. Campbell, T. C. and Hayes, J. R., Fed. Proceedings 35, Page 2470, 1976.

25.  Wade, A. E. and Norred, W. P., Ibid Ref. 23, Page 2475.

26.  Becking, G. C., Ibid Ref. 23, Page 2480.

27.  Falk, H. L., Prog. Exp. Tumor Research 14, Page 105, 1971.

28.  Crabtree, H. G., British Medical Bulletin 4, Page 345, 1947.

29.  Schramm, T., Wiss., Z., der Humboldt-University z Berlin,
     Math.-Natur. 11, Page 184, 1962.

30.  Miller, J. A., Annals New York Academy Science 49, Page 19,
     1947.

31.  Fouts, J. R., Kamm, J. J. and Brodie, B. B., J. Pharmacol.
     Exp. Therapy 120, Page 291, 1957.

32.  Miruish, S. S., Wallcave, L., Eagen, M. and Shubik, P.,
     Science 177, Page 65, 1972.

33.  Fan, T. Y. and Tannenbaum, S. R., J. Food Science 38, Page
     1067, 1973.

34.  Greenblatt, M., J. National Cancer Institute 50, Page 1055,
     1973.

35.  Edgar, J. A., Nature 248, Page 137, 1974.

36.  Arrhenius, E., Cancer Research 28, Page 264, 1968.

37.  Hultin, T. and Arrhenius, E., Cancer Research 25, Page 124,
     1965.

38.  Bieri, J. G., Nutrition Review 33, Page 161, 1975.

39.  Haber, L. and Wissler, R. W., Proceedings Soc. Exp. Biol.
     Med. 111, Page 774, 1962.

40.  Harris, L. J., Irmes, J. R. M. and Griffith, A. S., Lancet
     2, p. 614, 1932.

41.  Chu, E. W. and Malmgren, R. A., Cancer Research 25, Page
     884, 1965.

42.  Saffiotti, U., Montesano, R., Sellakumur, A. R. and Borg,
     S. A., Cancer 20, Page 857, 1967.

43.  Sanitzki, I. and Goodman, S., Cancer Research 34, Page 1564,
     1974.

44.  Bollag, W., Experientia 30/10, Page 1198, 1974.

45.  Sporn, M. B., Clamon, G. H., Dunlop, N. M., Newton, D. L.,
     Smith, J. M. and Saffiotti, U., Nature 253, Page 47, 1975.

46.  Moore, T., J. Clinical Nutrition 22, Page 1017, 1969.

47.  Stevenson, J. W. and Earle, I. P., J. Animal Science 15,
     Page 1036, 1956.

48.  Saraswat, R. C. and Arora, S. P., Indian J. Animal Science 42,
     Page 358, 1972.

49.  Smith, J. C., Brown, E. D., McDaniel, E. G. and Chan, W.,
     J. Nutrition 106, Page 569, 1976.

50.  Schwartz, M. K., Ibid Ref. 8, Page 3481.

51.  Petering, H. G., Buskirk, H. H. and Crim, J. A., Cancer Res.
     27(I), Page 1115, 1967.

52.  De Wys, W. D., Pories, W. J., Richter, M. C. and Strain, W. H.,
     Proceedings Soc. Exp. Biol. Medicine 135, Page 17, 1970.

53.  McQuity, J. T., De Wys, W. D., Monaco, L., Strain, W. H.,
     Rob, O. G., Apgar, J. and Pories, W. J., Cancer Research 30,
     Page 1381, 1970.

54.  McGlashan, N. D., Lancet 1, Page 578, 1972.

55.  Stocks, P. and Davies, R. I., British J. Cancer 18, Page 14,
     1964.

56.  Poswillo, D. E. and Cohen, B., Nature 231, Page 447, 1971.

57.  Duncan, J. R., Dreosti, I. E. and Albrecht, C. F., J. National
     Cancer Institute 53, Page 277, 1974.

58.  Duncan, J. R. and Dreosti, I. E., J. National Cancer Institute
     55, Page 195, 1975.

59.  Duncan, J. R. and Dreosti, I. E., S. African Medical Journal
     50, Page 711, 1976.

60.  Yamane, Y. and Sakai, K., Gann 64, Page 563, 1973.

61.  Kamamoto, Y., Makiura, S., Sugihara, S., Hiasa, Y., Arai, M.
     and Ito, N., Cancer Research 33, Page 1129, 1973.

62.  Schrauzer, G. N., Bioinorganic Chemistry $\underline{5}$, Page 275, 1976.

63.  Burnet, F. M., Science $\underline{133}$, Page 327, 1961.

64.  Berenblum, M. C., British Medical Bulletin $\underline{20}$, Page 159, 1964.

65.  Axelrod, A. E., Modern Nutrition in Health and Disease, Chapter $\underline{15}$, R. S. Goodhart and M. E. Shils, Editors, Lea & Febiger, Philadelphia, Page 493, 1973.

66.  Scrimshaw, N. S., Taylor, C. E. and Gordon, J. E., WHO Chronicle $\underline{23}$, Page 369, 1969.

67.  Law, D. K., Dudrick, S. J. and Abdou, N. F., Annals Internal Medicine $\underline{79}$, Page 545, 1973.

68.  Chandra, R. K., British Medical Journal $\underline{3}$, Page 608, 1974.

69.  Fernandes, G., Yunis, E. J. and Good, R. A., Nature $\underline{263}$, Page 504, 1976.

70.  Mertin, J. and Hunt, R., Proceedings National Academy Science $\underline{73}$, Page 928, 1976.

71.  Weinberg, E. D., J. American Medical Association $\underline{231}$, Page 39, 1975.

72.  Chandra, R. K., Nutrition Review $\underline{34}$, Page 129, 1976.

73.  Joynson, D. H. M., Walker, D. M., Jacobs, A. and Dolby, A. E., Lancet $\underline{2}$, Page 1058, 1972.

74.  Hemphill, F. E., Kaeberle, M. L. and Buck, W. B., Science $\underline{172}$, Page 1031, 1971.

75.  Cook, J. A., Marconi, E. A. and Diluzio, N. R., Tox. and Appl. Pharmacology $\underline{28}$, Page 292, 1974.

76.  Cook, J. A., Hoffman, E. O. and Diluzio, N. R., Proceedings Soc. Exp. Biol. Medicine $\underline{150}$, Page 741, 1975.

CHAPTER 16

THE EFFECTS OF IRON DEFICIENCY AND THE QUALITY AND QUANTITY OF FAT

ON CHEMICALLY INDUCED CANCER[1]

Joseph J. Vitale,* Selwyn A. Broitman,** Eva Vavrousek-Jakuba,*

Pamela W. Rodday,* and Leonard S. Gottlieb*


*Department of Pathology and **Department of Microbiology,
Boston University School of Medicine, Nutrition-Pathology Unit,
Mallory Institute of Pathology, Boston City Hospital,
Boston, Massachusetts  02118

## I.  INTRODUCTION

Iron deficiency has been shown to affect a number of systems including the immune system, the gastrointestinal system, the erythron, and the utilization of at least one essential nutrient and perhaps others.  A number of studies have indicated that in iron-deficient animals and humans there is decreased killing by polymorpholeucocytes[1,2], but phagocytosis may not be altered. Additionally, in iron-deficient humans, it is shown to depress the response of T cells to mitogens.[3]

Gastric atrophy in rats[4,5] as well as gastric atrophy and intestinalization of the stomach in humans[6] has been reported to occur in chronic iron deficiency with anemia.

The metabolism of folic acid has also been shown to be affected in iron deficiency.  Several of the features of folic acid deficiency such as increased formiminoglutamic acid excretion in the urine, the appearance of hypersegmented polymorphonuclear leucocytes in peripheral blood smears and megaloblastic changes in the bone marrow have been reported in iron deficiency and corrected by the administration of iron.[7,8,9,10]

[1]  Supported in part by Grants CA16750 from the National Cancer
     Institute, and 508 from the Nutrition Foundation, Inc., New York.

More recently, iron deficiency with anemia has been shown to abrogate what has been referred to as delayed erythropoiesis.(11) When marrow stem cells are infused into lethally irradiated histocompatible mice, they repopulate the hemopoietic tissues after seeding into reticular organs. As the proliferation of the infused marrow cells proceeds, discrete hemopoietic colonies appear on the surface of the host spleen. In the mouse, these colonies appear between seven and nine days after marrow grafting, and both erythropoiesis and granulopoiesis occur.(12,13) Hematopoiesis should be quantitated either by gross colony counting or by measuring the incorporation of the splenic DMH precursor, 5-iodo-2'-deoxyuridine I (IUdR) in the recipient spleens. Using this latter technique, we have found that erythropoiesis in spleens of lethally irradiated rats grafted with syngeneic marrow cells is inhibited or delayed during the five-day test period.(11,14) This is in marked contrast to observations in the mouse.(15,16)

We have found that we can enhance graft proliferation or abrogate what we have termed delayed erythropoiesis in the rat by prior induction of iron-deficiency anemia.(11)

Each of these effects of iron deficiency have been shown to be associated with either metastases or with premalignant lesions. For example, defects in immune incompetency has been suggested as playing a role, either in the pathogenesis of neoplasia, or in metastases.(17) Furthermore, spontaneous remissions of tumors have been associated with the return of the immune competency.(17)

Gastric atrophy and certainly, intestinalization of the gastric mucosa can be considered premalignant lesions.

The defects in folate and perhaps vitamin $B_{12}$ metabolism as a result of iron deficiency in or by themselves may not be considered premalignant, but it has been demonstrated that deficiencies of these essential nutrients, and particularly folic acid are associated with enhanced experimental chemical carcinogenesis.(18,19)

Finally, the effect of iron deficiency in abrogating delayed erythropoiesis in syngeneic recipients may be mediated through some host defense system. Teleologically, delayed erythropoiesis may be one manifestation of a complex host defense system. Incoming syngeneic bone marrow stem cells may appear to be aberrant cells to the host, and iron deficiency may abrogate this "guardian system", allowing these cells to proliferate.

Thus, in several instances, iron deficiency is associated with changes that can be linked to neoplasia, and it was of interest to us to determine how animals deficient in iron might respond to a known chemical carcinogen, dimethylhydrazine (DMH). The use of

this chemical carcinogen was the result of studies being performed
in our laboratory on the effects of the quality and quantity of fat
in animals given this chemical carcinogen.

## II.   METHODS

Twenty-one-day-old Lewis male rats were divided into four
groups of 12 and fed one of two diets, *ad libitum* (below).   The
animals were weighed once a week, provided deionized water, and
housed individually in stainless steel cages.   Whole milk was used
as the diet to produce iron deficiency.   The control diet was one
in which iron (as Fe $SO_4 \cdot 7H_2O$) was added to the whole milk diet
to provide 50 mg of iron per kilogram of diet.   Copper (as copper
sulfate) was also added (5 mg/kg diet) to both diets.   DMH was given
subcutaneously (10 mg/kg body weight) twice weekly, starting at
four weeks of age.

Six animals from each group were sacrificed at the end of 17
weeks, and complete autopsies were performed.   The animals were
anesthetized with ether and bled from the abdominal aorta.   The
liver, the entire gastrointestinal tract (small and large), kidney,
lungs, ear canals were examined.   The hematocrit was 8 to 20%, and
37% to 47% for iron deficient and control rats, respectively, regardless of DMH administration.

## III.   RESULTS AND DISCUSSION

At autopsy, all of the sacrificed iron-deficient, DMH-treated
rats showed identical changes.   Externally, all animals showed evidence of nutritional deficiency including poor grooming of fur,
some hair loss, and edematous eyes.   Internally, the abdominal vis-
cera showed decreased pigmentation of musculature and enlarged, pale
livers.   The fat deposits were pale and partially translucent.   Both
stomach and colon were distended and showed decreased muscular tone
and decreased rugae formation.   The hearts were not atrophic, but
the wall was thin and showed no muscular contraction.   The hearts
were increased in size.   On gross examination, the livers were pale
and enlarged, and showed from one to four nodules per liver.   The
nodules ranged from 1 to 2 mm in diameter. were white, appeared
discrete and rounded, and were slightly bulging on cut surface.

Microscopy of the livers showed a spectrum of changes.   The
general lobular architecture was intact.   There was a slight increase in fat content, primarily of a reticular and finely vacuo-
lated nature.   There was a diffuse, but mild nuclear pleomorphism
with an occasional hepatocyte being frankly dysplastic.   Occasional
hepatocytes showed degenerative features with isolated eosinophilic
hyalin bodies (dead hepatocytes).   Other hepatocytes showed a granular, eosinophilic, perinuclear material.   Scattered portal tracts

and lobules showed an increase of bile ducts, suggesting hyperplasia.
Although inflammation was not a prominent feature, occasional foci
of round cells and isolated intrasinusoidal polymorphonuclear leucocytes were present.

The grossly described nodules consisted of discrete foci of
pleomorphic hepatocytes with apparent compression of surrounding
liver tissue.  There was some increase of reticular fat, with hyper-
chromatic dysplastic nuclei.  Although sinusoids were present, the
cords were markedly distorted by increased cell thickness, pseudo-
papillary formation and apparent autonomous growth from the surrounding liver.  Several intracytoplasmic inclusions including round
globular structures and granular, congealed material were present.
The exact nature of these lesions is not clear from the preliminary
evidence, but certainly lies between foci of atypical hyperplasia
and hepatoma.  The biological behavior of the lesions can be asses-
sed only through longer follow-up studies.  The ability of cells
isolated from these hepatic lesions to grow as a tumor in syngeneic
rats remains to be determined.

Control rats and control rats given DMH showed no gross or
microscopic changes and appeared healthy.  Iron-deficient animals
not given DMH were also anemic and their livers were moderately
fatty on gross examination.  *They were, however, devoid of any
neoplastic lesions.*

Of perhaps important interest is the observation that all iron-
deficient DMH-treated rats developed what appeared to be neoplastic
changes within four months and only in the liver.  This is in contrast to other observations in which the median induction time of
malignant tumors following similar DMH administration procedure was
180 days, with tumors developing in the other organs as well.(20)

1, 2-Dimethylhydrazine (DMH) has been utilized in a number of
studies for the induction of colonic carcinoma in rats.  According
to J. H. Weisburger,(21) the procarcinogen is converted to a reactive intermediate in the following manner:

$$CH_3-NH-NH-CH_3 \qquad\qquad \text{1,2-dimethylhydrazine}$$
$$\downarrow \qquad\qquad\qquad \text{(absorbed from the GI tract)}$$

$$CH_3-N{=}N-CH_3 \qquad\qquad \text{azomethane}$$
$$\downarrow$$

$$CH_3-N{=}N-CH_3 \qquad\qquad \text{azoxymethane}$$
$$\text{liver} \qquad\qquad \overset{\downarrow}{O}\downarrow$$

$$CH_3-N{=}N-CH_2OH \qquad\qquad \text{methylazoxymethanol}$$
$$\text{liver} \qquad\qquad \overset{\downarrow}{O}\downarrow$$

CH$_3$-N=N-CH$_2$O-β-glucuronide          methylazoxymethanol-
                                          glucuronide

via bile          O
into colon
CH$_3$-N=N-CH$_2$OH          methylazoxymethanol

          O          reactive intermediate
                     in carcinogenesis

Following the intestinal absorption of 1, 2-dimethylhydrazine, oxidation to azo- and azoxymethane occurs.  Hydroxylation of azoxymethane to methylazoxymethanol takes place within the endoplasmic reticulum of the hepatocytes, followed by conjugation with glucuronic acid at the same site.  The glucuronide is secreted via the bile into the gut.  Relatively poor intestinal absorption of the glucuronide enables it to reach the terminal ileum and colon where glucuronidase contributed by the host flora hydrolyzes the methylazoxymethanol glucuronide to the reactive intermediate, methylazoxymethanol.  In addition, a side reaction may occur in an acid environment, namely, the spontaneous conversion of a relatively small percentage of methylazoxymethanol to alkylating methyl carbonium ion which contributes to toxicity, but not to carcinogenicity.

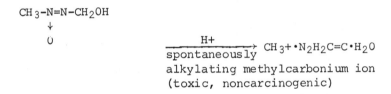

CH$_3$-N=N-CH$_2$OH

          O          $\xrightarrow[\text{spontaneously}]{\text{H+}}$ CH$_3$+·N$_2$H$_2$C=C·H$_2$O
                     alkylating methylcarbonium ion
                     (toxic, noncarcinogenic)

Thus, according to the route of DMH metabolism, one could expect that liver injury might result in some defect in its ability to conjugate an active intermediate to DMH.  This could result in the development of neoplastic lesions in the liver as indeed occurred in our first experiments.  In a more recent experiment, we measured serum and liver β-glucuronidase activity.  The data are reported in Table 1.

Iron deficiency obviously caused some changes in liver function that we were not able to detect by light microscopy.  It remains to be shown that the increase in glucuronidase activity in serum and in liver of iron-deficient rats is associated with enhancement of DMH-induced lesions.

## TABLE 1

### SERUM AND LIVER β-GLUCURONIDASE ACTIVITY[1] (MEAN ± S.D.)

| DIET | WEEKS ON DIET | HCT (%) | HB (g/100 ml) | SERUM β-GLUCURONIDASE (μg phenolphthalein/ 1 hr/ml) | LIVER β-GLUCURONIDASE (μg phenolphthalein/ 1 hr/mg wet weight) soluble | | |
|---|---|---|---|---|---|---|---|
| | | | | | total | supernatant | %total |
| CONTROL | 5 | (6) 51 ± 3 | (5) 15.2 ± 1.0 | (5) 75.0 ± 37.3 | | | |
| | 7 | (5) 48 ± 2 | (4) 15.6 ± 0.6 | (3) 78.3 ± 9.0 | | | |
| | 9 | (1) 48 | | (1) 51.0 | (1) 582 | 55 | 9.5 |
| | 15 | (3) 46 ± 2 | (3) 16.2 ± 1.1 | (3) 51.7 ± 7.6 | | | |
| FE DEFICIENT | 5 | (5) 29 ± 5 | (5) 7.8 ± 1.7 | (5) 112.8 ± 23.5 | | | |
| | 7 | (5) 25 ± 4 | (3) 6.1 ± 1.5 | (5) 103.8 ± 19.7 | | | |
| | 9 | | | (1) 126 | (1) 780 | 104 | 13.3 |
| | 15 | (4) 28 ± 2 | (4) 8.8 ± 2.5 | (4) 123.0 ± 4.2[2] | | | |

[1] *Enzyme activity expressed as μg phenolphthalein liberated from phenolphthalein-glucuronide acid per hour at 56° C. Serum enzyme was determined as described in the Sigma Tech. Bulletin #325 (1-75). Total hepatic β-glucuronidase activity was measured in aliquots of fresh homogenate prepared in 0.375 M sucrose - 0.05 M Tris - 0.005 M MgCl2 - 0.025 M KCl solution, pH 7.4 at 4° C. Soluble supernatant fraction was prepared by centrifugation of the homogenate at 1000,000 x g for 90 minutes, at 4° C in a Beckman Model L3-50 ultracentrifuge.*

[2] *Significantly different from control of the same age, P< 0.01*

In another seemingly unrelated set of experiments dealing with the quality and quantity of fat on DMH-induced cancers, we observed the following:

Weanling male rats were fed the various diets listed in Table 2. Safflower oil (20%) or coconut oil (hydrogenated) 20% were the saturated and polyunsaturated fats, respectively, used in the preparation of high-fat diets. The low-fat diets contained 5% of each of the above fats, with an appropriate addition of sucrose to compensate for the lowered fat content. All diets contained cholesterol and cholic acid. After a three-week interval, rats in each diet group were subdivided, and one-half were given DMH i.m., 10 mg/kg weekly, for a period of 20 weeks. Feeding was then continued for an additional 15 weeks, at which time animals were killed and autopsied, and tissues prepared for histology.

Animals fed the 5% safflower oil diet high in cholesterol did not thrive on this diet; all died within the first three months of the experiment. Weight gain in the group fed 5% coconut oil was considerably reduced when compared to animals fed the 20% coconut oil diet. Animals fed the 20% safflower oil diet exhibited the same weight gains as those fed the 20% coconut oil diet. Administration of DMH did not appreciably influence the weight gain in any group.

TABLE 2

DIETS

| INGREDIENTS | PERCENTAGE COMPOSITION |
|---|---|
| Safflower oil or Coconut oil (hydrogenated) | 20.0 |
| Casein, (vitamin free) | 18.0 |
| Sucrose | 50.3 |
| Cholesterol | 1.0 |
| Cholic acid | 0.3 |
| Choline chloride | 0.3 |
| Salt mixture | 4.0 |
| Vitamin mixture | 1.1 |
| Alphacel | 5.0 |

The vitamin powder and salt mixture contains the known vitamins and minerals for adequate maintenance of these animals, and has been used previously in this laboratory.(22)

The distribution of tumors throughout the GI tract is shown in Table 3. Rats fed either the 20% coconut oil or 20% safflower oil diets exhibited a similar distribution pattern, with the greatest number of tumors appearing in mid-colon, and approximately 10% appearing in the small intestine. Decreasing the fat content to 5% coconut oil (or increasing the sucrose content) significantly altered the tumor distribution. Approximately one-third were tumors of the small intestine and another one-third appeared in the descending colon.

TABLE 3

DISTRIBUTION OF TOTAL NUMBERS OF TUMORS
IN SMALL INTESTINE AND COLON OF RATS
FED HYDROGENATED COCONUT OR SAFFLOWER OIL DIETS
AND TREATED WITH DMH

| DIET | #RATS | PERCENTAGE DISTRIBUTION | | | | |
|------|-------|------------------|-------|-------|------------|--------|
|      |       | SMALL INTESTINE | CECUM | COLON | DESCENDING | RECTUM |
| 5% coconut | 11 | 28.6 | 14.2 | 23.6 | 28.6 | 0 |
| 20% coconut | 14 | 8.8 | 5.9 | 64.7 | 14.7 | 5.9 $P<0.001$ |
| 20% safflower | 8 | 10.5 | 2.6 | 65.8 | 15.8 | 5.3 $P<0.001$ |

Table 4 illustrates the numbers of large bowel tumors detected in each group. In the group fed 20% coconut oil and given DMH, a total of 31 tumors were found in the 14 rats, for an average of 2.2 tumors per rat. Reducing the fat content to 5% decreased the incidence of large bowel tumors by 52%. Substituting 20% polyunsaturated fat in the diet increased the tumor yield by 84%.

Histologic studies carried out to date indicate the following distribution of tumors induced by DMH:

Invasive adenocarcinoma - 38%

Invasive mucinous adenocarcinoma - 24%

Sessile polypoid carcinoma with and without
superficial invasion - 14%

Adenoma with Ca *in situ* - 10%

Villous adenoma with malignant degeneration - 5%

TABLE 4

NUMBER OF LARGE BOWEL TUMORS INDUCED BY DMH IN RATS
FED SATURATED AND POLYUNSATURATED FAT DIETS HIGH IN CHOLESTEROL

| DIET | #RATS | % OF RATS WITH ONE OR MORE COLONIC TUMORS | TOTAL # OF LARGE BOWEL TUMORS/ GROUP | AVERAGE# OF TUMORS PER RAT | % OF CHANGE |
|---|---|---|---|---|---|
| 20% coconut (C) | 14 | 93.0 | 31 | 2.2+0.41 | -- |
| 5% coconut (C) | 10 | 50.0 | 10 | 1.00+0.42 | 52% decrease |
| 20% safflower (S) | 8 | 100.0 | 34 | 4.25+0.96 | 84% increase |

5% C vs. 20% C  $P<0.025$

20% C vs. 20% S  $P<0.025$

5% C vs. 20% S  $P<0.005$

From these preliminary studies, it would appear that:  (1) iron
deficiency results in liver injury; (2) the quality of fat affects
the incidence of DMH-induced colon tumors; and (3) iron deficiency
alters the site of DMH-induced lesions (possibly hepatoma) and enhances its carcinogenicity (126 days for liver lesions in iron deficient rats versus 245 days for colon cancer in the nondeficient
rat).

That high-fat diets are linked to the pathogenesis of cancer
seems reasonable.(23,24,25)  That the quality of fat makes a difference in the induction of colon cancer remains a moot question, not-
withstanding the results of Reddy et al.(20) and Wilson et al.(26)
which contrast with our own observations; however, we did incorporate another dietary variable, cholesterol, and with added dietary

cholic acid we were able to manipulate serum cholesterol levels and most likely sterol excretion into the gut by varying the quality of fat. Eight rats fed the unsaturated fat diets (20% safflower oil) had mean serum cholesterol level of 173 mg% ($\pm$ 11) compared to 454 mg% ($\pm$ 89) in eight rats fed 20% coconut oil. Bile acid and steroid metabolite excretion in the gut is increased with the feeding of unsaturated fat diets; the increase is associated with an increased susceptibility to DMH-induced colon cancer, and bile acids are considered cocarcinogens.(27) *Pari passu*, it should be pointed out that the diets used in our experiments with added cholesterol and cholic acid are, and have been, used to study atherogenesis or the induction of atheromatous plaques in experimental animals.(22) The degree of atheromatous lesions can be graded on a 1 to 4+ basis.(22) In these studies, there was an inverse correlation between tumors in the colon and degree of atheromatous lesions in the ascending and descending aorta of the animals; the more tumors, the less vascular lipidosis.

How does iron deficiency relate to the studies dealing with the quality of fat on DMH-induced cancer? In the first instance, dietary iron deficiency is associated with lipidemia and fatty infiltration of the liver.(28,29,30) Secondly, iron deficiency does result in hepatic injury, which could conceivably alter bile acid and sterol excretion into the gut. Hepatic injury,(29,30) lipidemia,(28,31) fatty infiltration of the liver,(29,30) alterations in gut flora,(32,33) may all play some role in changing the usual target organ, the colon, to the liver of DMH-treated, iron-deficient rats.

It would seem reasonable in attempting to sort out some of the variables and their relative role in carcinogenesis to include in one's study the addition of other chemical carcinogens and other nutritional deficiencies that share some common features.

It would be of interest to study the relationship between iron deficiency and quality of fat on the induction time and site of tumors in rats treated not only with DMH but with aflatoxin $B_1$, the latter being a potent hepatocarcinogen under normal (nondeficient) conditions.

Aflatoxin $B_1$, which usually results in hepatomas was shown to cause a significant number of colon tumors in rats fed diets low or marginal in vitamin A.(32,33) The authors concluded that a significant change in the target organ occurred (liver to colon) in vitamin A deficiency. In view of some of the effects of vitamin A deficiency (e.g., metaplasia of intestinal epithelial tissue), it might be expected that aflatoxin $B_1$-treated animals fed a vitamin A-deficient diet might have as much if not more colon tumors than liver tumors. The authors also rightfully point out that other changes can occur in vitamin A deficiency, which might account for the change in the usual aflatoxin target organ of liver to colon.(33)

Thus, the administration of DMH and aflatoxin can result in cancer or neoplastic changes in both liver and colon, but the organ affected is obviously influenced by dietary variables.

Iron, $B_6$, and $B_2$ deficiencies also share some common features including anemia and liver injury. Pyridoxine deficiency is usually associated with microcytic, hypochromic anemia (similar to iron deficiency) but in the presence of a hyperferremia. Riboflavin deficiency is usually associated with erythroid hypoplasia in marked contrast to the hyperplastic marrow of iron deficiency.(34, 35)

Also not generally appreciated is the observation that riboflavin deficiency results in hepatocyte injury and ultrastructural changes.(36, 37, 38, 39) These changes consist principally of fat infiltration, disarray of rough endoplasmic reticulum and vesiculation of cisternae, increased numbers of free ribosomes, abnormal mitochondria (mega) with decreased function, and lysosomal damage. Indeed, these changes may be more specific for liver injury, per se, than for any specific insult.

There are other possibilities by which any hepatic injury might render the liver more susceptible to further insults; e.g., DMH or aflatoxin. In liver injury, following liver injury, and during hepatic regeneration following injury, serum alpha-fetoprotein levels are raised.(40) Perhaps more important and more relevant to our own observation is the fact that serum alpha-fetoprotein levels have been associated with the growth of primary hepatoma and it has also recently been found to be increased in nonmalignant hepatic disorders such as viral hepatitis and alcoholic cirrhosis.(41,42) Thus, increased hepatic and/or serum alpha-fetoprotein, as a result of iron deficiency, for which we have only limited observations, may play a major but secondary role in altering the site of DMH-induced lesions.

The two major leading causes of death in this country are cancer and atherosclerosis. Diet, and particularly dietary fat, has been implicated in their pathogenesis. Also appreciated is the observation that one of the more prevalent nutritional deficiencies in all age groups is iron. Further, we have evidence that iron deficiency as well as the ingestion of highly unsaturated fats and sterols is associated with enhanced chemical carcinogenesis. It would seem appropriate, then, to investigate the interaction between these dietary components and to determine to what extent they alter the onset, site, incidence, and type of tumor. The use of two chemical carcinogens whose target organ is affected by nutritional insults that have some common features and differ in other aspects could be useful. This approach should help clarify possible mechanisms of action whereby neoplasia can be shifted from one organ to another.

## IV.  SUMMARY

The effect of iron deficiency as well as the quality of fat
has been studied in chemically induced carcinogenesis in the rat.
Dimethylhydrazine (DMH) has been shown to produce colon cancer in
the nondeficient rat.  In these studies, the quality of fat altered
the incidence of colon tumors; highly unsaturated fat diets promoted
colon carcinogenesis, whereas highly saturated fat diets reduced
the risk to colon cancer; however the degree of atheromatous lesions
on aortic vascular lipidosis was significantly greater in rats fed
the unsaturated fat diet.  Iron deficiency not only altered the site
of DMH-induced tumors from colon to liver, but induced liver tumors
much sooner (126 days for iron-deficient rats versus 245 days for
colon tumors in nondeficient rats).  This effect of iron deficiency
may have resulted from changes in liver enzymes involved in the inactivation of DMH intermediates and/or aberrations in organelles
wihin the hepatocyte involved in conjugation of DMH intermediates
with glucuronic acid.

*REFERENCES*

1.   Chandra, R. K., Arch. Dis. Child 48, Page 864, 1973.

2.   Arbeter, A., Echeverri, L., Franco, D., et al., Symposium, Fed.
     Proceedings 30, Page 142, 1971.

3.   Joyson, D. H. M., Jacobs, A., Walker, D. M. and Dolby, A. E.,
     Lancet 2, Page 1058, 1972.

4.   Jacobs, A., British J. Haemat. 16, Page 1, 1969.

5.   Jacobs, A., Gerent. Clin. 13, Page 61, 1971.

6.   Vitale, J. J., "Deficiency Diseases," in Pathologic Basis of
     Disease, S. L. Robbins, Editor, Edition 1, W. B. Saunders
     Company, Philadelphia, pp. 475-508, 1974.

7.   Chanarin, I., Bennett, M., Berry, V. and V., J. Clinical Path.
     15, Page 269, 1962.

8.   Vitale, J. J., Restrepo, A., Velez, H., et al., J. Nutrition
     88, Page 315, 1966.

9.   Velez, H., Restrepo, A., Vitale, J. J., et al., American J.
     Clinical Nutrition 19, Page 27, 1966.

10.  Chanarin, T., Rothman, D., Berry, V. and V., British Medical
     Journal 1, Page 480, 1965.

11.  Rodday, P., Bennett, M. and Vitale, J. J., Blood 48, Page 435, 1976.

12.  Bennett, M., Cudkowicz, G., Foster, R. S., Jr., Metcalf, D. and D., J. Cell Physiology 71, Page 221, 1968.

13.  Rauchwerger, N. M., Gallagher, M. T. and Trentin, J. J., Transplantation 15, Page 610, 1973.

14.  Rodday, P. and Bennett, M., submitted to Transplantation, 1977.

15.  Comas, F. V. and Byrd, B. L., Radiation Research 32, 355, 1967.

16.  Sztanyik, B. L. and Elson, L. A., Haematologia (Budapest) 3, Page 401, 1969.

17.  Editorial: "Immunosuppression and Human Cancer," British Medicine 31, Page 713, 1972.

18.  Rogers, A. E., Cancer Research 35, Page 2469, 1975.

19.  Rogers, A. E. and Newberne, P. M., Nature 246, Page 491, 1973.

20.  Reddy, B. S., Marisawa, T., Vutusich, D., et al., Proceedings Society Experimental Biology 151, Page 237, 1976.

21.  Weisberger, J. A., Cancer 28, Page 60, 1971.

22.  Hellerstein, E. E., Nakamura, M., Vitale, J. J., et al., J. Nutrition 71, Page 339, 1960.

23.  Haenszel, W., Berg, J. W., Segi, M., et al., J. National Cancer Institute 51, Page 1765, 1973.

24.  Wynder, E. L., Cancer Research 35, Page 3388, 1975.

25.  Armstrong, B. and Doll, R., Intern. J. Cancer 15, 617, 1975.

26.  Wilson, R. B., Wideman, D. P. and L., American J. Clinical Nutrition 30, Page 176, 1976.

27.  Reddy, B., Weisburger, J. H. and Wynder, E. L., J. National Cancer Institute 52, Page 567, 1974.

28.  Amine, E. K. and Hegsted, D. M., J. Nutrition 101, 927, 1971.

29.  Folch, M. H., Sherman, D. Y. C., Herskovic, T., et al., Arch. Pathology 87, Page 526, 1969.

30.  Dollman, P. R. and Goodman, J. R., J. Cell Biology 48,
     Page 79, 1971.

31.  Amine, E. K. and Hegsted, D. M., J. Nutrition 101, Page 1576,
     1976.

32.  Newberne, P. M. and Rogers, A. E., J. National Cancer Institute
     50, Page 439, 1973.

33.  Newberne, P. M. and Rogers, A. E., Fundamentals in Cancer
     Prevention, P. N. Magee, et al., Editors, University of Tokyo
     Press, Tokyo and University Park Press, Baltimore, pp. 15-40,
     1976.

34.  Ghitis, J. and Vitale, J. J., Post Graduate Medicine 34, Page
     300, 1963.

35.  Foy, H., Kondi, A. and Verjee, Z. H. M., J. Nutrition 102,
     Page 571, 1972.

36.  Hoppel, C. L. and Tandler, B., J. Nutrition 105, 562, 1975.

37.  Hoppel, C. L. and Tandler, B., J. Nutrition 106, Page 73, 1976.

38.  Tandler, B. and Hoppel, C. L., Experimental Molecular
     Pathology 21, Page 88, 1974.

39.  Tandler, B., Erlandson, R. A. and Wynder, E. L., American J.
     Pathology 52, Page 69, 1968.

40.  Abelev, G. I., Perova, S. D., Khramkova, N. I., et al.,
     Transplantation 1, Page 174, 1963.

41.  Silver, H. K., Gold, P., Shuster, J., et al., New England
     J. Medicine 291, Page 506, 1974.

42.  Silver, H. K., Gold, P., Shuster, et al., Clinical Research
     21, Page 525, 1973.

## CHAPTER 17

IMPLICATIONS OF THE INHIBITION OF ANIMAL TUMORS

BY DIETARY ZINC DEFICIENCY

Walter J. Pories

Department of Surgery, Case Western Reserve School of Medicine,
Cleveland Metropolitan General Hospital, Cleveland, Ohio

William D. DeWys

Department of Medicine, Northwestern University Medical School,
Chicago, Illinois

Arthur Flynn, Edward G. Mansour, and William H. Strain

Department of Surgery, Case Western Reserve School of Medicine
Cleveland Metropolitan General Hospital, Cleveland, Ohio

## I.  INTRODUCTION

Experiments with mice and rats have been carried out to determine whether the growth of malignant tumors can be controlled by
dietary manipulation of zinc, an essential element for growth and
repair.  Although it is well established that growth rates of bacterial and tissue cultures, and indeed, of whole organisms and populations, can be reduced by the limitation of a critical nutrient,
application of this technique does not seem to have been made to the
study of experimental tumors.  The experiments were designed to develop a system without the hazard of a known carcinogenic agent.

The experiments were conducted by maintaining male mice and
rats on zinc deficient or sufficient diets, implanting with tumor
suspensions, and statistical analysis of tumor growth and animal survival.  Young adult CDF and C 57 BI/6 male mice and weanling male
Sprague-Dawley rats were used.  The test groups of animals were maintained on the zinc-deficient diets for periods of time ranging from
7 to 21 days prior to inoculation.  Lewis mouse carcinoma, mouse
leukemia L 5178gt, mouse leukemia L 1210, and mouse leukemia B 388
were administered to the mice, and Walker 256 carcinosarcoma to the

rats, all as suspensions in Hanks' solution.  Tumor growth was measured at appropriate time intervals, and deaths on the day of demise.

The growth rates of bacterial and tissue cultures, and indeed,
of whole organisms and populations, can be reduced by the limitation
of a critical nutrient.  This is a report of a series of experiments
that demonstrate that the growth of mouse and rat malignant tumors
can be similarly controlled by the manipulation of the essential
element, zinc.

## II.  MATERIALS AND METHODS

The tumor models, species, tumor dosages, routes of administration, and zinc deficiency pretreatment periods are shown in
Table 1.

### TABLE 1

TUMOR MODELS, SPECIES, TUMOR DOSAGES, ROUTES OF ADMINISTRATION, and
PRETREATMENT PERIODS OF ZINC DEFICIENCY USED IN THESE STUDIES

| Tumors | Species | Tumor Dosage | Route | Pretreatment Periods |
|---|---|---|---|---|
| Lewis Lung Carcinoma | C57BI/6 Male Mice | $10^6$ | IM | 11 days |
| Mouse Leukemia (L5178yf) | CDF, Male Mice | $10^5$ | IP | 7 days |
| Mouse Leukemia (L1210) | CDF, Male Mice | $10^5$ | IP | 7,14,21 days |
| Mouse Leukemia (P388) | CDF, Male Mice | $10^5$ | IP | 7 days |
| Walker 256 Carcino-sarcoma | Sprague-Dawley Male Rats | $10^7$ | IM, IP | 7 days |

Mice were used at six weeks of age (18-24 g) and rats at three
weeks of age (35-55 g).  Tumors were obtained from A. D. Little,
Inc., Cambridge, Massachusetts, and carried by serial transplant
passage in our laboratory.  Ascites transplants involved sterile
collection of ascites from a tumor-bearing animal, dilution of the

ascites cells in Hanks' balanced salt solution, and inoculation of experimental animals with known numbers of tumor cells.  For solid tumor transplants, tumor fragments were minced through a cytosieve (U. S. Standard Sieve Series, 100 mesh inch, Dual Manufacturing Co., Chicago, Illinois), and the cells suspended in Hanks' balanced salt solution.  In carrying out both types of transplant, cells were

TABLE 2

COMPOSITION OF ZINC-DEFICIENT DIET*

| Dietary Constituent | Percent Composition |
|---|---|
| Egg Albumin | 26.40 |
| Glucose monohydrate | 56.00 |
| Corn oil | 10.00 |
| Mineral Mix+ | 5.36 |
| Vitamin mix† | 1.00 |
| DL-Methionine | 0.50 |
| L-Histidine hydrochloride | 0.50 |
| Santoquin antioxidant (dry) | 0.02 |
| Choline chloride | 0.22 |

\* Zinc content of 1.3 ppm determined by atomic absorption spectrometry.

+ Mineral mix supplied the following minerals in mg/100 g diet:  $NaH_2PO_4 \cdot H_2O$, 1730; $KH_2PO_4$, 680; $CaCO_3$, 2172; $MgCO_3$, 400; $MgSO_4$, 255; $FeSO_4 \cdot 7H_2O$, 102; $MnSO_4 \cdot H_2O$, 16.8; $CuSO_4 \cdot 5H_2O$, 5.5; KI, 0.3.  This mix differs from that used previously (2,3) because other studies indicated a lower level of potassium and sodium could be used and fluoride could be omitted.

† One gram mix supplied the following vitamins per 100 g diet: inositol, 25 mg; niacin, 5 mg; Ca pantothenate, 2.0 mg; thiamine HCl, 1.0 mg; riboflavin, 1.0 mg; pyridoxine HCl, 0.45 mg; folic acid, 0.40 mg; biotin, 0.43 mg; vitamin A, 500 IU; vitamin D (Delstrol), 150 IU; vitamin $B_{12}$, 2.0 µg; vitamin K (Klotogen F), 0.1522 mg; vitamin E (Rovimix), 6.6 IU.

counted in a hemocytometer, the concentration was adjusted, and the animals were inoculated with the indicated number of cells as given in the tables and figures, in a volume of 0.2 ml per animal. The time of tumor transplant is designated "0" in the tables and text figures.

An experimental zinc-deficient diet, meeting all nutritional requirements of rats and mice except for zinc(1) was formulated in collaboration with the U. S. Plant, Soil, and Nutrition Laboratory, Ithaca, New York (Table 2). In each experiment, a zinc-deficient group received the diet ad libitum and deionized distilled water. Groups designated "zinc adequate" or weight-matched" received the diet plus deionized distilled water, supplemented with 50 parts per million (ppm) zinc ion as zinc acetate. The zinc-adequate animals were fed ad libitum, and the weight-matched animals received the diet in amounts planned to result in weight changes equal to those of a matched member of the zinc-deficient group (average about 0.5 g per day for mice, and 7 g per day for rats). All animals were housed individually in stainless steel suspension cages and fed the diet in glass feed cups. Water, zinc free or zinc supplemented was presented in clear, glass bottles with Neoprene stoppers having stainless steel spouts. These glass containers had been tested for zinc exchange and no significant leaching or adsorption of zinc was found. Frequent determinations of animal weight, anteroposterior and mediolateral tumor diameters, and daily survival were recorded. Differences in survival were evaluated by the Mann-Whitney two-sample rank test for nonparametric data. (4)

## III.   RESULTS

### A.   Lewis Lung Carcinoma in Mice

The tumor growth and survival results for the Lewis lung carcinoma are presented in Figures 1 and 2. Zinc deficiency markedly reduced the growth of tumor. The great difference between the weight-matched and zinc-deficient groups emphasizes that the effect was due to zinc deficiency and not due to caloric restriction.

The tumor grew in only 4 of 10 implanted zinc-deficient mice (data shown are the average of these 4 mice), but in all of the 19 mice in the other two groups. All zinc-supplemented mice had palpable tumors by day 11, but zinc-deficient group tumors appeared between days 11 and 17.

The median survival for the zinc ad libitum and weight-matched groups was similar (29.5 and 29 days, respectively), whereas the survival of the zinc-deficient group was significantly prolonged (33 days; p<0.02).

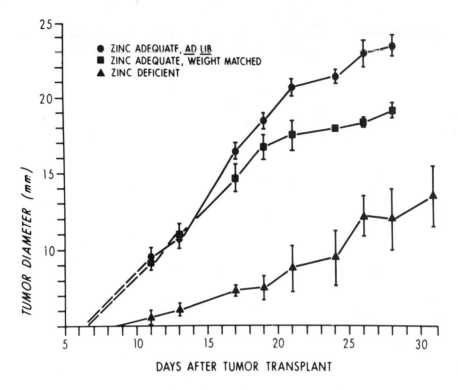

Figure 1

Growth of Lewis Lung Carcinoma in Male Mice

Tumor growth was markedly reduced in the zinc-deficient group.  The
difference in tumor growth in the zinc-deficient and weight-matched
groups indicates that the tumor inhibition was not attributable to
reduced caloric intake, but was an effect of zinc deficiency.


B.    Leukemia in Mice

The survival response in the three experiments with the different mouse leukemias is shown in Table 3.

In all experiments, the zinc-deficient group demonstrated a
one-day increase in median survival over the zinc-adequate control
group.  In two of the three experiments, the difference in survival
was statistically significant (see Table 3).

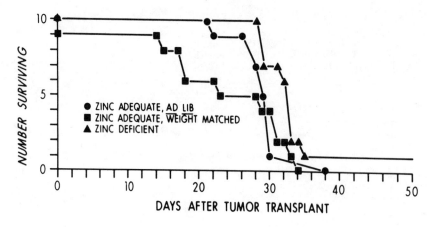

Figure 2

Survival of zinc-deficient mice with Lewis lung carcinoma was significantly prolonged (p<0.02), compared with the other two groups.

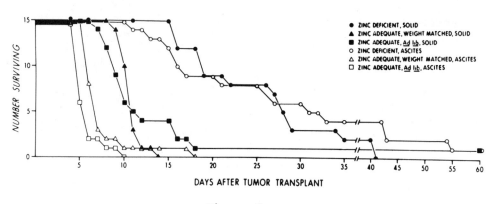

Figure 3

Survival of Sprague-Dawley male rats receiving $10^7$ Walker 256 carcinosarcoma cells intraperitoneally or intramuscularly into the
hind leg. For both types of tumor growth, survival was significantly
prolonged in the zinc-deficient groups (p<0.001).

C.    Walker 256 Carcinosarcoma in Rats

The experiments with Walker 256 carcinosarcoma in rats were
devised to answer two questions:   (1) whether the effect of zinc
deficiency on tumor occurred in other species; and (2) whether the

TABLE 3

SURVIVAL RESPONSE OF MICE WITH LEUKEMIA

| Tumor* | Diet | Mean Survival | Median Survival | Individual P+ Survival |
|--------|------|---------------|-----------------|------------------------|
| L5178yf | Control | 13.5 (16.3)† | 16 | 3, 7, 16, 16, 16,16, 17, 17, <0.01 |
|  | Zinc-Deficient | 17.1 | 17 | 13,14,17,17,17 17,17,19,19,19 |
| L1210 | Control | 11.0 | 11 | 9,11,11,11,11, 11,11,12,12 <0.01 |
|  | Zinc-Deficient | 12.6 | 12 | 11,12,12,12,12, 12,14,14,14 |
| P388 | Control | 9.1 | 9 | 9, 9, 9, 9, 9 9, 9, 9 >0.05 |
|  | Zinc-Deficient | 9.3 | 10 | 77, 9, 9,10 10,10,10 |

* CDF$_1$ male mice received $10^5$ cells ip of the designated leukemia after seven days of dietary pretreatment.

+ Significance testing with the Mann-Whitney two-sample rank test for nonparametric data.(4)  Although the difference between mean or median survival of the deficient and control groups is not great, this statistical test based on sequence of deaths yields significant differences for L5178yf and L1210.

† Mean excluding two unexplained early deaths.

effect was related to the mode of tumor growth.  A cell suspension was prepared from the minced solid tumor and $10^7$ cells were injected intraperitoneally (ip) or intramuscularly (im).  The survival response is presented in Figure 3.

The effect of zinc deficiency on inhibiting tumor growth was as profound in rats as in mice, and was equally significant (p<0.001) in the ascites and solid tumor groups.

D.   Effect of Duration of Diet on Leukemia L1210 in Mice

Mice were fed the zinc-deficient diet for 7, 14, or 21 days before tumor transplantation to determine the effect of duration of the pretreatment diet on tumor growth (Table 4). The longest median survival prolongation by zinc deficiency occured in the seven-day group, and the least occurred in the 21-day group. These results probably reflect the adverse effects of prolonged zinc deficiency.

IV.   DISCUSSION

Zinc is essential for growth and normal development.(5,6)   In the absence of adequate amounts, rapidly growing tissues suffer: wounds fail to heal;(7) testes stop producing sperm;(8) skin becomes scaly and fragile;(9,10,11) and severe abnormalities develop in fetal tissues.(12,13,14)

This intense essentiality for growth and development is probably due to the dependence of protein synthesis and metabolism on zinc enzymes, and perhaps even more subtle mechanisms of control, dependent on variation in the concentration of zinc. Over 70 zinc metallo enzymes have now been identified in various species including aldolases, dehydrogenases, peptidases, and thymidine kinase, and in each of these, the zinc atom is located on the active site for the catalytic process.(15)

Zinc is also required for DNA and RNA synthesis and catabolism and thus plays a central role in mitosis and cell division. Both DNA and RNA polymerases contain zinc; RNA-ase is inhibited by the presence of zinc. There is a large body of evidence (2,3,5,15,16) that zinc-deficient organisms have impaired nucleic acid synthesis.

This intimate dependence of growth, development, mitosis, protein, and nucleic acid synthesis on the presence of appropriate amounts of zinc indicates that zinc is also essential for the growth and maintenance of cancer. Our own studies (2,3,17) strongly support this thesis. In two species, a variety of cancers, and with both solid and ascites forms of tumor, we found zinc to be essential not only for growth of tumor but also for tumor "take" and survival. Others have found similar effects. Petering et al.(18) first noted this phenomenon during a study of the effect of mineral supplements on the antitumor activity of 3-ethoxy-2-oxobutyraldehyde bis (thio-semicarbazone) on Walker 256 carcinosarcoma, and found zinc to be essential for tumor growth. Duncan et al.(19) reported inhibition of a 3-methyl-4-dimethylaminoazobenzene-induced hepatoma in rats by diets low in zinc (0.4 mcg/g), and of great interest, by diets with considerable zinc excess (above 500 mcg/g).

The inhibition of tumor growth by zinc deficiency may simply be due to deprivation of an essential nutrient, reflecting the great demand for zinc by the growing tumor. We(20) have observed that Walker 256 sarcomas in rats preferentially concentrate zinc in comparison to the tissues of the host organism, similar to the phenomenon observed in healing wounds.(21) Hirayama(22) reported radiozinc-65 localization in prostatic tumors to be two or three times higher than in normal prostate of rats. Schwartz et al.(23) similarly noted that the mean zinc concentration of malignant breast-tissues was five to seven times greater than that of normal breast tissue in nine patients undergoing radical mastectomy.

There is, however, a growing body of evidence that the systemic effects of zinc metabolism indirectly acting on tumors are also of considerable importance. The various studies by Flynn, et al.(24) and Pories, et al.(7) demonstrate the complexity of zinc metabolism and the close relationship between the element and various endocrine functions. The changes in the rate of tumor growth associated with changes in zinc nutrition may well be an expression of an altered endocrine milie.

Although zinc is essential for the growth of tumors, there is virtually no evidence that the element is carcinogenic. Blot and Fraumeui(25) reported increased lung cancer mortalities in 36 counties with copper, lead, and zinc industries, compared with 2,985 counties without smelting and refining activities. All evidence, however, points to carcinogenesis as an effect of arsenical pollution rather than of zinc. Eisenbud and Walter(26) reported a case of cancer developing at the site of long-term injection of zinc-insulin (Lente), but attributed this to repeated trauma rather than zinc.

The evidence, on the contrary, is that zinc has a protective effect, especially against tumors induced by cadmium and other carcinogens. Gunn et al.(27) reported that the administration of zinc reduced the incidence of cadmium-induced interscapular sarcomas in rats from 41% to 12%. The same workers(28) were also able to prevent cadmium-induced interstitial cell tumors of rat and mice testes by the injection of zinc. Both Edwards(29) and Poswillo and Cohen(30) have documented that zinc, as a dietary supplement, inhibited the development of dimethylbenzanthracene-induced tumors in the pouches of hamsters.

Our knowledge about zinc metabolism in human malignancies remains fragmentary. A series of early studies were reviewed by Prasad(31) in 1966. Since then, there have been a series of reports, many of which demonstrate significant changes in serum zinc levels with different tumors.(32,33,34) For example, Fisher et al.(35) reported that patients with primary osteosarcomas had elevated serum

TABLE 4

EFFECT OF DURATION OF ZINC-DEFICIENT DIET ON SURVIVAL RESPONSE WITH LEUKEMIA L1210

| Group* | Duration of Diet Before Tumor Transplant | Mean Survival | Median Survival | Individual Survival | P values Compared with Ad Libitum Control | P values Compared with Respective Weight-matched Control |
|---|---|---|---|---|---|---|
| Control, ad libitum | — | 9.2 | 9 | 9, 9, 9, 9, 9, 9, 9, 9,10, 10 | | |
| Zinc-deficient | 7 | 11.1 | 11 | 10,10,11, 11,11,11, 11,12,12, 12 | < 0.001 | < 0.001 |
| Weight-matched | 7 | 9.4 | 9.5 | 8, 9, 9, 9, 9,10, 10,10,10 10 | | |
| Zinc-deficient | 14 | 10.4 | 10.5 | 7, 9,10, 10,10,11, 11,12,12, 12 | < 0.02 | < 0.05 |
| Weight-matched | 14 | 9.2 | 9 | 8, 9, 9, 9, 9, 9, 9,10,10, 10 | | |
| Zinc-deficient | 21 | 9.8 | 10 | 5, 9, 9, 10,10,10, 11,11,11, 12 | < 0.1>0.05 | > 0.1 |
| Weight-matched | 21 | 9.8 | 10 | 9, 9, 9, 9,10,10, 10,10,10,12 | | |

* CDF1 male mice received $10^5$ L1210 leukemia cells ip after the indicated dietary pretreatment. Groups were started on diet at 6, 7, or 8 weeks of age, respectively, and then all were inoculated with leukemia cells at 9 weeks of age.

zinc levels, those with metastases showed depressed levels, and amputated patients who were clinically tumor-free had newly normal serum zinc levels. Zaun and Gall(36) found a decreased zinc content in all of a series of patients with mycosis fungoides, internal malignant neoplasia, and malignant melanomas with metastases. Recently, we(37) completed a study of 279 patients and found a profound fall in zinc levels compared to controls (78.3 $\pm$ 18.3 mcg/ml versus 108.0 $\pm$ 12.3 mcg/ml) and marked elevation of the Cu/Zn ratio from 1.01 to 2.19. Of particular interest was the finding that the Cu/Zn ratios were markedly different between responders to chemotherapy and nonresponders.

Only 15 years ago there was little evidence that zinc was of any importance in human nutrition and homeostasis. Now there is a torrent of information demanding an intensive study of the applications of zinc metabolism in oncology. The elegant zinc balance studies in patients with neoplasia carried out by Spencer et al. (38) need to be extended. Additional investigations of the role of zinc in cellular and subcellular mechanisms, especially in the areas of nucleic acid catabolism and synthesis, enzymology, energy production and transfer, and genetic control need to be done.

Our observations that tumor growth can be controlled by zinc deficiency in two species and with several types and modes of tumor, and review of the literature imply that the manipulation of zinc nutriture, and indeed, of other essential trace elements, can be used in the diagnosis and treatment of human tumors. The ability of tumors to compete successfully for zinc may allow the use of the radioisotopes zinc-65 or zinc-69m to localize in primary or metastatic lesions. Zinc-65, given to patients in severe zinc deficiency, may concentrate in the tumors, and similar to $^{131}$I, may allow for long-term intracellular radiation of appropriate cancers. The induction of zinc deficiency by dietary withdrawal, natural chelates such as phytates, therapeutic ligands such as tetracycline, hormonal manipulation, or the administration of other trace elements after "debulking" of tumor may sharply decrease metastatic implantation and increase patients' ability to cope with their remaining tumor.

The application of zinc metabolism and nutrition to oncology promises to open new horizons in cancer therapy. Finally, and equally promising, is the possible use of zinc therapy to stimulate tumor growth so as to make it more vulnerable for chemotherapy and radiotherapy.

## V.  SUMMARY

Because zinc is an essential nutrient for tissue growth, cellular division, protein synthesis, and DNA and RNA replication, it
also ought to play a critical role in the growth of tumors.  To
test this thesis, a series of experiments were performed to test
the effect of zinc deficiency on the lethality of a variety of solid
and ascites tumors in mice and rats.  Specifically, the following
models were tested:  Walker 256 carcinosarcomas, solid and ascites
forms in rats; three mouse leukemias (L5178yf, L1210, and P388) in
CDF, male mice; and Lewis lung carcinoma in C57BI/6 male mice.

Rats receiving a zinc-deficient diet showed marked reduction
of tumor growth, both of solid or ascites models, and this was
accompanied by striking increase in survival.  Survival of mice
with transplanted leukemias was also significantly prolonged by
zinc deficiency.  In addition, growth of the Lewis lung carcinoma
was inhibited, but the survival though increased, was probably limited by the adverse effects of zinc deficiency.  The results suggest that tumor inhibition is a general effect of zinc deficiency,
irrespective of cell type, cell growth rate, species, or site of
growth.  There are numerous potential applications of zinc metabolism to the diagnosis, therapy, and understanding of cancer.

## REFERENCES

1.   National Research Council, Committee on Animal Nutrition,
     Nutrient Requirements of Laboratory Animals, 990, Washington,
     D. C., 1972.

2.   McQuitty, J. T., Jr., DeWys, W. D., Monaco, L., Strain, W. H.,
     and Pories, W. J., Inhibition of Tumor Growth by Dietary Zinc
     Deficiency, Cancer Research 30, Page 1387, 1970.

3.   DeWys, W. D., Pories, W. J., Richter, M. C. and Strain, W. H.,
     Inhibition of Walker 256 Carcinosarcoma Growth by Dietary Zinc
     Deficiency, Proceedings Soc. Exp. Biol. Med. 135, Page 17, 1970.

4.   Goldstein, A., Biostatistics.  An Introductory Text, New York,
     MacMillan Co., 1964.

5.   Prasad, A. S. and Oberleas, D., Editors, Trace Elements in
     Human Health and Disease, Vol. 1, Zinc and Copper, Academic
     New York, 1976, Page 470.

6.   Pories, W. J., Strain, W. H., Hsu, J. M. and Woosley, R. L.,
     Editors, Clinical Applications of Zinc Metabolism, Charles
     C Thomas, Springfield, Illinois, 1974.

7.  Pories, W. J., Mansour, E. G., Plecha, F. R., Flynn, A. and Strain, W. H., "Metabolic Factors Affecting Zinc Metabolism in the Surgical Patient," A. S. Prasad and D. Oberleas, Editors, Trace Elements in Human Health and Disease, Vol. 1, Zinc and Copper, Academic Press, New York, Page 115, 1976.

8.  Lei, K. Y., Abbasi, A. and Prasad, A. S., Function of Pituitary-Gonadal Axis in Zinc-Deficient Rats, American J. of Physiology, 1976.

9.  Hsu, J. M., "Current Knowledge of Skin Lesions in Zinc Deficiency," J. M. Hsu, R. L. Davis and R. W. Neithamer, The Biomedical Role of Trace Elements in Aging, Echerd College Gerontology Center, St. Petersburg, Florida, pp. 41-53, 1976.

10. Thyressen, N., Zinktherapie Bei Akrodermatitis Enteropathica, Der Hautarzt 26, Page 408, 1975.

11. Tucker, S. B., Schroeder, A. L., Brown, P. W., Jr. and McCall, J. T., Ph.D., Acquired Zinc Deficiency, J. A. M. A. 235, Page 2399, 1976.

12. Blamberg, D. L., Blackwood, V. B., Supplee, W. C. and Combs, G. F., Effect of Zinc Deficiency in Hens on Hatchability and Embryonic Development, Proceedings Society Exp. Biol. Med. 104, Page 217, 1960.

13. Hambidge, K. M., Neldner, K. H. and Walravens, P. A., Zinc, Acrodermatitis Enteropathica and Congenital Malformations, Lancet, March 8, 1975, Page 577.

14. Hurley, L. S., Trace Elements and Teratogenesis, Med. Clin. N. A. 60, Page 771, 1976.

15. Prasad, A., "Zinc in Human Studies," J. M. Hsu, R. L. Davis, and R. W. Neithamer, Editors, The Biomedical Role of Trace Elements in Aging, Echerd College Gerontology Center, St. Petersburg, Florida, pp. 15-40, 1976.

16. Burch, R. F. and Sullivan, J. F., Biochemistry of Zinc, Med. Clin. N. A. 60, Page 661, 1976.

17. DeWys, W. D. and Pories, W. J., Inhibition of a Spectrum of Animal Tumors by Dietary Zinc Deficiency, J. National Cancer Institute 48, Page 375, 1972.

18. Petering, H. G., Buskirk, H. H. and Crim, J. A., The Effect of Dietary Mineral Supplements of the Rat on the Antitumor Activity of 3-Ethoxy-2-Oxobutyraldehyde Bis (thiosemicarbazone), Cancer Research 27, Page 1115, 1967.

19. Duncan, J. R., Dreosti, I. E. and Albrecht, C. F., Zinc Intake and Growth of a Transplanted Hepatoma Induced by 3-Methyl-4-Dimethylaminoazobenzene in Rats, J. National Cancer Institute 53, Page 277, 1974.

20. Pories, W. J. and Strain, W. H., Unpublished Data.

21. Savlov, E. D., Strain, W. H. and Huegin, F., Radiozinc Studies in Experimental Wound Healing, J. Surgical Research 2, Page 209, 1962.

22. Hirayama, M., Experimental Studies of Zinc Metabolism in the Prostatic Gland, Part III, Experimental Neoplasm of the Prostatic Gland, Acta Urol. Japan 10, Page 584, 1964.

23. Schwartz, A. E., Ledicotte, G. W., Fink, R. W. and Friedman, E. W., Trace Elements in Normal and Malignant Human Breast Tissue, Surgery 76, Page 325, 1974.

24. Flynn, A., Pories, W. J., Strain, W. H. and Hill, O. A., Jr., Mineral Element Correlation with Adenohypophyseal-Adrenal Cortex Function and Stress, Science 173, Page 1035, 1971.

25. Blot, W. J. and Fraumeui, J. F., Arsenical Air Pollution and Lung Cancer, Lancet 2, Page 142, 1975.

26. Eisenbud, E. and Walter, R. M., Cancer at Insulin Injection Site, J. A. M. A. 233, Page 985, 1975.

27. Gunn, S. A., Gould, T. C. and Anderson, W. A., Effect of Zinc on Carcinogenesis by Cadmium, Proceedings Soc. Exp. Biol. Med. 115, Page 653, 1964.

28. Gunn, S. A., Gould, T. C. and Anderson, W. A., Cadmium Induced Interstitial Cell Tumors in Rats and Mice and Their Prevention by Zinc. J. National Cancer Institute 31, Page 745, 1963.

29. Edwards, M. B., Chemical Carcinogenesis in the Cheek Pouch of Syrian Hamsters Receiving Supplementary Zinc. Arch. Oral Biol. 21, Page 133, 1976.

30. Poswillo, D. E. and Cohen, B., Inhibition of Carcinogenesis by Dietary Zinc, Nature 231, Page 447, 1971.

31. Prasad, A. S., Zinc Metabolism, Charles C Thomas, Springfield, Illinois, Page 465, 1966.

32. Davies, I. J. T., Musa, M. and Dormandy, T. L., Measurements of Plasma Zinc, J. Clinical Pathology 21, Page 359, 1968.

33.  Halstead, J. A. and Smith, J. C., Jr., Plasma Zinc in Health
     and Disease, Lancet 1, Page 322, 1970.

34.  Strain, W. H., Mansour, E. G., Flynn, A., Pories, W. J.,
     Tomaro, A. J. and Hill, O. A., Jr., Plasma Zinc Concentration
     in Patients with Bronchogenic Cancer, Lancet 1, Page 1021, 1972.

35.  Fisher, G. L., Byers, V. S., Shifrine, M. and Levin, A. S.,
     Copper and Zinc Levels in Serum from Human Patients with
     Sarcomas, Cancer 37, Page 356, 1976.

36.  Zaun, H. and Gall, S., The Zinc Content of Leukocytes in
     Cutaneous Neoplasia and Non-Malignant Skin Disease, Arch.
     Klin. Exp. Dermatology 238, Page 285, 1970.

37.  Mansour, E. G., Flynn, A., Plecha, F. R. and Pories, W. J.,
     Plasma Cu and Zn Determinations in Cancer Screening and
     Therapy, Submitted for Publication.

38.  Spencer, H., Osis, D., Dramer, L. and Noms, C.,"Intake,
     Excretion, and Retention of Zinc in Man," A. S. Prasad,
     Editor, Trace Elements in Human Health and Disease, Vol. 1,
     Zinc and Copper, Academic Press, New York, pp. 345-361, 1976.

CHAPTER 18

THE ARSENIC PROBLEMS

Douglas V. Frost

Consultant - Nutrition Biochemistry
17 Rosa Road, Schenectady, New York 12308

## I.   INTRODUCTION

Arsenophobia has held sway over civilized governments through-out this century.  Because of the still unproven association between arsenic (As) and cause of cancer, arsenophobia has gained strength to the point that many safe uses of arsenicals have been abandoned. Even the production of arsenic trioxide ($As_2O_3$) is in jeopardy.  No arsenical has been shown to cause cancer, but arsenicals have proven anticancer value.  Evidence suggests that As is an essential nutri-ent and that the level of As in the United States' and Canadian diets may be too low.  Due to the long history of errors in judg-ment about "arsenic" and the strength of the traditional dogmas, there are many problems to be solved; hence, the above title.

This review will attempt to place some of the historic errors about As into perspective in terms of the current situation.  Un-doubtedly, As has played a catalytic role in biology since life be-gan.  Evidence that As stimulates phosphorylations seems secure, even though little understood.  The historic "alterative" improve-ment in appearance, stamina, and sense of well-being from traces of inorganic As is apt to be viewed as folklore, but may reflect the first nutrient effect of a trace element.  The name arsenic, from the Greek ARSENIKON, meaning potent, reflects its very early uses in human medicine and as an economic poison.  Although there are many more potent toxins than any arsenical, As developed its "poor press" in part because it could be used surreptitiously to poison people without destroying appetite.  For centuries it was the tool of professional poisoners.  At the same time, the "arsenic eaters" were finding health benefits from ingesting small amounts of arsenic, and As was used in human medicine.  In 1786, Fowler introduced the

259

use of small doses of potassium arsenite for relief of various ail-
ments.  By 1912 it was recognized as the best agent in the Pharma-
copoeia.  About that time, arsphenamine became the first "magic
bullet" for control of venereal disease.  Thousands of people were
so treated, until arsenicals were replaced by antibiotics in the
1940's.  The idea of "arsenic cancer" kept gaining strength to the
point that Fowler's solution and most other medical uses of arsenicals have been finally abandoned.

Arsenic's sister element, selenium (Se), was also impugned as
a cause of cancer from 1943 until very recently.  Last year, it
seemed appropriate to cite(19) for the Se situation, L. S. Kubie's
questioning statement, "The primary achievement of science is the
humility and honesty with which it corrects its own errors.  Is
this what makes science the greatest of all humanities?"  The As
problems pose even more room for correction of historic errors than
is the case with Se.

Lasagna, writing in terms of medical progress, stated that
preference for simple falsehoods over more complex truths is a
major weakness of our times.(1)  He quoted a prediction of a century ago, indicating that "...our times would be the age of the great
simplifiers and that the essence of tyranny would be the denial of
complexity".  The tenaciously held dogmas relating As and Se to
cause of cancer reflect such simple preferences.

## II.  HISTORIC ERRORS

Examples of blame falsely assigned to As include:

1.    Henry Butlin expanded in the 1880's on Percival Potts'
epidemiologic association of chimney sweeps' scrotal cancer with
exposure to something in soot.(2)  Butlin rejected J. A. Paris's
popularly accepted notion of "arsenic cancer" to prove that good
hygiene and protective clothing sufficed.  This led to discovery of
the carcinogenic polycyclic aromatic hydrocarbons (PAH) in soot and
tar.  Similarities in the historic association between PAH and As
cancer suggests that As was blamed for cancers due to PAH.(3)

2.    J. A. Paris's fanciful writings are still cited as the
first evidence for the carcinogenicity of As.(17,51)  Discovery
that Paris's description of 1820 actually fits Se and not As toxicity has failed to change things.  As a citation[1] from Paris shows,

---

[1] Paté Arsenicale.  This favorite remedy of the French surgeons
consists of 70 parts cinnebar, 22 sanguis craconis, and 8 of
arsenious acid, made into paste with saliva, at the time of apply-
ing it.  This combination, observes a periodic writer, is similar,
with the exception of the ashes of the soles of old shoes, to that
recommended by Father Cosmo, under the name "Pulvis Anti-
carcinomatosa."  Paris, J. A., Pharmacologia, London, 1820.

there was as much confusion about how As affects cancer in 1820 as there is now.

3.   Sir Ernest Kennaway worked unceasingly to learn the role of As in relation to cancer.  His bitter polemic with Wilhelm Hueper as to the meaning of J. A. Paris's writings of 1820 stands as mute testimony to the unacceptability of arsenic cancer to him.(5) Dr. Hieger, who worked with Kennaway, told me that Kennaway never subscribed to the carcinogenicity of As.  Hieger simply noted that evidence for the carcinogenicity of As is "hard to find".(6)

4.   Woglom(7) reported that coal tars low in As proved carcinogenic, whereas tars high in As failed to induce experimental cancers.  This followed similar work.(8)  To my knowledge, this important finding has not been confirmed or denied.

5.   Although I could find no mention of an association between As and cancer in the British Beer Poisoning of 1900, Satterlee in a retrospective study incorrectly cited that incident to try to prove the carcinogenicity of As.(9)

6.   The weakness of the association between prolonged arsenite therapy and cancer induction can be seen in the fact that, whereas, millions of people were so treated from 1786 on, fewer than 143 cases of so-called "arsenic cancer" were rounded up from the world's literature.(10)  Close scrutiny of the cases showed that some of these patients clearly never had As therapy.(10)  An example is entitled "Arsenic Cancer, a Case of".  Careful reading of the paper reveals no evidence that the patient in question was ever treated with an arsenical.(11)  The belief was so strong that anyone who developed cancer was simply assumed to have had arsenical therapy, which was then assumed to have caused the cancer.

7.   The calculated arsenite intake of 16 patients for whom Neubauer(11a) found records averaged 28 g $As_2O_3$, thousands of times more As, and in quite a different form from that ingested in foods.

TABLE 1

CHRONOLOGY BY WOODHOUSE(3) OF OCCUPATIONAL CANCER
AND LATENCY OF EXPOSURE

| Agent | Originator | Year | Latency in Years |
|-------|-----------|------|------------------|
| Soot | Pott | 1776 | Many Years |
| Arsenic | Paris | 1820 | 3-46 |
| Coal Tar | Volkman | 1875 | 1-50 |
| Paraffin Oil | Bell | 1875 | 3-25 |

A.    Unresolved Problems Relating to As and Se

Palmar and plantar keratoses and abnormal pigmentation were
occasional sequelae of massive arsenite therapy.  In such uses to
control leukemia, Goodman and Gilman(12) and the Merck Manual note
that beginning signs of arsenicism are overlooked in its application.  In the use of oxophenarsine hydrochloride to aid in the
regression of cancer, the acute toxicity is monitored.(13)  Both
agents have been discarded in medicine and are no longer available
in the United States.  Their safe return can come only via better
understanding of how arsenicals act in biology.  Because of the
close nutritional and biochemical interrelation between As and Se,
misunderstandings about them must first be clarified.

I referred a decade ago(10) to arsenophobia as the most virulent form of chemophobia.  We have yet to find a cure.  When I
wrote that review, the validity of these discoveries seemed clear.
They are even more clear now.

1.    J. A. Paris's 1820 imputation of cancer of the rumps in
horses and cattle do not fit toxicity of As, but do fit Se toxicity.(4)

2.    Both As and Se were reported at toxic levels in the beer,
brewing sugar, and the $H_2SO_4$ used to invert the brewing sugar in the
British Beer Poisoning of 1900.(10,15,16)  Yet sole blame was
assigned to As by the Royal Commission on Arsenical Poisoning in
1903.  This led to the setting of the world's first tolerance and
to later tolerances for As residues in food.

3.    Despite about 40 attempts to induce cancer experimentally
in animals with arsenicals, all have failed.(10,10a,17)  Nevertheless, the hope was expressed(17) that with luck, someone would be
able to do so.  Hueper assigned carcinogenicity to Se as irration-
ally as to As.  In doing so, he failed to discover that, if any-
thing, cancer mortality is inverse to the ambient bioavailability
of Se.(18,19,79,80)  The same may be true for As.(79a)

From an element nearly as firmly entrenched as a proven carcinogen as As, Se has emerged as of probable anticancer value.
Under some conditions, compounds of As and Se counteract each other's
toxicity.(21)  Under other conditions, toxicity may be aggravated.(22)
Under most conditions, excesses of Se are exhaled as dimethyl selenide, but in the presence of enough As, excretion is via the bile.
(23,24)  When toxicity is accentuated, the detoxification mechanisms
may be blocked.  Much remains to be learned along this line.

Excess arsenite is known to speed the respiratory decline of
excised tissues from animals deficient in Se and vitamin E.(25)
Yet research at this university showed inhibition of spontaneous
mammary tumor incidence in susceptible mice by high levels of either

Se or As.(*26,20*)  Such findings led to the concept that supplementary Se with vitamin E may protect against too much arsenite.(*19,27*)

The possibility that inhalation of $As_2O_3$ may predispose toward lung cancer, as cited by Pinto and Nelson(*28*) may be reflected in depletion of the Se-dependent enzyme, glutathione peroxidase. Such a sequence could be studied in animals using isotopically labeled As and/or Se and a technique such as that described by Bencko and Symon.(*29*)

## III. DO ARSENICALS HAVE VALUE AGAINST CANCER?

The inability to induce cancer experimentally with arsenicals seems to be accepted.  But the evidence in animals, indicating that arsenicals may decrease susceptibility to cancer(*10,16,27*) has been accorded little attention.  To my knowledge, there have been no research efforts to confirm or deny such unexpected value.  The possible value of lifeterm arsenical feeding to decrease the incidence of spontaneous lung cancer(*30*) seems to deserve consideration. No hazard was assigned to As from cigarette smoking.(*31*)  Lung cancer rate accelerated after the voluntary surcease in the use of arsenical pesticides by tobacco growers in the early 1950's.  Lung and other cancer rates were recently reported to be inverse to dietary As intakes.(*79a*)

## IV. IS ARSENIC AN ESSENTIAL NUTRIENT?

Evidence that arsenic deficiency could be induced in rats came in a preliminary way in 1975, in work by Nielsen, Givand, and Myron(*32*) at the USDA Human Nutrition Laboratory.  A diet with about 30 ppb As on dry basis was fed to rats in plastic cages.  Offspring from the As-deficient dams grew at reduced rates and had enlarged black spleens with greatly increased iron content.  The erythrocytes from such offspring at 12-15 weeks showed poor osmotic fragility, with lowered hematocrit.  An apparent hematopoietic effect of As was reported by Hove et al. (*33*) and by Skinner and McHargue.(*34*)

Anke, Grun, and Partschefeld made a manuscript available at the 1976 Missouri Trace Substances in Environmental Health Conference entitled "The Essentiality of Arsenic for Animals."  According to Dr. Anke of the University of Leipzig, this appeared in Archiv fur Tierernahrung, 1976, and is in press in Trace Substances in Environmental Health-X, University of Missouri, Columbia, 1977.  It reports that second generation female goats on a semisynthetic ration of less than 50 ppb As grew poorly and had reduced skeletal bone ash. Female minipigs on the As-low diet bore significantly smaller piglets than control minipigs on the diet supplemented with 350 ppb As. Only 58% of the As-deficient goats and 62% of the As-deficient minipigs were reported to give birth.  The spleens of the As-deficient goats were reported to contain more iron than those of the controls. The abstract ended with "Altogether we cannot help pointing out the essentiality of As for animals".

In a study by Leibscher and Smith(35) of the essentiality of trace elements, only in the way in which it was excreted was As judged as possibly essential. In this regard, it should be real- ized that As is one of the most ubiquitous of elements. As its natural distribution shows (see Table 2), whereas Se is avidly accumulated by animal tissues from the environment, arsenic is taken up sparingly. While Se is needed only by animals and certain microbes, As appears to be needed as much by plants as by animals. Arsenic follows phosphorus (P) closely in biology, and evidence(36,37) suggests that it may play an essential role in phosphorylations.

TABLE 2

DISTRIBUTION IN ROUGH APPROXIMATION
(Except for sea water, values are in ppm dry matter)

| Element | Sea Water | Earth's Crust | Animals | Plants |
|---------|-----------|---------------|---------|--------|
| As | 0.003 | 2-5 | 0.1-4.0 | 0.01-10 |
| Se | 0.0001-0.004 | 0.05 | 0.4-4 | 0.01-1 |
| P | 0.07 | 1,200 | 6,000-10,000 | 1,000-5,000 |
| S | 900 | 600-5,000 | 5,000-10,000 | 600-9,000 |

Seafood and fish have higher levels of As than shown.
Sea plants may contain up to 100 ppm As , as may seafood.
Rare Se-accumulator plants may have up to 10,000 ppm Se.

---

Although the use of food-additive arsenicals is limited to three species and a large part of their effectiveness is via disease con- trol, evidence that they also exert positive effects on food effic- iency seems secure.(10,38,39) Whether this is due to the As they contain remains to be learned.

Beneficial effects of As on plant growth have been long repor- ted(40,41) and confirmed by USDA studies.(42) Goldschmidt wrote eloquently(43) of the geochemistry of As, noting that forest humus may contain up to 300 ppm of As. He hypothesized that over time, this had led to the high content of As in fossil fuels. Coal, met- al ores and phosphorites all contain high levels of As. During years when the safe uses of arsenicals were in vogue, Greaves des- cribed the role of As in stimulating nitrogen-fixing organisms in the soil.(44) A little understood benefit of a single spraying of

lead arsenate is to hasten the maturation and sweetening of grape-
fruit and temple oranges in Florida.(45)

## V.  THE SUDDEN AND INEVITABLE VICTORY
## OF SUPERSTITION OVER SCIENCE

Because of blind fears, the use of arsenicals for the control of
undesirable grasses is little known except among turf specialists.
This useful effect was discovered only two decades ago(46,47) and
led to widespread control of POA ANNUA and crabgrass in fine turf,
such as golf courses and home lawns.  That there were no ill effects
to humans was testified to in a court case between the PAX Company
and the U. S. government, with PAX the temporary winner.(48)  In a
later incident, grass clippings treated with the PAX Company product were fed inadvertently to horses, resulting in their death.
This led to formation of an EPA PAX Company Arsenic Advisory Committee via NAS recommendation.  This committee reviewed the matter
carefully and reported to the EPA that with labeling to avoid mis-
use, such as the feeding of treated grass clippings to animals, the
product appeared safe and should be reregistered.  The EPA has not
published this report.  Soon thereafter, reports appeared alleging
carcinogenic hazards from exposure to inorganic arsenicals.(49,50)
Symposia relating adverse health effects to occupational exposure
to As and other pollutants followed.(51)  These furthered official
antagonism toward arsenicals and the demise of many arsenicals followed, with major producers withdrawing from arsenical manufacture.

The great disparity in the way government officials of different
training and interest view the toxic trace elements came clearly to
me in a letter from one government official who wrote in part:  "It
appears arsenophobia will outlast us all.  Selenium hasn't the same
poor press, and has a better chance for rational treatment.  I feel
as you do, that once we know more about the nutritional biochemistry
of arsenic and selenium and their interrelation, solutions for some
important human and animal health problems will become evident".

## VI.  ENVIRONMENTAL AND FOOD ASPECTS
## THE FDA TOTAL DIET STUDIES

A few reports have described As cycles in nature.(10,52,53)  A
concept of the As cycle (see Figure 1) with no attempt at quantita-
tion was prepared for the OST Panel on Arsenic of 1970-72, but not
previously published.  It should be considered in the light of
others(52,53) and of reports showing the mobility of As as volatile
arsines.(53)  Fossil fuel burning puts much $As_2O_3$ in particle form
into the air.  This is reflected in the high content of As in house-
hold dust, ranging from 0.2 to 618 ppm in one area.(35)  The very
high level of As from coal burning in Prague has been extensively
studied.(29)  It has not been positively associated with ill effects

in humans, even though the average was reported as 0.019 mg/m   of
air, well above the proposed limit for As in workroom air in the
United States.  Prior to the recent OSHA concern about "arsenic
cancer", little official concern was expressed concerning air pollution aspects of arsenic.(54)  However, despite the many causes
suggested to account for the rapid increase in lung cancer in recent years, preoccupation with As as a likely contributor persisted.(55)

## Arsenic Ecodiagram

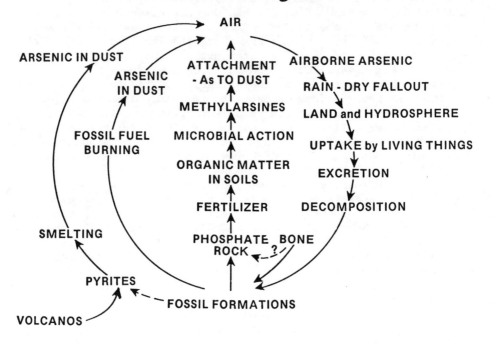

Figure 1

Vast amounts of As are distributed by Nature and by man's
activities.  None of these seems to account for the
apparent decrease in the level of As in American and
Canadian diets of recent years.  Reduction in the As
content of food phosphates may be a factor.  The use
of sulfuric acid made from Frasch process sulfur, rather
than from pyrites, in making phosphate fertilizers, will
have reduced this source of As in soil.  Frost, 1970.

Stokinger stressed the need for more reasonable governmental guidelines than now apply, using the limit for As in water as an example.(56)  Hueper and Payne(17) failed to cause any adverse effects in rats with 14 months of feeding of about 25 times the EPA limit for As in water.  Kanisawa and Schroeder(30) reported an actual reduction in lung cancer in animals getting 100 times the EPA limit for As in water as sodium arsenite lifeterm.  No difference in cancer mortality rate was reported among people in high-arsenic water areas in Lane County, Oregon, as compared with people in arsenic-low areas.(57)  The mayor of Fallon, Nevada wrote that people in Churchill County, Nevada, where arsenic-high wells abound, were found to have a better health record than people in other counties with nonarsenical water.

If As is an essential nutrient, the question becomes whether American diets provide enough.  Governmental objectives have been to minimize the level of As in foods in all possible ways.  Besides the imposition of tolerances for arsenicals in food and water, the level of As in food phosphates was reduced in the Food Chemical Codex from 10 to 3 ppm in the early 1960's.(10)  No significant residue of As in food has been reported for many years.(58,59)

The FDA Total Diet Study, representing foods from about 30 to 35 market baskets from 30 cities, is in its ninth year, and provides the FDA with an index to the levels of many pesticide residues and contaminants in major foods.  Dr. P. E. Cornelliusen of the FDA Bureau of Foods kindly sent me a report of the Total Diet Studies to 1973.  It was surprising to note from these that the calculated average intake of As from representative diets fell from about 63 $\mu$g As per day in the 1965-1970 period, to 10.1 $\mu$g As per day in the 1971-1973 period.  This is a surprising decrease.  According to Anke et al., a level of 100 ppb of As suffices to meet the needs of goats and pigs for reproduction and growth.  This would represent 100 $\mu$g of As in a kilo of dry diet, considerably more than is calculated for the Total Diet Studies in the United States.  The FDA report showed meats contributed more than half the estimated 10 $\mu$g daily intake of As, with dairy products, cereal grains and potatoes contributing lesser amounts.  By comparison, Se was reported to be present in the same dietary ingredients at 149.7 $\mu$g per day.  Lead and cadmium intakes were calculated to be 60 and 51 $\mu$g per day, with mercury about 8 $\mu$g.

When in Lund, Sweden in 1975, I was summoned to Germany to help toward acceptance of the safe feed additive use of four phenylarsonic acids by the EEC countries.  This was noted along with discussion of the reason that strict avoidance of As may be leading toward As deficiency in our diets.(60)

Canadian pesticide residue studies(60a) indicated that "...the

arsenic in the total diet would amount to no more than 30 μg per
person per day". As in the FDA Total Diet Studies analyses were
made of composites of foods representing normal Canadian diets.
All As levels were low and close to the limit of detection, which
was 0.01 mg/kg. Fish or seafood was not included. The Canadian
samplings were taken in 1970. The FDA Total Diets of 1974 were
reported to provide an average of 21 μg As per day.

Rarely, if ever, has public exposure to even very high levels
of As in the environment caused measurable toxicity in humans.
During the extreme local contamination with $SO_2$ and $As_2O_3$ around
Anaconda in the early 1900's, frank toxicity and liver levels of
63 ppm $As_2O_3$ were reported in horses and cattle.(61) The hair of
one horse had 460 ppm As and dust from a haystack had 9,190 ppm
$As_2O_3$. Similarly, toxicity in animals was reported for another
smelter indiscretion involving the uncontrolled emission of $As_2O_3$.(62)
In neither case was toxicity to humans reported.

Arsenicism from ingestion of water from mine tailings was reported.(63,63a) Study of blackfoot disease, with reports of high
cancer rate in people on As-high water in Taiwan became a cause
celebré, with National Cancer Institute support for many years.(64)
The Taiwan water which came via bamboo pipe, was reported to have
had enough impurities to fluoresce. Animals in New Zealand's geo-
thermal area, where the content of As in water, soil, and plants is
very high, showed signs of toxicity from undue ingestion of arsenical muds(65) but the people in that area were reported to have a
relatively low cancer rate.(10)

## VII. THE "ARSENIC CANCER" MYSTIQUE

It is impossible here to review all instances in which As has
been impugned of carcinogenicity. In most instances, alternate
causes appear. Lisella et al.(66) developed reasons why exposure
to arsenicals could not account for the many ills ascribed to them.
Durham(67) noted the reason that exposure to lead arsenate sprays
does not pose a hazard toward cancer. This was later proved to be
true in studies by the EPA Health Effects Group.(68) Orchardists long
exposed to lead arsenate sprays were found to have a better health
record, including lower cancer mortality, than others of the state
of Washington not so exposed. In reviewing the occurrence of As in
marine organisms, Penrose(69) reviewed the unreasonableness of tag-
ging arsenicals with unproven guilt. Pelfrene(70) provided a careful evaluation of the question regarding arsenic and cancer, calling
it still unanswered.

Pelfrene, a research oncologist, wrote that "...the arsenic
problem is not seen with a cold enough eye. The idea that arsenic
is a carcinogen remains uppermost and hence the attitude seems to
be that all data must tend to prove it. This myth has now plagued

scientific research on arsenic for 150 years". His review(70) cited
many of the vagaries and inaccuracies that led to the original idea.
He cited work by Samuels and Howarth(71) questioning the validity
of the conclusions of the retrospective study by Ott et al. (49)
He noted also that Fraumeni's(52) imputations involving As are
clouded by the concurrent exposure of workers to $SO_2$ and PAH, as
well as other known carcinogens. In short, "arsenic" has served
as not only the convenient, but the inevitable culprit. This
pattern fits Lasagna's(1) criterion of our tendency to prefer simple falsehoods to more complex truths. Kennaway referred to acceptance of the idea of "arsenic cancer" as "the strange viability of
the false".(5)

Rachel Carson's Silent Spring cited Hueper's(17) unshakable
acceptance of "arsenic cancer" as real evidence against the element.
In his book, Before Silent Spring, Whorton(72) provided a history of
the Congressional battle of some 50 years over the safety of arsenical pesticides. His review provides a realistic account of the
conflict between medical and consumer critics versus entomologists
and farmers, particularly over the safe use of lead arsenate.
Strange as it may seem, concern about the possible carcinogenicity
of inorganic arsenical pesticides did not become an issue until the
report by Ott et al. (49) This came 12 years after concern about
the safety of the organic arsenical food additive residues as possible hazards toward cancer.(73) All organic arsenicals studied
were shown to be noncarcinogenic; but concern about their tissue
residue continues unabated. This applies, even though research has
established that the phenylarsonic acids are excreted with little
or no change.(73)

By 1974, the fear of cancer, coupled with the arsenic mystique
as applied to inorganic arsenicals, had gained the support of many
agencies of government.(50) As Dr. Herman Kraybill graphically put
it, the Dow and Allied Chemical companies' retrospective allegations
concerning work exposure to arsenicals "put the last nail in the
coffin". Dr. Kraybill spoke at various OSHA hearings and symposia
as Scientific Coordinator for Environmental Cancer of the National
Cancer Institute.(50,51) As a long-time friend, I noted to Kraybill
that he mistakenly assigned carcinogenicity to trout for carbarsone
via early studies by John Halver. Halver's work and that of others
uncovered the powerful carcinogenicity of aflatoxin for trout. The
idea of involvement of carbarsone was then discarded as meaningless.
Such failures by prominent scientists to correct the mistakes of
science permits the "arsenic cancer" mystique to prevail, making
progress crawl. Rather than admitting that the association of As
with cause of cancer is pure speculation, those who call the shots
for government hedge their bets. This reflects the semantic power
of arsenophobia. Coupled with ignorance of the basic causes of
cancer and the role of As in biochemistry, it has slowed research
progress, and may have indeed "put the last nail in the coffin" for
the safe uses of arsenicals.

## VIII.  DISCUSSION

Schwarz' tabulation(14) of the essential trace elements shows As to be under special consideration.  Clearly, we need to be right about elements, especially those we fear without really knowing why.

Tabulation of the chronologic discovery of the essentiality of trace elements (Table 3) shows how fast this field is unfolding.

TABLE 3

ESSENTIAL ELEMENTS

Need Known By

| 1930 | C HOPKINS Ca Fe Mg Na Cl |
| 1940 | Mn Zn Cu Co F |
| 1950 | Mo |
| 1960 | Se Cr |
| 1970 | Vd Ni Sr? |
| 1975 | Si As? |
| 1976 | Cd Pb? |

Under Study

B Br Al Hg Li Ag

Au W Be Ti Rb Cs Ba

---

It was startling to discover in doing this review that As levels of United States and Canadian Total Diets have fallen to levels at which one may question their adequacy in terms of nutrition.  The samples of diet ingredients, beginning with meat, fish, and poultry, were from Atlanta, Baltimore, Boston, Buffalo Chicago, Cincinnati, Dallas, Denver, Kansas City, Los Angeles, Minneapolis, New Orleans, Newark, New York, Philadelphia, San Juan, San Francisco, and Seattle,  Within and between cities, the calculated As intake from Total Diets varied greatly.  For instance, 55.9 $\mu$g As per day was estimated for samples taken in January 1973, with none detectable for February and March samples.  The December San Francisco sampling was estimated to provide 29.2 $\mu$g As per day, but for the October and February samplings, none was detected.  No detectable As was reported for single samplings from five cities, for two samplings from three cities, and zero to traces for three cities.  New York and Philadelphia samples were reported to provide 26-28 $\mu$g As per day in single samplings.  By contrast, all samplings of meat, fish, and poultry from all cities provided from

27 to 88 μg per day of Se, with an average of 56.3. Although meat
was calculated to make up only 8% of the diet, it provided more than
half the As estimated from the diets. The AOAC official method of
analysis (11th Edition, 25.016 silver diethyldithiocarbamate) was
used, with sensitivity of 0.1 ppm $As_2O_3$ and results reported to the
nearest 0.1 ppm.

As noted above, As intakes of only about 10-30 μg per day would
represent deficiency judging from the animal studies cited. Certainly, such very low levels of As indicate that the traditional
goal to minimize the As intake has been achieved. This finding is
so recent that there has been little time to check it out with Dr.
Cornelliusen at the FDA, or with others. If the analyses are correct, the As level of this representative diet is very low. Earlier
information indicated that most plant and animal materials had app-
reciable levels of As.(81,82) Because arsenical pesticides were
used for so many years, data are provided in many instances compar-
ing treated versus nontreated samples in the NAS-NRC arsenic panel
report.(74) For more than 25 years, arsenicals have played a dim-
inishing role as pesticides. The 1973 Total Diet Study reflects
this avoidance of arsenicals, but there may be undiscovered factors
making for the apparent low level of As in human diets.

The 1973 WHO report on Trace Elements in Human Nutrition
accepted the traditional view that legal limits should be placed on
As in food and beverages. It stated, "Until further data are obtained, the maximum load of arsenic can be tentatively placed at
0.05 mg/kg bodyweight per day". For a 70 kg person, this means 3.5
mg As per day, far above the estimated As intake noted above.

That the value of Se to minimize the toxicity of mercury and
methyl mercury was enhanced by concurrent administration of As was
noted by Ganther.(45,76) Evidence that the As in lead arsenate
greatly reduced its toxicity, as compared with other lead salts,
was noted.(10) The noncarcinogenicity of lead arsenate was clearly
established.(77) The relatively low toxicity of lead arsenate was
shown long ago.(77a)

That excessive levels of arsenites and other arsenicals, far
beyond the physiological range, uncouple phosphorylations, poison
sulfhydryl- and Se-dependent enzymes, and cause teratogenic changes
and other metabolic lesions is well known. These ill effects of
too much As have dominated scientific attitudes toward the element.
Despite this, outstanding arsenical medications have gradually emerged. Recently, Zingaro(78) described dimethylarsino derivatives of
thio or seleno sugars that proved active against lymphoid leukemia
in National Cancer Institute studies. Related compounds repressed
carcinoma cells in culture systems.

Arsenicals have not caused mutagenesis against mammalian cells in Ames-type tests employing Salmonella and Saccharomyces indicator organisms.  Vitamin A, Se and other nutrients are known to cause teratogenic changes more dramatic than those reported for excess arsenicals.  Until we know far more about nutrition and cancer than we do now, it is futile to continue to speculate about such matters.

The complexity of the situation is illustrated by the findings of Schrauzer et al. (20) noting that arsenite inhibited spontaneous tumor incidence, but enhanced tumor growth, once started.  Excess zinc abolished the cancer-protecting value of Se and increased tumor incidence above that reported in Se-deficient mice.(79)  A recent communication from Schrauzer's laboratory(79) stated: "It should be noted that the age-correlated female breast cancer mortalities in 28 countries correlate with the apparent dietary arsenic intakes inversely, but not significantly (0.1)".  Significant correlation of breast cancer mortality with dietary zinc intake was observed for the same countries.  Most recently published epidemiological work revealed statistically significant inverse association of dietary arsenic intake with lung cancer mortality.(79a)

The vagaries of the As cycle in terms of man's activities seem as complex as for the Se cycle.(10,80)  Results to date of the FDA Total Diet Studies indicating constant Se intake but diminished As intake, suggest that more problems may reside in the As cycle than in that of Se.  Considering their in vivo reactivity, one may ask whether As and Se interact in emissions from fossil fuel burning.(19)  Little attention has been paid to the effects of geographic distribution or soil pH on the uptake of As by plants.  Unlike Se, As was found to be taken up by the air plant, Spanish moss.(80)

The estimated FAO/WHO daily tolerated doses of Hg, Pb, and Cd are all well above the estimated intake of As.  In terms of abundance of elements, arsenic ranks 18th in the universe, 20th on the earth's crust, 14th in sea water and 12th in the human body.  Considering its reactivity, one may ask whether the apparent decrease in the level of As in food may be due to its binding in inert form by one or more of the polluting elements.  Has a net loss in available As in the agricultural ecosystem over time resulted in a declining level of As in agricultural products?(53)

As noted many times, our tendency to be wrong about As has persisted so long that some event is needed to provide the liberating concept that As is more friend than foe.  The preface to one symposium(51) gave as basis for the meeting, "...and that the questions of what constitutes a safe level for carcinogens, such as arsenic, would also be considered".  At his luncheon talk at this

symposium, Dr. Russell Peterson of the Council on Environmental
Quality praised the Allied Chemical and Dow Company disclosures(49)
indicating that their work finally confirmed the Lee and Fraumeni(55)
evidence of "arsenic cancer". He noted that OSHA would propose a
new workroom standard of no more than 4 µg As/m$^3$ of air. Correspondence with Dr. Peterson and his staff failed to elicit much concern regarding whether or not As had really caused cancer. Considering the level of As in phosphates, one wonders if they can be
produced without exceeding that proposed limit for As in air.(83)

The position of As in the periodic chart, with properties like
those of P and N, assure its importance in biology. More organic
arsenicals, above 10,000, have been made than for any other trace
element. Despite arsenophobia, new uses continue to emerge. If
we will let it happen, As will prove to be as beneficial as Se is
proving to be. If we taboo As further, the consequences may be
more tragic than race prejudice has been.

## IX.   CONCLUSION

Adversary attitudes toward As have permeated society and are
supported by irrational bans and limits. None of these regulations
are scientifically justified. One result is that we may be nearing
deficiency levels of As in human diets. Action programs needed
include:

1.   Change attitudes toward arsenic. Consider As as a
     nutrient.

2.   Clarify the role of As in plant and animal nutrition.

3.   Clarify the As cycle with emphasis on explaining the
     apparent decrease in the As level in foods.

4.   Learn why arsenicals both diminish and accentuate the
     susceptibility to some forms of cancer. Do nutrient
     levels of As, Se, and antioxidants reduce suscepti-
     bility to cancer and other chronic disease?

5.   Remove the EPA limit for As in public drinking water.
     This costly and troublesome limit serves no useful
     purpose.[2]

---

[2] Dr. O. A. Levander of the USDA noted at a recent international
meeting on arsenic that the EPA limit for As in drinking water
appears to be below its nutrient need.

6.    Remove the tolerances for As in foods and the five-day re-
      moval stipulations regarding the safe uses of arsenical
      food additives.[3]  The tiny residues of these additives,
      which improve the well-being of the animals, cannot en-
      danger consumers.

7.    Advance the safe use of arsenicals in agriculture and
      industry.  Return the safe use of arsenicals to human
      and veterinary medicine.

*ADDENDUM*

The level of As in the FDA Total Diet Survey from 1965 to 1974
were reported by K. R. Mahaffey et al. (Environmental Health Perspectives 12, Page 63, 1975).  This noted that WHO/FAO tolerances had
not been set for As; also, that increased levels are undesirable.

The 1976 International Conference on Environmental Arsenic
prepublications dealt mainly with massive damage and threat of such.
W. R. Penrose, of Environment Canada, and E. A. Woolson, of USDA
described how aquatic forms of life evolved ways to metabolize "this
moderately toxic element" without biomagnification.  G. Lunde noted
how differently aquatic animals handle As from land animals.  A significant, positive report by S. Milham, Jr., found no health abnormalities among children living near the ASARCO smelter in Tacoma,
despite increased levels of As in hair and urine.  R. S. Braman
outlined advances in analytical methods to measure inorganic and
organic arsenicals (see also, ACS Symposium Series 7. E. A. Woolson,
Editor, American Chemical Society, Washington, 1975).

The NAS-NRC ARSENIC report(74) reflected the final environmental Impact Statement — INORGANIC ARSENIC, by the Department of
Labor's OSHA, which was issued in February 1977.  Both supported
the view that lowered exposure to As is in order as a health measure.  One EPA letter published with the OSHA pronouncement expressed
"environmental reservations", noting that no information was provided on possible effects on the nonoccupational environment.
R. L. Schauer's letter, published with the impact statement, noted
its complete lack of consideration of most environmental consequences.  Both of these very influential publications became so pre-

---

[3] One of the arsenical food additives has been used for decades
    in human medicine as Carbarsone[R] at levels far above any
    residues in animal tissues.

occupied with the possible adverse effects of some arsenicals that they overlooked the problems that society may face if further avoidance of As results. A more realistic appraisal of inorganic arsenic in relation to cancer is found in D. B. Clayson and P. Shubik (Cancer Detection and Prevention 1, Page 60, 1976).

*REFERENCES*

1.   Lasagna, L., Perspectives Biol. Medicine, Page 537, Summer,1976.

2.   Butlin, H., British Medical Journal 2, Page 66, 1892.

3.   Woodhouse, D. L., Progress in the Biological Sciences in Relation to Dermatology, A. Rock, Editor, University Press, Cambridge, England, Page 356, 1960.

4.   Frost, D. V., Nutrition Review 18, Page 129, 1960.

5.   Kennaway, E., Lancet 2, Page 769, 1942; 1, Page 599, 1943; Hueper, W. C., Lancet 1, Page 538, 1943.

6.   Heiger, I., Carcinogenesis, Academic Press, New York, 1961.

7.   Woglom, W. H., Arch. Path. Laboratory Medicine 2, Page 533,1926.

8.   Bierich, R., Klin. Wchnschr. 1, Page 2272, 1922.

9.   Satterlee, H. S., New England J. Medicine 263, Page 676, 1960.

10.  Frost, D. V., Federation Proceedings 26, Page 194, 1967.

10a. IARC Monograph-Evaluation of Carcinogenic Risk to Man, World Health Organization, Geneva, 1973.

11.  Nutt, W. H., Beattie, J. M. and Pye-Smith, R. J., Lancet 2, pp 210 and 282, 1913.

11a. Neubauer, O., Brit. J. Cancer 1, Page 192, 1947.

12.  Goodman, L. S. and Gilman, A., Pharmacologic Basis of Therapeutics, MacMillan, New York, 1935.

13.  Knock, F. E., et al., JAMA 224, Page 129, 1973; Oncology 30, Page 1, 1974.

14.  Schwarz, K., Federation Proceedings 33, Page 1748, 1974.

15. Frost, D. V., World's Poultry Science Journal 21, Page 139, 1965.

16. Frost, D. V., World Rev. Pest Control 6, Page 9, 1970.

17. Hueper, W. C. and Payne, W. W., Arch. Environmental Health 5, Page 445, 1962.

17a. Hueper, W. C., Occupational and Environmental Cancer of the Respiratory System, Springer-Verlag, New York, 1966.

18. Shamberger, R. J. and Frost, D. V., Canadian Medical Association Journal, 100, Page 682, 1969; Shamberger, R. J. and Willis, C. E., CRC Critical Review, Clinical Laboratory Science 2, Page 211, 1971.

19. Frost, D.V. and Ingvoldstad, D., Chemica Scripta 8A, Page 96, 1975.

20. Schrauzer, G. N., Bioinorganic Chemistry 5, Page 275, 1976.

21. Hill, C. H., Federation Proceedings 34, Page 2096, 1975.

22. Frost, D. V., Proceedings Cornell Nutrition Conference, Page 31, 1967.

23. Levander, O. A. and Bauman, C. A., Toxicology Appl. Pharmacology 9, pp 98 and 106, 1966.

24. Levander, O. A. and Argrett, L. C., Toxicology Applied Pharmacology 14, Page 308, 1969.

25. Schwarz, K., Vitamins and Hormones 20, Page 463, 1962.

26. Schrauzer, G. N. and Ishmael, D., Annals Clinical Laboratory Science 4, Page 441, 1974.

27. Frost, D. V., Feedstuffs 47(14), Page 20, 1975.

28. Pinto, S. S. and Nelson, K. W., Annual Review Pharmacology 16, Page 95, 1976.

29. Bencko, V. and Symon, K., Atmos. Environment 4, Page 157, 1970.

30. Kanisawa, N. and Schroeder, H. A., Cancer Research 27, Page 1192, 1967; 29, Page 892, 1969.

31. Smoking and Health, PHS Publication 1103, USGPO, Washington, 1974.

32. Nielsen, F. H., et al., Federation Proceedings 34(3), Abstr.3987, 1975.

33. Hove, E., et al., American J. Physiology 124, Page 205, 1938.

34. Skinner, J. T. and McHargue, J. S., American J. Physiology 145, Page 500, 1946.

35. Liebscher, K. and Smith, H., Arch. Environmental Health 17, Page 881, 1968.

36. Chan, T., et al., J. Biolog. Chemistry 244, Page 2883, 1969.

37. Dilley, R. A., Arch. Biochem. Biophysics 137, Page 270, 1970.

38. Peoples, S. A., The Use of Drugs in Animal Feeds, National Academy Science, Washington, D. C., Page 77, 1969.

39. Sullivan, T. W. and Al-Timimi, A. A., Poultry Science 59, Page 1582, 1972.

40. Stoklasa, J., Annals Agronomy 23, Page 471, 1897.

41. Stewart, J. and Smith, E. S., Soil Science 14, Page 111, 1922.

42. Woolson, E. A., et al., Soil Science Society America 37, Page 254, 1973.

43. Goldshmidt, V. M., Geochemistry, Oxford-Clarendon Press, Oxford, 1954.

44. Greaves, J. E., J. Agricultural Research 6, Page 389, 1916.

45. Reitz, H. J., Proceedings Florida Horticultural Society 49, 1949; 83, Page 15, 1970.

46. McNulty, I. R. and Rhodes, E. A., Utah Academy Proceedings 32, Page 125, 1955.

47. Hiltbold, A. E., Report to EPA Arsenic Advisory Committee, 1973.

48. Done, A. H. and Peart, A. J., Clinical Toxicology 4, Page 343, 1971.

49. Ott, M., et al., Arch. Environmental Health 29, Page 250, 1974.

50. Criteria for a Recommended Standard-Occupational Exposure to Inorganic Arsenic, NIOSH, Washington, 1973; Federal Register 40, Page 3391, 1975.

51. Carnow, B. W., Editor, Health Effects of Occupational Lead and Arsenic Exposure, USGPO, Washington, D. C., 1976.

52. Ferguson, J. F. and Gavis, J., Water Research 6, Page 1259, 1974.

53. Sandberg, G. R. and Allen, I. K., ACS Symp. Series 1975 (Arsen-
    ical Pesticide Symposium 1974), Page 70; CA 82, 119631Q, 1975.

54. Sullivan, R. J., et al., Air Pollution Aspects of Arsenic and Its
    Compounds, NAPCA Project, National Tech. Information Service,
    Springfield, Virginia, 1969.

55. Fraumeni, J. F., J. National Cancer Institute 55, 1039, 1975.

56. Stokinger, H. E., Science 174, Page 662, 1971.

57. Morton, W., et al., Cancer 37, Page 2523, 1976.

58. Duggan,R.E. and Weatherwax,J.R.,Science 157, Page 1006, 1967.

59. Johnson, R. D. and Manske, D. D., Pesticide Monitor Journal 9,
    Page 157, 1976.

60. Frost, D. V., Feedstuffs 58(14), Page 55, 1976.

60a. Smith, D. C., et al., Pesticide Science 3, Page 207, 1972.

61. Harkins, W. D. and Swain, R. E., J. American Chemical Assoc-
    iation 30, Page 928, 1908.

62. Birmingham, D. J. and Key, M. M., Arch. Dermatology 91,
    Page 457, 1965.

63. Borgono, J. M. and Greiber, R., Trace Substances in Environ-
    mental Health, V. D. Hemphill, Editor, University Missouri,
    Columbia, Page 13, 1971.

64. Yeh, S., National Cancer Institute Monograph 10, Page 81, 1963;
    Tseng,W.P.,et al.,J. National Cancer Institute 40,Page 453, 1968.

65. Grimmett, R. E. R., et al., New Zealand J. Science Technology
    21(3A), Page 137, 1939.

66. Lisella, F. S., et al., J. Environmental Health 34, 511, 1972.

67. Durham, W. F., Residue Reviews 4, Page 33, 1963.

68. Nelson, W. C., et al., J. Chron. Disease 26, Page 105, 1973.

69. Penrose, W. R., CRC Crit. Review Environmental Control 4,
    Page 465, 1973.

70. Pelfrene, A., J. Toxicology Environmental Health 1, Page 1003,
    1976.

71.  Samuels, S. and Howarth, C., Arch. Environmental Health 30,
     Page 423, 1975.

72.  Wharton, J. C., Before Silent Spring, Princeton University
     Press, 1974.

73.  Symposium "Feed Additives and Significance of Their Residues
     in Animal Tissues," J. Agr. Feed Chm. 11, Page 362, 1963.

74.  Arsenic, EPA 600/1-76-036, National Technology Information
     Service, Springfield, Virginia, 1976.

75.  Ganther, H. E., Nutrition Notes 11(3), Page 4, 1975.

76.  El-Begiarmi, M., et al., Poultry Science 53, Page 1921, 1974.

77.  Kroes, R., et al., Food Cosmetic Toxicology 12, Page 671, 1974.

77a. Groves, K., et al., J. Agricultural Research 73, Page 159, 1946.

78.  Zingaro, R. A., Chemica Scripta 8A, Page 51, 1975.

79.  Schrauzer, G. N., et al., Bioinorganic Chemistry 6, Page 265, 1976.

79a. Schrauzer, G. N., White, D. A. and Schneider, C. J., Bio-
     inorganic Chemistry 7, Page 35, 1977.

80.  Frost, D. V., CRC Critical Review Toxicology 1, Page 467, 1972.

81.  Schroeder, H. A. and Balassa, J. J., J. Chron. Dis. 19,
     Page 83, 1966.

82.  Stevens, L. J., et al., Pesticide Monitor Journal 4,
     Page 145, 1970.

83.  Tremarne, T. H. and Jacobs, H. D., USDA Tech. Bulletin 781,
     USGPO, Washington, D. C., 1941.

CHAPTER 19


THE INFLUENCE OF NUTRITIONAL FACTORS

ON PULMONARY ADENOMAS IN MICE

Frederic A. French

Mount Zion Hospital and Medical Center
San Francisco, California   94115

I.   INTRODUCTION

This research had its inception two decades ago in an interest
in the possibility that heterocyclic nitrogen bases in cigarette
tobacco smoke might be carcinogens or cocarcinogens.  An abbreviated
schematic diagram of the enzymatic, bacterial, and pyrolytic degradation of nicotine in tobacco is shown in Figure 1.  A number of
these substances have an unmethylated pyridine ring that is C substituted in the 3 position; hence, they are potential candidates
for the *in vivo* formation of pseudo NAD and NADP, and could lead
to metabolic perturbations via this mechanism.  The compounds en-
closed in dotted or solid lines may be regarded as potential carcinogens.  Interestingly, the concentration of nicotinic acid and
its vitamin-like derivatives (indicated on the right side of Figure 1) is quite low in cigarette tobacco, while cigar tobacco is
the richest known natural source of nicotinic acid.

In mammals, tryptophane can serve as a precursor of nicotinic
acid and the functional derivatives of nicotinamide.  This well-
known pathway becomes critically important when the dietary supply
of niacin becomes inadequate.  The metabolism of tryptophane toward
NAD is also subject to a number of modifications, depending on the
nutritional status of the animal.  The aspects of tryptophane metabolism pertinent to this study are shown in Figure 2.  Allen et
al.(1) showed that 3-hydroxyanthranilic acid, 3-hydroxykynurenine,
3-hydroxy-2-aminoacetophenone, and xanthurenic acid 8-methylether
are active bladder carcinogens in mice.  8-Hydroxyquinaldic acid
may be regarded as a candidate on a structural basis.  More recently,
Kuznezova(2) noted the potent mutagenic effects of 3-hydroxykynuren-
ine and 3-hydroxyanthranilic acid on cell suspensions from seven- to

nine-week-old human embryos.  Hence, it may be hypothesized that in mammals, there is a complex built-in carcinogenic system that would be activated by a niacin deficiency and suppressed by adequate or by pharmacological levels of niacin.

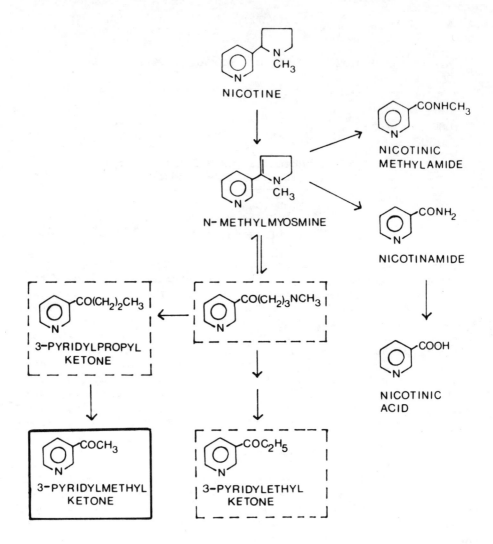

Figure 1

Some Products of Degradation of Nicotine

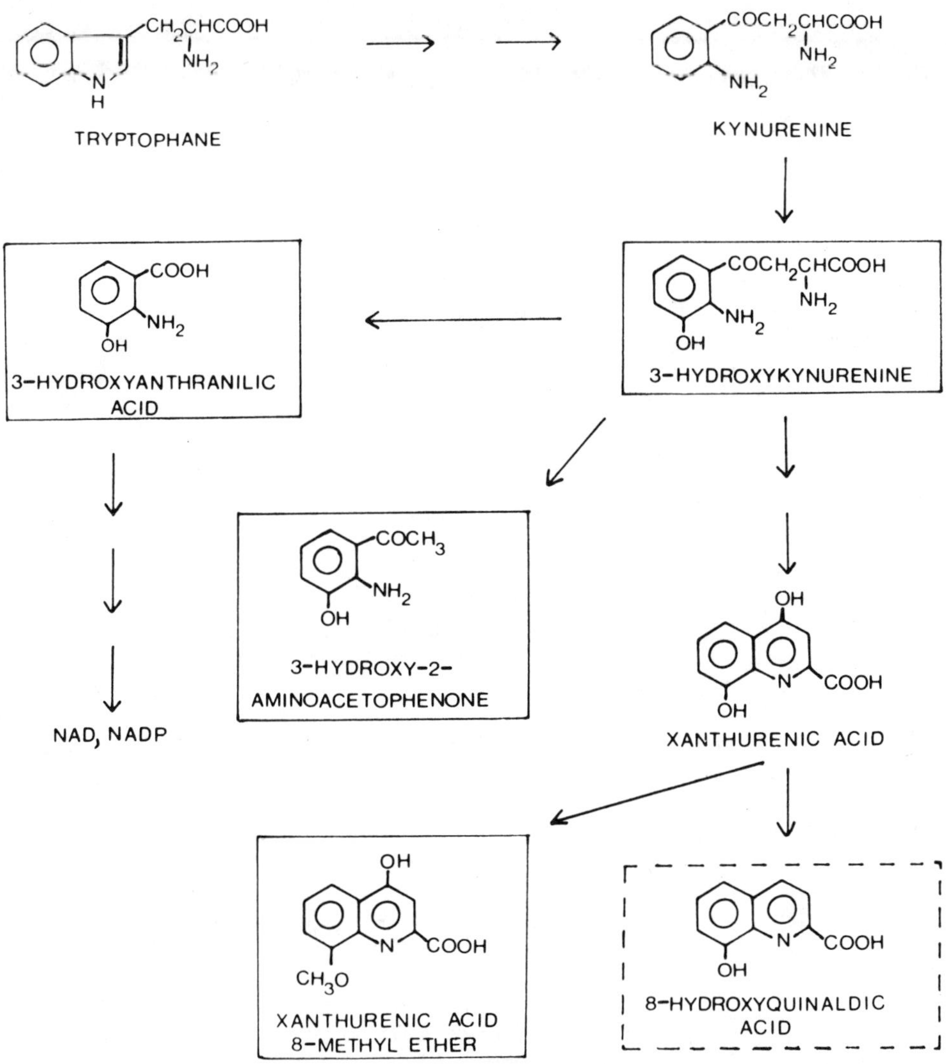

Figure 2

Some Metabolites of Tryptophane

The next step was to select and develop an experimental test system for the study of these and other potential carcinogens and anticarcinogens. It was necessary to choose a system of sufficient duration for these effects to become manifest. The urethane-induced pulmonary adenoma system in mice (particularly A/He) was selected for study. Extensive basic studies had been conducted by Nettleship

et al.(*3*), by Rogers(*4, 5*), by Shimkin and Polissar(*6-8*), and by
Tannenbaum and Silverstone.(*9*)  Rogers noted in his first paper
that fasting did not affect the yield of tumors.  He also noted that
high age-dependent effects observed in weanling mice became relatively slight in mice who were 10 or more weeks old at the time of urethane injection.

## II.  METHODS

Over a period of time, with considerable preliminary experimentation, a system suitable for extensive screening was developed.
It was generally difficult to procure large groups of A/He mice with
narrow birthdate ranges.  This source of variation was held to a
practical minimum.  Each treated and each control group contained
approximately 40 mature mice.  A single dose of 1,000 mg/kg urethane
was given ip to all the mice at the start of the experiment.  The
periods of therapy usually ranged from 11 to 16 weeks.  At the termination of the experiments, the mice were autopsied and the lungs
fixed in Fekete's modification of Tellyeniczky's fluid.(*3*)  Surface
tumors with diameters equal to or greater than 0.25 mm were counted,
using a binocular microscope at 10X.  From these data, the average
number of tumors per mouse was computed.  A few experiments were
also conducted on Swiss mice.  Groups of 80 were required to reduce
the variance to a tolerable level.

Kevin McCarty, of this laboratory(*10*), made an extensive study
of statistical approaches to handling these data.  For both strains
of mice, a negative binomial distribution (NBD) gave a much better
fit to the data than a Poisson distribution.  His NBD method was
used to compute the values given herein.  The t test, F test, and
$\chi^2$ test were used where applicable.  The index of evaluation was a
percent reduction in mean tumors per mouse relative to controls.

## III.  RESULTS AND DISCUSSION

In very preliminary experiments(*11*) it appeared that a niacin-
deficient diet increased the number of pulmonary adenomas in A/He
mice and that the niacin analogs, 3-pyridylmethylketone and 3-
pyridylethylketone reduced this effect.  3-Pyridylmethylketone forms
a pseudo DPN that is both more and less functional in particular enzyme systems than is DPN.  Additionally, some of it is oxidized *in
vivo* to nicotinic acid.  In these experiments, no lower size limit
was used in tumor counting.  The mice on these regimes were frequently fragile, in poor thrift, and mortality was often in the 10% to
25% range.  Consequently, these effects can be only regarded as in-
dicative and not statistically significant.  Because of the diffi-
culty in handling mice over long periods of time on niacin antagonists or niacin-deficient diets, this line of study was abandoned and
attention was directed to the effect of excess nicotinamide.  In this

early work it was found that excess nicotinamide sharply reduced
the number of pulmonary adenomas per mouse.  This finding withstood
the test of time, more precise experimental techniques, and adequate
statistical evaluation.

The effect of nicotinamide on urethane-induced pulmonary adenomas in Swiss, A/He, and A/Jax mice at 0.25% and 0.4% in the drinking water is remarkably constant in spite of the wide range of base
lines, as shown in Table 1.  It is especially noteworthy that nicotinic acid is inactive in this system.  The control values increase
with the level of inbreeding from Swiss to A/Jax mice.  The data
were insufficient to define a dose-response relation.  In toxicity
studies, nicotinamide could be given at levels as high as 8% for a
few days, but for periods of many weeks, the practical upper limit
is 2% in the diet.  In Table 2 , the data show that pretreatment with
nicotinamide has no effect, and that the observed effect is proportional to the duration of treatment post urethane.  The expression,
$y = 6.24-0.217x$ (where y = mean tumors per mouse, x = weeks of
treatment) was derived by regression analysis.  The correlation co-
efficient is -0.974.  Consequently, the validity of a treatment
time-effect relationship appears to be definite.  An additional
experiment was carried over four generations with Swiss mice receiving 0.25% nicotinamide in the drinking water from the 4th to the
20th week, giving urethane at nine weeks.  The average reduction in
the number of pulmonary adenomas was 42.6%, with no significant difference among generations.

Originally, the mechanism of the nicotinamide effect was obscure.  Nicotinamide plays so many roles in intermediary metabolism
that it was not possible to single out any process that might be a
key to its carcinostatic role.  It was suggested that it might be
acting through methyl group depletion.  This is clearly disproved
by the first experiment in Table 4.  In this experiment, 2.5% choline
dihydrogen citrate in the diet had no significant effect on the
therapeutic effect of 0.25% nicotinamide in the drinking water.  The
basic investigations of Kerr(12,13),Craddock(14) , and particularly,
of Halpern and colleagues(15-18) led to the discovery by Halpern's
group that nicotinamide, in addition to a nondialyzable factor, is
a potent inhibitor of tumor-derived tRNA methylase.  I feel that at
least part of the carcinostatic activity of nicotinamide in our experiments is due to this mechanism.  It is interesting to note that
the nicotinamide-treated mice were exceptionally thrifty and healthy.

A number of metabolites and other compounds were negative at
the following doses and modes of administration:

| | | |
|---|---|---|
| Calcium d-pantothenate | 0.02% | drinking water |
| Pyridoxine hydrochloride | 0.05% | "        " |
| Chromium(III)hexaurea chloride | 0.0033% | "        " |
| Ascorbic acid | 0.5% | "        " |

| | | |
|---|---|---|
| Sodium ascorbate | 2% | diet |
| Calcium ascorbate | 1, 2, and 4% | " |
| Thiamin hydrochloride | 0.05% | " |
| Riboflavin | 0.05% | " |
| p-Aminobenzoic acid | 0.25% | " |
| Cod liver oil | 1% | " |
| Mixed tocopherols | 0.24% | " |
| Ammonium dihydrogen phosphate | 3.4% | " |
| D-glucoronolactone | 0.5% | " |
| Betaine (anhydrous) | 1.5% | " |
| Methionine | 1% | " |
| Cyanocobalamin | 7 mg/kg | ip ( x week) |
| Disodium calcium EDTA | 250 mg/kg | ip (1 x day) |

The negative findings for betaine and methionine are particularly interesting in view of the positive results obtained with choline.

The results of experiments with choline and inositol are given in Table 3. The mechanism of action of choline in these experiments is not known, but the tumorigenic effect of choline deficiency is well documented. The early study by Copeland and Salmon(19) showed that prolonged choline deficiency in rats led to the appearance of a variety of neoplasms including primary carcinoma of the lung. Malachovskis(20) noted an inhibitory effect of choline against sarcoma M-1 in rats. Stein-Werblowsky(21) found the tumor inhibitory factor in post-coital fluid to be phosphorylcholine. Tyihak(22) found high concentrations of choline and betaine in red beets. He attributed the clinical benefits observed in cancer patients fed high levels of red beets and red beet juice to these components. In our laboratory, we noted that dietary choline dihydrogen citrate could be raised to 25% to 40% before ill effects were observed. When the dosage was reduced to 16%, normal eating, drinking and weight gain returned. Whatever the mechanism or mechanisms of action may be, supra-adequate choline would be helpful in the maintenance of cellular integrity.

myo-Inositol, in toxicity studies, was tolerated at levels as high as 40% in the diet; 10 times the maximum dose used in these experiments. As in the case of choline, the mechanism of action is not known. myo-Inositol is in a complex relation to carbohydrate metabolism and via myo-inosose-2 is in balance with scyllo-inositol in many tissues. The maintenance of cellular and subcellular membranes appears to be a primary role. Laszlo and Leuchtenberger(23) found that inositol had an inhibitory effect on sarcoma 180 in female Rockland mice when given intravenously at approximately 5-50 mg/kg.

TABLE 1

EFFECT OF NICOTINAMIDE AND NICOTINIC ACID ON URETHANE-INDUCED PULMONARY ADENOMAS IN MICE

| Experiment | Mouse Strain | No. Mice | Dose[a] | Weeks Treated[b] | Weight Change (g) | Mort. | Mean Lung Tumors per Mouse (±SE) | % Reduction | P |
|---|---|---|---|---|---|---|---|---|---|
| Nicotinamide | Swiss | 80 | 0.25% | 15 (-4) | +12.9 | 3 | 3.17 ± 0.33 | 42.3 | <<0.001 |
| Controls | | 80 | | | +11.9 | 3 | 5.49 ± 0.53 | | |
| Nicotinamide | A/He | 41 | 0.25% | 16 (-5) | +1.9 | 0 | 4.37 ± 0.57 | 39.3 | 0.005 |
| Nicotinic acid | A/He | 41 | 0.25% | 16 (-5) | +2.2 | 3 | 7.24 ± 0.79 | -0.6 | >0.90 |
| Controls | | 41 | | | +2.7 | 0 | 7.20 ± 0.82 | | |
| Nicotinamide | A/He | 40 | 0.25% | 13 (-2) | -0.7 | 3 | 3.40 ± 0.37 | 42.0 | <<0.001 |
| Controls | | 42 | | | +0.1 | 0 | 5.86 ± 0.42 | | |
| Nicotinamide | A/Jax | 37 | 0.4% | 17 (-1) | +3.7 | 1 | 5.97 ± 0.61 | 44.5 | <<0.001 |
| Controls | | 36 | | | -0.3 | 2 | 10.76 ± 0.70 | | |
| Nicotinamide | A/Jax | 40 | 0.4% | 14 (-1) | +1.9 | 1 | 7.56 ± 0.63 | 41.5 | <<0.001 |
| Controls | | 50 | | | +2.4 | 4 | 12.93 ± 0.80 | | |
| Nicotinamide | A/Jax | 30 | 2.0% | 14 (-3) | +2.0 | 6 | 3.63 ± 0.48 | 65.5 | <<0.001 |
| Controls | | 32 | | | +3.4 | 0 | 10.53 ± 0.89 | | |

a Nicotinamide or nicotinic acid given in the drinking water except in the last experiment in which nicotinamide was mixed with the powdered diet.

b No. in parentheses: weeks started before urethane.

TABLE 2

EFFECT OF VARYING TREATMENT SCHEDULE OF NICOTINAMIDE
ON URETHANE-INDUCED PULMONARY ADENOMAS IN MICE
(0.25% in Drinking Water)

| Treatment Period[a] (Started Relative to Urethane) | Weight Change (g) | Mort. | Mean Lung Tumors per Mouse (±SE) | % Reduction | P |
|---|---|---|---|---|---|
| 13 weeks (2 weeks before) | -0.7 | 3 | 3.40 ± 0.37 | 42.0 | ≪0.001 |
| 10 weeks (2 days after) | +1.9 | 2 | 3.78 ± 0.39 | 35.5 | <0.01 |
| 9 weeks (2 weeks after | -0.6 | 1 | 4.51 ± 0.39 | 23.0 | <0.05 |
| 4 days (2 days before to 2 days after) | +0.4 | 0 | 6.48 ± 0.59 | +10.6 | >0.10 |
| Controls | +0.1 | 0 | 5.86 ± 0.42 | | |

[a] 40 mice used in each treated group and 42 in controls.

A few experiments were conducted with combinations of choline, inositol, and nicotinamide at the lower dose levels. These data are presented in Table 4. All of the combinations were active per se. The data are not sufficient for making positive assertions about the efficacy of combinations; however, the question is open about the combined effects of optimum levels of nicotinamide, inositol, and choline, singly or in various combinations.

In summary, individually, nicotinamide, choline, and inositol in protracted treatment are potent inhibitors of pulmonary adenomas in mice. The effect of nicotinamide is specific and not shared by nicotinic acid. The presence or absence of pharmacological levels of methyl donors is not involved. Numerous other vitamin and vitamin-like factors are not active in this test system. In view of the results, it would appear desirable to conduct further investigations in this specific area. Many metabolites and trace metal effects were not explored. Summed over a large number of control values, it was noted that mice on natural chows had significantly

TABLE 3

EFFECT OF CHOLINE AND INOSITOL IN THE DIET ON URETHANE-INDUCED PULMONARY ADENOMAS IN MICE

| Experiment | Mouse Strain | No. Mice | Dose | Weeks Treated[a] | Weight Change (g) | Mort. | Mean Lung Tumors per Mouse (±SE) | Reduction | P |
|---|---|---|---|---|---|---|---|---|---|
| Choline dihydrogen citrate | A/He | 40 | 2.5% | 13(-2) | -1.3 | 0 | 3.40 ± 0.37 | 42.0 | <<0.001 |
| Controls | | 42 | | | +0.1 | 0 | 5.86 ± 0.42 | | |
| Choline bitartrate | A/He | 40 | 2.5% | 14(-3) | +2.2 | 0 | 7.60 ± 0.57 | 24.4 | <0.001 |
| Controls | | 40 | | | +2.3 | 0 | 10.05 ± 0.59 | | |
| myo-Inositol | A/He | 40 | 0.25% | 15(-4) | +2.8 | 0 | 7.10 ± 0.52 | 36.0 | <<0.001 |
| Controls | | 40 | | | +4.1 | 0 | 11.10 ± 0.71 | | |
| myo-Inositol | A/He | 37 | 0.25% | 15(-4) | +7.6 | 1 | 7.33 ± 0.66 | 29.9 | <0.001 |
| Controls | | 38 | | | +6.2 | 1 | 10.46 ± 0.63 | | |
| myo-Inositol | A/Jax | 31 | 4.0% | 14(-3) | +4.0 | 0 | 4.84 ± 0.47 | 54.0 | <<0.001 |
| Controls | | 32 | | | +3.4 | 0 | 10.53 ± 0.89 | | |

a No. in parentheses: weeks started before urethane.

TABLE 4

EFFECT OF COMBINATIONS OF NICOTINAMIDE, INOSITOL, AND CHOLINE
ON URETHANE—INDUCED PULMONARY ADENOMAS IN A/He MICE

| Experiment | No. Mice | Dose [a] | Weeks Treated [b] | Weight Change (g) | Mort. | Mean Lung Tumors Per Mouse (±SE) | % Reduction | P |
|---|---|---|---|---|---|---|---|---|
| Nicotinamide Choline dihydrogen citrate | 40 | 0.25% 2.5% | 13(-2) | -1.3 | 3 | 3.59 ± 0.40 | 38.7 | <0.001 |
| Controls | 42 | | | +0.1 | 0 | 5.86 ± 0.42 | | |
| Nicotinamide myo-Inositol | 39 | 0.25% 0.25% | 13(-2) | +0.6 | 0 | 5.69 ± 0.56 | 53.6 | <<0.001 |
| Choline bitartrate myo-Inositol | 39 | 2.5% 0.25% | 13(-2) | +0.8 | 1 | 6.59 ± 0.53 | 46.2 | <<0.001 |
| Nicotinamide Choline bitartrate myo-Inositol | 40 | 0.25% 2.5% 0.25% | 13(-2) | +0.7 | 0 | 5.88 ± 0.67 | 52.0 | <<0.001 |
| Controls | 40 | | | +2.0 | 0 | 12.25 ± 0.67 | | |

[a] Nicotinamide given in the drinking water; choline and inositol in the powdered diet.

[b] No. in parentheses: weeks started before urethane.

fewer adenomas than mice on synthetic (casein-based) diets. One may ask the question: Are there missing factors or balances of possible importance to our understanding of carcinogenic and anti-carcinogenic processes?

Some of the material in this paper was published in abstract form in the following:

F. A. French, IRCS (73-5) 6-8-4, 1973.

F. A. French, IRCS (73-9) 8-12-3, 1973.

*ACKNOWLEDGEMENTS*

The early portions of this research were supported by the Tobacco Industry Research Committee, the American Cancer Society, and the Damon Runyan Memorial Fund; later portions were published by the National Cancer Institute (Grant CA-03287).

The author gratefully appreciates the excellent technical assistance of June French, Arvia Hosking, Douglas French, and Kevin McCarty.

*REFERENCES*

1.  Allen, M. J., Boyland, E., Dukes, C. E., Horning, E. S. and Watson, J. G., British J. Cancer 11, Page 212, 1957.

2.  Kuznezova, L. E., Nature 222, Page 484, 1969.

3.  Nettleship, A., Henshaw, P. S. and Meyer, H. C., J. National Cancer Institute 4, Page 309, 1943.

4.  Rogers, S., J. Exp. Medicine 93, Page 427, 1951.

5.  Rogers, S., Ibid 105, Page 279, 1957.

6.  Polissar, M. J. and Shimkin, M. B., J. National Cancer Institute 15, Page 377, 1954.

7.  Shimkin, M. B. and Polissar, M. J., Ibid 16, Page 75, 1955.

8.  Ibid Ref. 7, 21, Page 595, 1958.

9.  Tannenbaum, A. and Silverstone, H., Cancer Research 18, Page 1225, 1958.

10.  McCarty, K. IRCS (73-11) 8-12-5, 1973.

11.  French, F. A. and Freedlander, B. L., Proceedings American Society Cancer Research 3, Page 21, 1959.

12.  Kerr, S. J., Biochemistry 9, Page 690, 1970.

13.  Kerr, S. J., Proceedings National Academy Science 68, 406, 1971.

14.  Craddock, V. M., Nature 228, Page 1264, 1970.

15.  Chaney, S. Q., Halpern, B. C., Halpern, R. M. and Smith, R. A., Biochemistry and Biophysics Research Comm. 40, Page 1209, 1970.

16.  Halpern, R. M., Chaney, S. Q., Halpern, B. C. and Smith, R. A., Ibid. 42, Page 602, 1971.

17.  Buch, L., Streeter, D., Halpern, R. M., Simon, L. N., Stout, M. G. and Smith, R. A., Biochemistry 11, Page 393, 1972.

18.  Murai, J. T., Jenkinson, P., Halpern, R. M. and Smith, R. A., Biochemistry and Biophysics Research Comm. 46, 999, 1972.

19.  Copeland, D. H. and Salmon, W. D., American J. Pathology 22, Page 1059, 1946.

20.  Malachovskis, A., Tr. Inst. Onkol. Lit. SSR 2, Page 43, 1961.

21.  Stein-Werblowsky, R., European J. Cancer 6, Page 445, 1970.

22.  Tyihak, E., Naturwiss. 51, Page 315, 1964.

23.  Laszlo, D. and Leuchtenberger, C., Science 97, Page 515, 1943.

CHAPTER 20

IODINE AND MAMMARY CANCER

Bernard A. Eskin

Medical College of Pennsylvania
Philadelphia, Pennsylvania  19129

## I.  INTRODUCTION

While iodine has been found in lower prechordates, no identi-
fiable physiologic influence of the element is recognized until the
level of amphibians.  Organified iodine is required for the meta-
morphosis of the tadpole to the adult frog.  Iodinated compounds
are essential to growth and development of most vertebrates, and
iodine levels temper these metabolic changes.

In order to properly function and form the characteristic iodinated secretions of thyroxine ($T_4$) and triodothyronine ($T_3$), iodine must be adequately present in the circulating blood.  Iodine
deficiency is expressed by the development of a "goiter", which is
hypertrophy or hyperplasia of the thyroid parenchyma.  The formation
of a "goiter" is an effort of the body to conserve the available
iodine stores and secrete the $T_4$ and $T_3$ needed to maintain a euthyroid state.  Kidney excretion of iodine is minimized and recycling of the precious element, in various forms, continues until
iodine is made available again to the system.  Activity of the thyroid gland is controlled by pituitary thyroid-stimulating hormone
(TSH).  Release of $T_4$ from the pituitary is, in turn, dependent on
the levels of free $T_4$ and $T_3$.  The pituitary/thyroid axis is unique
in that there is greater intrinsic pituitary control than in other
endocrine systems.  TSH secretion is inversely proportional to metabolic effects of $T_4$ and $T_3$.  The hypothalamic effluent, thyroid-
releasing hormone (TRH), exerts only a modulatory influence on the
pituitary and is not the final regulator of feedback.

In the higher vertebrates, it was thought that the synthesis of iodinated compounds was limited to the thyroid gland. Since the thyroid gland can trap the greatest load of iodine into its cell transport system, it normally serves as the active reservoir for iodine. Currently, the biochemical and physiological action of the iodinated compounds have been studied at end organs as well.(1) In addition, iodine has now been found, in measurable amounts, in the salivary glands, gastric mucosa, liver, certain tumors, and in the ovaries and testes.(2)

In several laboratories, including our own, iodine has been shown to be present in breast tissues. Using tissue slices,(3) autoradiography,(4) and radioactive iodine uptakes,(5,6) iodine has been measured and found to be present, in moderate amounts, but not in the abundance seen in the thyroid gland. The biochemical transport and metabolism of iodine by the breasts resemble, at a quantitatively lower level, those seen in the thyroid gland.

Laboratory experiments show that an inadequate supply of iodine, due to an iodine-deficient diet or perchlorate blockade, results in focal atypia and dysplasia of the breast in rodents.(6,7,8) It thus appears that maintenance of the optimum structure and function of the breast requires the presence of continuous and specific amounts of iodine. This *iodine effect* has been shown to depend on a secretion of TSH from the pituitary and responds negatively to relative and absolute reduction in TSH.(5)

From this basic information, it became apparent that iodine serves not only as an incidental element, responsible for growth and development, but may in itself, be involved in the intracellular metabolism of certain tissues, and hence, in the normalcy of these structures. The research from our laboratory concerns the activities of iodine in mammary glands and, specifically, the carcinogenicity and cocarcinogenicity of the conditions caused by modifications in iodine availability. The work to be reviewed and presented will be divided into (1) the experimental histology; (2) metabolic activity; and (3) clinical responses in altered iodine conditions.

## II.   EXPERIMENTAL HISTOLOGY

### A.   Carcinogenicity

Basic research performed in our laboratory, and since confirmed by others, has shown that iodine deficiency from dietary restriction produces specific changes in pubertal rat breasts.(7,8) The results have consisted of dysplastic changes, either atrophic or hyperplastic, and sometimes atypical. In the presence of estrogen treatment, the responding histology approaches that of a neoplastic state. Concomitantly with this work, the possibility that the dysplastic changes are secondary to hypothyroidism caused by iodine deprivation

was tested by inducing hypothyroidism in the presence of iodine.(7)
The histologic changes seen in the mammary glands of the hypothyroid
rats appeared to be distinctly different from those that were seen
in the breasts of the iodine-deficient animals which were euthyroid,
as indicated by serum thyroid function measurements.  The results
of this work suggested the probability that iodine itself directly
influences breast histology.

Further confirmation of these conclusions are presented by the
utilization of perchlorate to prevent iodination of the affected
tissues in rats.(6)  Breast changes were related to the percentage
of the effectiveness of the blockade, increased atypia occurring
with reduced iodine availability.  These histologic changes were
greatest in those breasts rendered euthyroid by thyroxine replacement, thus clearly indicating the necessity of iodine itself for
maintenance of normal breast development.

Recent research from our group employed animals whose ages
corresponded to mature human adults.  With increasing age of the
rats, in iodine-deficient breasts, even more evidence of atypical
changes in the epithelium occurred.(9)  This is seen in many foci
in the "menopausal" age group.  With the use of perchlorate and,
hence, the iodine blockade, statistically significant increases in
periductal fibrous overgrowth in trapping adjacent lobules with
aberrant ductular proliferation, sclerosing adenosis, and microcyst
formation takes place.  All are strongly reminiscent of the analogous fibrocystic disease in the human.

But further, there are areas in this group of atypical lobules
showing hyperchromatism, enlargement of nuclei, altered nuclear-
cytoplasmic ratios, increased mitosis, and loss of polarity of the
epithelium.  Some of the lobules exhibited papillomatosis with poorly polarized epithelium.  In one breast from this menopausal group,
there is a focus of a lobule to a histologically malignant pattern,
completely apart from the adenosis.

In all these studies, termination of either dietary iodine restriction or perchlorate results in variable modest return toward
the normal tissue structure.  Use of thyroxine ($T_4$) results in enhancement of the already existing abnormal changes, particularly if
the amount given is greater than maintenance requirements.(10) Parallel replacement of iodine with the several iodine-deficient diets
used results in normal control breast histology.(5)  Additional iodine levels (2-6 x normal) show no measurable change.

Steroidal estrogen therapy as estradiol-17β($E_2$) causes hyperplasia of the mammary gland ducts in normal estrus rats; however,
$E_2$ enhances the glandular dysplasias seen in iodine deficiency, and
to a lesser extent, in iodine blockade therapy.(11)  The consideration of estrogen-iodine interaction in breast tissue will be dis-

cussed later.

Thus, breast iodine inadequacy by itself causes disturbing changes in the rat tissues that, once formed, are not reversed completely by replacement methods.

## B.  Cocarcinogenicity

Basic research findings indicate that there is an earlier onset of breast cancer in prepubertal rats, due to a carcinogen (DMBA), as well as an increase in size and numbers of lesions when the carcinogen is administered after an iodine-deficient or hypothyroid state is reached.(12,13,14)  The growth of the cancers in size and numbers is greater in the iodine-deficient than in the hypothyroid rats.(12)  The onset of lesions and tumor responses to DMBA appear to differ(12,14) according to techniques used and whether the carcinogen is given before or after the animals have become hypothyroid or iodine deficient.  All rats used were pubertal before medications were given.

These results are seen also in long-term perchlorate therapy. Again, the dysplastic and neoplastic changes occur more rapidly in perchlorate-treated DMBA rats than in the control groups.  Perchlorate treatment is supplemented by replacement thyroxine therapy, in order to maintain a euthyroid condition.  The blockade remains at the breast tissue level; hence, the changes seen would represent only cellular effects of the breast, not affected by any perpheral reduction in available thyroxine.

## C.  Autoradiography

The histologic presence of breast iodine was confirmed by the utilization, in our laboratory, of autoradiography employing $^{125}$I. Findings indicate that in iodine deficiency there is a decrease in the iodine in the breast tissues and intracellular iodine, diminished further in the chronic deficiency state, leading to the dysplastic changes described.  The same response occurs when perchlorate is given where iodine, again, does not enter the breast tissue itself.(4)

Particularly exciting in these studies was the fact that not all glandular cells showed the iodine-effect simultaneously.  The response appeared to be randomized, which may permit some speculation on the cause of the *focal* atypia that was described in iodine-deficiency carcinogenesis.

The histologic evidence of both carcinogenesis and cocarcinogenesis that has been presented relates to a requirement for intracellular iodine.  How the iodine is biochemically employed within the cells has received some recent attention.

## III.   METABOLIC ACTION

### A.   Radionuclide Studies

Radioactive iodine uptakes were determined in rat breasts under varying physiologic and pharmacologic conditions of iodine
availability.(17)   This utilized the fact that when radioactive
iodine is given, uptake is greatest where iodine is deficient; the
exception would be in total blockade.   In rat breast tissues with
dysplasia, the uptake was increased, a finding that was employed in
our clinical diagnostic research project(18) as described later.

Total breast $^{125}I$ uptake results are the sum of both vascular
and cellular radioactive content.   The breast parenchyma $^{125}I$ uptake can be calculated by subtracting the $^{125}I$ count in blood present in the breast from the total $^{125}I$ breast count.   The amount of
blood in the breast tissue has been determined by $^{51}Cr$ serum dilution studies in our laboratory.   Preliminary $^{51}Cr$ studies have confirmed the feasibility of measuring this absolute breast parenchyma
uptake.

The results of these most recent calculations have permitted
us to compare the amount of iodine contained in the breast tissues
with the related histologic findings.   From these data we hope to
construct a quantitative level required for breast normalcy in our
rat model.

### B.   Intracellular Studies

Several biochemical studies have been performed to understand
how iodine acts within the breast cells.   By using the experimental
rat model and modifying iodine therapies, our laboratory has shown
variations in DNA/RNA, estrogen receptor protein (ERP), and cytosol
radionuclide uptakes.   Changes in these moieties with added thyroid
and estrogen were also studied.

When total body iodine levels are lowered, breast DNA/RNA ratios
increased threefold over normal values, and the DNA/RNA ratios shift
contrary to those of the hypothyroid state (p<.001).(5,19)

The aggregation properties of estrogen receptor protein (ERP)
is altered in iodine deficiency.(19)   Sucrose density gradient pro-
files were employed and showed the protein significantly less aggre-
gated in iodine deficiency and the 4-58 form remarkably increased in
the deficient group as compared with the controls.   The ERP of breast
tissue is used as a diagnostic test for assessing the dependence of
tumor tissue on the presence of estrogen for growth and development.(20)   A consideration of our findings permits speculation on
estrogen interaction with the iodine present.   The increase in receptor may enhance the tumorigenesis of breast tissues when estrogen
is present.

In mice, the uptake of [125]I iodine by transplanted hormone responsive (HR) mammary tumors has been shown to be significantly greater than the uptake of [125]I iodide by transplanted hormone independent (HI) mammary tumors.(21)  As anticipated, uptake of [125]I by HR mammary tumors was greatly reduced by the simultaneous injection of an excess of nonradioactive iodide.  In addition, perchlorate treatment blocked the uptake in the breasts.

This interaction between iodine and estrogen has been described in castrated female rats made iodine deficient.(11)  In these animals, breast [125]I uptake was greater than in intact rats, and when given estrogen, the breast dysplasia resulting was significantly greater than in the ovariectomized controls.  When both iodine and estrogen were given to these animals, the breast tissues approached normalcy. It would appear, then, that estrogen activity in the breast requires the presence of an adequate level of iodine.

When rat breast cells are fractionated by ultracentrifugation, the content of iodine in the soluble portion can be determined by [125]I uptakes.(19)  The soluble blood fraction is calculated by the [51]Cr method previously described.  Under these circumstances, the uptakes of both iodine deficiency and perchlorate blockade are significantly lower than the uptake found in the control animals and in certain altered thyroid states.  These findings show that cytosol iodine has been reduced by dietary and blockade methods, while the levels obtained by hypothyroidism, hyperthyroidism, and additional iodine are not significant.  These intracellular results offer evidence that iodine acts at the breast tissue level and that biochemical homeostasis is disturbed when iodine is reduced.

## IV.  CLINICAL

### A.  Epidemiology

While a correlation between thyroid/iodine and breast cancer has been considered and presumably investigated since 1890, no definitive statements about a relationship between iodine and mammary gland physiology were published until 1956.(3)  Consideration of the relationship of iodine metabolism to breast neoplasia was first described in 1967(7) and reviewed in 1970.(5)

Published statistics by others and by us indicate high rates of breast cancer in regions of known endemic goiter and lower rates where iodine is adequate.(22)  The incidence of breast cancer is high in Mexico and Thailand, both of which are regions of endemic goiter, while the incidence of breast carcinoma is low in Japan and Iceland where goiter is not endemic.(23)  Higher incidence rates of breast cancer have been published in localized pockets of endemic goiter in Poland, Switzerland, Australia, and the Soviet Union.(24,25)

In the United States, close correspondence exists between regions of high mortality rates due to breast cancer (American Cancer Society statistics) and areas of endemic goiter described by literature from several sources including the World Health Organization.(26,27)

A recent report from a radiology screening program in a United States metropolitan area with known iodine deficiency(26) provoked much controversy concerning the safety of thyroid medication for women by concluding that thyroid therapy increases the incidence of breast cancer, particularly in nulliparous women.(28)  The authors stated that the increased incidence of breast cancer in their patients was either a function of hypothyroidism itself or of the thyroid supplements.  The breast cancer morbidity described in the article was much higher than would be found in nongoitrous regions. Studies in rats have shown that l-thyroxine, in the presence of iodine deficiency, causes an increase in breast dysplasia.  These clinical data, however, lacked firm diagnostic evidence of the thyroid/iodine abnormality for which the patients were treated.

Variations in iodine-deficiency levels differ within given populations.  The evolution of the human organism permits the adaptation of thyroid function and structure to respond to a lower-than-normal supply of iodine.  Goiter formation serves only as a symptom of the deficiency and therapeutics that decrease the thyroid growth do not necessarily restore the body metabolic iodine balance.(29) The need for further epidemiologic studies in regions of endemic goiter is evident.

B.   Endocrinology

There has been a good deal of recent clinical interest in the thyroid/iodine axis as it relates to breast cancer.  It is suggested that breast cancer patients, as a group, have a level of thyroid function that is lower than that found in women in hospitals with conditions unrelated to the breast, and that this lowered function is of primary thyroid, and not of pituitary or hypothalamic origin as shown by TSH values.(30)  In addition, it has been shown that women with breast cancer may exhibit higher resting levels of TSH and a greater TSH response to TRH than women admitted with disorders unrelated to the breast.(31)

A hypothesis for dietary iodine and risk of breast cancer has been presented in which it is suggested that relatively low dietary iodine intake might produce an evanescent intermittent primary hypothyroidism that would lead to changes in the hypothalamic/pituitary pool.(32)  This, in turn, results in increased gonadotrophic stimulation, which in turn, may produce a hyperestrogenic state; a condition theorized as basic to increased risk of breast carcinoma. From these factors, it has been concluded that women in areas of the world where iodine intake is relatively low should be encouraged to increase their iodine intake.

## C.   Radionuclide Studies

Using a data base that we have obtained in our animal research, we have begun a clinical research program.  Initially, we have evaluated patients in our breast cancer screening unit to determine whether iodine uptakes and scans might be useful in the diagnosis of breast cancer.  The research program was designed to obtain the history, breast examination, xeromammography, radioiodine uptake of breasts and thyroid, and scan of the breasts.(18)

With data collated from the experimental design, we conclude that it is possible to determine the breast uptake of an administered tracer dose of radioactive iodine.  After experimenting with several techniques, reproducible results are being obtained.  Using our latest method in 181 cases, radioactive iodine uptakes were significantly greater in malignant or atypical breasts by tissue diagnosis than in normal breasts.  Statistical analysis also showed:

   1.   thyroid uptakes and breast uptakes appeared to be
        dependent and to vary directly with one another.

   2.   iodine and estrogen interacted by the fact that
        radioactive iodine uptake is higher in postmeno-
        pausal breasts than it is in premenopausal
        breasts ($p < 0.05$).

   3.   gestational status and breast feeding do not
        seem to change the uptake of the breasts by
        this method.

In other aspects of this clinical research, we have shown that $^{125}I$ or $^{99m}Tc$ radionuclide imaging shows reduced tracer in areas of the scans where clinically malignant or equivocal breast disease is diagnosed by breast examination, mammography, and/or tissue biopsy. Increased uptake of iodine in breast cancer tissue (biopsy or mastectomy) has been described.(33)

## D.   Estrogen and Estrogen Receptors

It has been suggested that the presence of estrogen receptor in a breast tumor in women would indicate whether the tumor was hormone dependent, and therefore might be made to regress following appropriate ablative therapy of estrogen-secreting glands.(20)  On the other hand, a large number of patients may thus be spared unrewarding major endocrine ablative surgery if estrogen-receptor assays are performed and the tumor is hormone resistant.  In mice, the uptake of iodine is much greater in hormone-responsive than in

hormone-independent breast cancer.(21)   Therefore, the effectiveness
of estrogen on growth and metastases of a given breast tumor may be
determined by iodine evaluation by uptakes or other methodology in
the parenchyma of the involved tissues.

Earlier work in rats showed that breast tissue radioiodine uptake increases in ovariectomized rats.  The presence of an increased
uptake of iodine in menopausal women may indicate that menopausal
women have become more estrogen responsive and that possibly, hormone resistance is lost.

The reciprocal actions between estrogen and iodine in the
breast are not clear.  Whether estrogen metabolism requires iodine
or whether iodine deficiency in itself prevents normal growth and
development of the breast tissues remains to be determined.  We are
continuing our present research on the effect of estrogen on the
uptakes of women at high risk for breast cancer.

E.   Therapeutic Use of Iodine

The use of iodine in therapeutics to prevent breast cancer has
been historically described since the late 19th century.(34)   However, as indicated by basic research, replacement of iodides to iodine-deficient animals after breast abnormalities have occurred,
seems to result in a relatively slow and incomplete return to normal.(5)   The utilization of thyroid medication, in lieu of iodine
replacement in these cases, seems ineffectual and perhaps harmful.
Large amounts of iodine do not seem to have any valid treatment
basis from the research that has been done.(35)

At present there are several medical groups who are studying,
by double-blind technique, treatment of fibrocystic disease and
other dysplasias and carcinoma of the breast with both iodides and
organic iodine forms.  The treatment of iodine deficiency per se
throughout the world is a huge, and presumably, almost impossible
task.  Publications by the World Health Organization and the Pan
American Health Organization have shown that the employment of various iodine therapeutic regimens has been successful in reducing
fetal and neonatal abnormalities due endemic goiter.(26,27)   However, as stated in all of these volumes, the problem of eradicating
endemic goiter seems insoluble at present.(27)

V.   SUMMARY

From laboratory studies presented, iodine appears to be a requisite for the normalcy of breast tissue in higher vertebrates.
When lacking, the parenchyma in rodents and humans show atypia, dysplasia, and even neoplasia.  Iodine-deficient breast tissues are
also more susceptible to carcinogen action and promote lesions earlier and in greater profusion.  Metabolically, iodine-deficient

breasts show changes in RNA/DNA ratios, estrogen receptor proteins, and cytosol iodine levels.

Clinically, radionuclide studies have shown that breast atypia and malignancy have increased radioactive iodine uptakes. Imaging of the breasts in high-risk women has localized breast tumors. The potential use of breast iodine determination to determine estrogen dependence of breast cancer has been considered and the role of io-dide therapy discussed.

In conclusion, iodine appears to be a compulsory element for the breast tissue growth and development. It presents great poten-tial for its use in research directed toward the prevention, diag-nosis, and treatment of breast cancer.

*REFERENCES*

1.   Dratman, M. B., "On the Mechanism of Action of Thyroxine...", J. Theoretical Biology 46, Page 255, 1974.

2.   Schiff, L., Stevens, C. D., Molle, W. R., Steinberg, H., Kimpe, S. W. and Stewart, P., "Gastric (and Salivary) Excretion...", J. National Cancer Institute 7, Page 349, 1947.

3.   Freinkel, N., Ingbar, S. H., "The Metabolism of $^{131}$I by Surviving...", Endoc. 58, Page 51, 1956.

4.   Eskin, B. A., Stamieszkin, I., "Iodine Localization in Mammary...", Abstract submitted Am. Ass. Ca. Res., 1978.

5.   Eskin, B. A., "Iodine Metabolism and...", Trans. New York Academy of Science 32, Page 911, 1970.

6.   Eskin, B. A., Shuman, R., Krouse, T. and Merion, J., "Rat Mammary Gland Atypia...", Cancer Research 35, Page 2332, 1975.

7.   Eskin, B. A., Bartuska, D. G., Dunn, M. R., Jacob, G. and Dratman, M. B., "Mammary Gland Dysplasia...", JAMA 200, Page 691, 1967.

8.   Aquino, T. I., Eskin, B. A., "Rat Breast Structure in Altered...", Arch. Pathology 94, Page 280, 1972.

9.   Krouse, T., Eskin, B. A., "Age-Related Changes in Iodine-Blocked...", Proc. Amer. Ass. Ca. Res. 18, Page 79, 1977.

10.  Eskin, B. A., Dunn, M. R., "Resistance by Hormone-Dependent Mammary...", Obst. Gynecology 33, Page 581, 1969.

11.  Eskin, B. A., Merion, J., Krouse, T. and Shuman, R.,
     "Blockade of Breast Iodine...", Thyroid Research, J. Robbins
     and L. Braverman, Editors, Excerpta Medica, Amsterdam, 1976.

12.  Eskin, B. A., Murphey, S. A. and Dunn, M. R., "DMBA Induction
     of Breast Cancer...", Nature 218, Page 1162, 1968.

13.  Jabara, A. G., Maritz, J. S., "Effects of Hypothyroidism and
     Progesterone," British Journal Cancer 28, Page 161, 1973.

14.  Kellen, J. A., "Effect of Hypothyroidism on Induction...", N.
     National Cancer Institute 48, Page 1901, 1972.

15.  Brown-Grant, K., "The Iodide Concentrating Mechanism of
     the...", J. Physiology 135, Page 644, 1957.

16.  Honour, A. J., Myant, M. B. and Rowlands, E. N., "Secretion
     of Radioiodide in...", Clinical Science 11, Page 447, 1952.

17.  Eskin, B. A., "The Influence of Estrogen and Testosterone
     on...", Proceedings Endoc. Society 53, Page A192, 1971.

18.  Eskin, B. A., Parker, J. A., Bassett, J. G. and George, D. L.,
     "Human Breast Uptake...", Obst. Gynecology 44, Page 398, 1974.

19.  Eskin, B. A., Jacobson, H. I., Bolmarcich, V., Murray, J.,
     "Breast Atypia in Altered..", Intracellular Changes,"
     Senologie 1, Page 51, 1976.

20.  McGuire, W. L., "Estrogen Receptors in Human...", J. Clinical
     Investigation 52, Page 73, 1973.

21.  Thorpe, S. M., "Increased Uptake of Iodide by Hormone...",
     International J. Cancer 18, Page 345, 1976.

22.  Finley, J. W., Bogardus, G. W., "Breast Cancer and Thyroid..",
     Quarterly Review Surg. Obst. Gyn. 17, 1960.

23.  Buell, P., "Epidemiological Study of Breast Cancer...", J.
     N. C. I. 51, Page 1479, 1973.

24.  Koszarowski, T., Gadomska, H., Warda, B. and Drozdzweska, A.,
     "Prevalence of Malignant Neoplasms of..." (1962-1965) Pel Tyg
     Lek. 23, Page 933, 1968.

25.  Shivetskii, A. V., "Distribution of Breast Cancer in a
     Goiter...", Vrach Delo 7, Page 37, 1968.

26.  Kelly, F. C., Snedden, W. W., "Prevalence and Geographic
     Distribution of...", WHO Monograph Series 44, Page 27, 1960.

27.  Dunn, J. T., Medetros-Neto, G. A., "Endemic Goiter and
     Cretinism...", Pan American Health Organization, 1974.

28.  Kapdi, C. C., Wolfe, J. N., "Breast Cancer:  Relationship
     to Thyroid...", JAMA 236, Page 1124, 1976.

29.  DeLange, F., Thilly, C. and Ermans, A. M., "Iodine Deficiency,
     A Permissive Condition...", J. Clinical Endoc. 28, Page 114, 1968.

30.  Mittra, I., Hayward, J. L., "Hypothalamic-Pituitary-Prolactin
     Axis...", Lancet 2, Page 885, 1974.

31.  Mittra, I., Hayward, J. L., Ibid., Page 889.

32.  Stadl, B. V., "Dietary Iodine and Risk of Breast,
     Endometrial...", Lancet 2, Page 890, 1976.

33.  Cancroft, E. T., Goldsmith, S. J., $^{99m}$Tc-pertechnetate
     Scintigraphy...", Radiology 106, Page 441, 1973.

34.  Beatson, G. T., "Adjuvant Use of Thyroid Extract in Breast...",
     Lancet 104: No. 2, Page 162, 1896.

35.  Eskin, B. A., Aquino, T. I., Dunn, M. R., "Replacement Therapy
     With Iodine...", International J. Obst. Gynecology 8, Page 232,
     1970.

## CHAPTER 21

GASTROINTESTINAL CANCER:

EPIDEMIOLOGY AND EXPERIMENTAL STUDIES

Birger Jansson, Maryce M. Jacobs, and A. Clark Griffin

University of Texas System Cancer Center
M. D. Anderson Hospital and Tumor Institute
Texas Medical Center, Houston, Texas   77030

## I.   INTRODUCTION

Cancer rates seem to be influenced by two counteractive types
of agents:

1.   carcinogens, that cause increasing rates for
increasing exposure

2.   anticarcinogens, that reduce the effects of
the carcinogens

In recent years, the interests of researchers in carcinogenesis
have turned increasingly toward the possibility of preventing cancer by the use of anticarcinogens.  Primarily, compounds with anti-
oxidative properties have been studied.  These include vitamin A
(Rogers et al. and Sporn et al.(1,2)); disulfiram (Wattenberg(3));
and selenium (Shamberger-Willis, and Shamberger).(4,5)  These antioxidants may work by reducing the amount of ultimate carcinogens
produced from a precarcinogen that needs oxidation for its metabolic transformation.

We shall concentrate on the trace element, selenium, by discussing some epidemiological findings and some new, experimental
results that illustrate the anticarcinogenic property of selenium.

## II.   BACKGROUND

Primarily, three approaches have been used for the study of

selenium as a cancer inhibitor.

a.  Geographical similarities have been pointed out between
    the distribution of selenium-deficient areas and the
    distribution of areas with high cancer rates, especially
    colorectal cancer and breast cancer.  For the United
    States, this has been effected with the selenium map
    presented by Kubota-Allaway(6) and with the detailed
    cancer mortality rates per county published by N. C. I.
    (Mason-McKay(7) which were later condensed into maps
    of cancer distribution (Mason et al. and Jansson et
    al.).(8,9)  The similarities are also evident on a
    global scale.  Selenium-deficient regions such as
    Denmark, the southern part of Sweden, New Zealand and
    South Australia have high colorectal and breast cancer
    rates, while selenium-adequate areas such as Japan,
    have low rates in these cancers.

b.  Selenium levels in human blood plasma have been
    measured in cancer patients.  McConnell et al. and
    Broghamer et al.(10,11) have reported significantly
    lower mean serum selenium levels in patients with
    gastrointestinal cancers compared to patients with
    other disorders.

c.  Laboratory experiments have been performed using
    selenium.  As early as 1949, Clayton and Baumann(12)
    reported that in rats, the induction of liver tumors
    by a carcinogen was decreased when selenium was added
    to the diet.  Harr et al.(13) made a similar obser-
    vation.  Schrauzer and Ismael(14) reduced the inci-
    dence rates of a spontaneous mammary tumor in virgin
    female $C_3H$ mice by adding selenium to the drinking
    water, and Jacobs et al.(15) reported a reduced rate
    of DMH-induced colon cancer in rats by using a selenium
    additive in the drinking water.

In addition to these animal experiments, two experiments on a
chromosomal level have been performed:  (1) the use of selenium to
reduce the rate of carcinogen-induced mutations in the Ames' test
(Jacobs et al.(16); and (2) the use of selenium in the reduction
of sister chromatid exchanges, caused by carcinogens, in cultured
human lymphocytes.

Indirect evidence of selenium as a cancer inhibitor also exists.
Comparisons have been made between two phenomena both related to
selenium deficiency.  Since a lack of selenium is known to reduce
the fertility in some animals such as sheep, in areas low in selenium one would expect low birth rates and high colorectal cancer rates.

Investigating this hypothesis, Jansson et al.(*17*) found a negative
correlation between human birth rates and colorectal and breast cancer rates in the United States.

## III.   TWO EPIDEMIOLOGICAL OBSERVATIONS

A.   Seasonal Variation of Selenium in Water

In a previously reported study (Jansson et al.(*9*), a high,
positive correlation was demonstrated between the geographical distribution of colon cancer and of rectum cancer within the United
States.  This similarity between the distributions permitted the
development of a procedure that reduced the statistical variation
of the mortality rates per county.  The refined distribution map
obtained this way shows very high rates in the Northeast and especially along the Atlantic coast from the Canadian border through
New Jersey.  The majority of the 100 counties in the United States
that have the highest colorectal cancer rates are situated in this
coastal strip(Jansson, et al. and Jansson and Jacobs).(*17,18*)   The
previous finding of a negative correlation between the geographical
distribution of selenium and of colorectal cancer initiated a more
detailed study of the selenium levels.  The United States Geological
Survey (U. S. G. S.) measures the selenium concentration in water in
the United States to detect toxic levels of this trace element with
a level of 10 ppb specified as toxic.  One thousand seventy-four
selenium measurements made during a period from 1972 to 1976 in
different places and at different times of the year show a clear
seasonal variation (see Figure 1), with a peak in the winter, a
trough in the summer, and a smaller peak in the fall.

In order to give more structure to these data, the section of
the Northeast that is north of the 40° latitude was divided into
four zones parallel to the coast.  These zones, each approximately
130 miles wide, are shown in Figure 2, together with some of the
300 counties with highest colorectal cancer rates in this country.
The year was divided into five time periods, each with a rather constant concentration of selenium.  The means of the selenium concentrations in each geographic zone and time period are compiled in
Table 1.  One may note:

a.   that the winter peak is a coastal phenomenon, while
     inland the fall peak dominates;

b.   that the selenium concentration in water over the
     year decreases as one moves inland.

The last point contradicts the hypothesis of a negative correlation between the prevalence of selenium and the colorectal cancer rates.  To study this contradiction, the means of the mortality
rates for colon and rectal cancer for males and females were calcul-

ated using all counties within each zone.  The results (shown in
Figure 3) show an almost linear relationship between selenium
concentration and mortality rates.  This raises some relevant
questions:

a.    Is there a corresponding seasonal variation of the
      selenium concentration over the year in soil, plants,
      animals, and humans?  If so, this must be taken into
      account, for example, in studies of the selenium
      levels in blood plasma.

b.    Is the selenium concentration in water over the
      year negatively correlated to the selenium concen-
      tration in soil, plants, animals, and humans?  That
      would explain the positive correlation between the
      cancer rates and the selenium levels in water.

c.    How can a quantitative model of the cycling of
      selenium over the year be constructed?  There is
      obviously a flow, with a period of one year, of
      selenium between compartments such as water, air,
      soil, plants, animals, and humans.

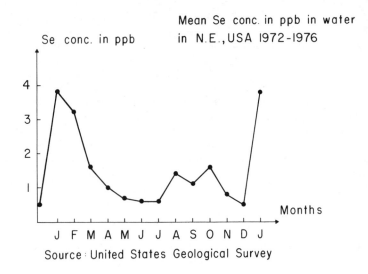

Figure 1

One of the authors (B. Jansson) in a yet unpublished study,
has determined the distribution of the month of birth for a group
of 180,000 cancer patients.  After adjustment for the well-known
seasonal variation of births, it is found that unexpectedly, many
cancer patients were born in the winter, and unexpectedly few in

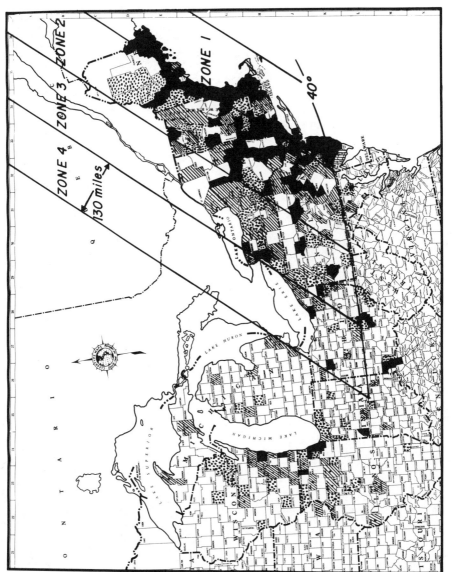

Figure 2

TABLE 1

MEAN Se CONCENTRATION IN ppb IN WATERS IN NEW ENGLAND

| Months Zone | Jan.-Feb. | March-April | May-June-July | Aug.-Sept.-Oct.- | Nov.-Dec. | All Year |
|---|---|---|---|---|---|---|
| 1 | 699/166<br>4.21 | 276/173<br>1.60 | 103/161<br>.64 | 134/106<br>1.26 | 37/59<br>.63 | 1249/665<br>1.88 |
| 2 | 25.2/30<br>.84 | 16.5/30<br>.55 | 36/52<br>.69 | 181.2/103<br>1.76 | 19/28<br>.68 | 277.9/243<br>1.14 |
| 3 | 6/14<br>.43 | 12/27<br>.44 | 19/43<br>.44 | 31/33<br>.94 | 20/21<br>.95 | 88/138<br>.64 |
| 4 | 3/3<br>1.00 | 0.6<br>.00 | 0/1<br>.00 | 0/11<br>.00 | 2/7<br>.29 | 5/28<br>.18 |
| 1-4 | 733.2/213<br>3.44 | 304.5/236<br>1.29 | 158/257<br>.61 | 346.2/253<br>1.37 | 78/115<br>.68 | 1619.9/1074<br>1.51 |

Source:  U. S. G. S.

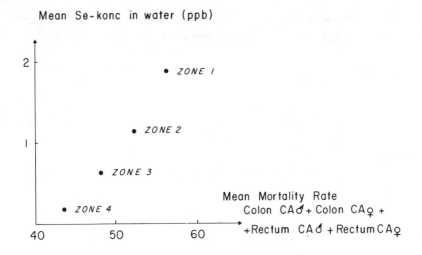

Figure 3

summer.  The graph of the month of birth for cancer patients is
strikingly similar to the graph of selenium concentration in the
water during the year.  Some hypotheses of carcinogenesis consider
the induction of a cancer as a multistep procedure in which the
first step might be a very early one.

    d.    Is it possible that a seasonal variation like the
        one observed for selenium plays a role in the
        seasonal variation in the month of birth for
        cancer patients?

B.   Negative Correlation Between Colon-Rectum Cancer and
     Stomach-Liver Cancer

    Many authors have observed a negative correlation between stom-
ach cancer and colon cancer.  Since cereals and fish are rich in
selenium, while muscular meat and sugar are low in this element, it
is of interest to compare the amounts of these food groups in the
diet of different regions of the world.  From a table published by
Schrauzer(19) we extract the data in Table 2 containing correlation
coefficients between colon, rectum, stomach, and liver cancer rates
on one hand and the intake of meat, sugar, cereals, and fish on the
other hand.  It is striking that colon and rectum cancer rates are
almost consistently positively correlated with the amount of meat
and sugar in the diet and negatively correlated with the amount of
cereals and fish, while the opposite is true for stomach and liver

cancer. Since toxic levels of selenium are known to cause damage
to the liver, one may question whether selenium protects against
colon, rectum, and breast cancer while contributing to increased
risks for stomach and liver cancer; or possibly selenium may be
only a weak or nonextent protector against stomach and liver cancer
and a strong protector against colon, rectal, and breast cancers. A
further illustration is given in Figure 4 in which rates for colon
and rectal cancer are plotted against rates for stomach and liver
cancer for about 40 regions of the world, with data obtained from
Doll-Payne-Waterhouse.(20)  To compare the rates, for each organ
site and for each sex, the rates were normalized to mean 1; then
the sums of the rates for colon-rectal cancer and for stomach-
liver cancer were also normalized to mean 1.  The six regions with
very low rates for all four cancers are the four African regions
in the study, Jamaica, and Singapore.  The region with an extremely
high rate of stomach and liver cancer is Japan, while the region
highest in colorectal cancer is Connecticut.

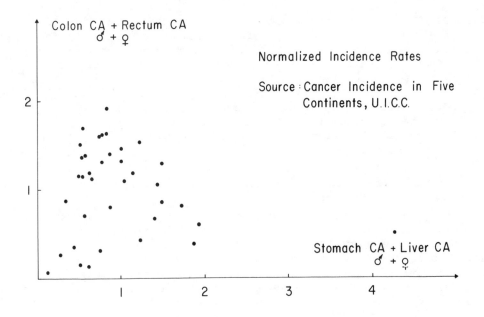

Figure 4

TABLE 2

CORRELATION COEFFICIENTS

Females

| | Meat | Sugar | Cereals | Fish |
|---------|-------|-------|---------|------|
| Colon | +.81 | +.68 | -.72 | -.52 |
| Rectum | +.39 | +.42 | -.38 | -.35 |
| | | | | |
| Stomach | -.77 | -.65 | +.77 | +.44 |
| Liver | -.36 | -.71 | +.44 | -.10 |

Males

| | Meat | Sugar | Cereals | Fish |
|---------|-------|-------|---------|------|
| Colon | +.91 | +.68 | -.69 | -.63 |
| Rectum | +.57 | +.57 | -.44 | -.45 |
| | | | | |
| Stomach | -.76 | -.67 | +.75 | +.44 |
| Liver | -.56 | -.92 | +.75 | +.18 |

From Schrauzer, Medical Hypotheses 2, 1976.

IV.   SOME EXPERIMENTAL EVIDENCE FOR THE
CANCER INHIBITORY ACTIVITY OF SELENIUM

Selenium has been reported to exhibit inhibitory effects on
selected carcinogens.  The proposition is set forth that selenium
either inhibits the activation of test compounds and/or deters carcinogenic or mutagenic events ascribed to the activated compounds.
These selenium activities are suggested by (a) human epidemiologic
studies as discussed previously in this paper; (b) experimental rat
assays; (c) mutagenesis assays; and (d) assays with human lymphocytes in culture.  Points b-d will be further discussed in the
following paragraphs.

A.   Experimental Rat Assays

As reported in Jacobs et al.(15) selenium inhibited 1,2-
dimethylhydrazine (DMH) and methylmethoxymethanol (MAM) induction of
colon tumors in rats.  Male Sprague-Dawley rats were injected weekly
with 20 mg/kg body weight for 18 weeks with either DMH or MAM.  The
animals, initially weighing about 200 grams each, were divided into
four groups of 15 rats.  Of the two groups receiving DMH, one was
provided with 4 ppm selenium ($Na_2SeO_3$) *ad libidum* in the drinking
water throughout the DMH administration, while the other group received DMH only.  Similarly, two groups received MAM injections,
with one group provided with supplemental selenium (4 ppm).

The rats receiving DMH with and without selenium gained 205 ± 8
and 206 ± 6 grams, respectively, with no measurable selenium effect
(P=0.8) between groups.  The weight gain of rats receiving MAM with
and without selenium was 184 ± 5 and 185 ± 7 grams, respectively,
also yielding no detectable selenium effect (P=0.8).  However, comparison of the growth curves between the two carcinogens yielded a
significant growth effect, P=0.001, in which rats receiving DMH
gained 20 grams more than rats receiving MAM.

Tumor incidence is expressed in percentage and refers to the
number of animals with tumors per total number of animals in a group.
As seen in Table 3, the colon tumor incidence with DMH is reduced
from 87% (13 rats with tumors in a group of 15) to 40% (6 to 15) in
rats receiving DMH and supplemental selenium.  The significance of
this reduction is reflected in a P value of 0.025.  No significant
selenium effect on the tumor incidence was evident between the
groups receiving MAM (100%) and the group administered MAM plus
selenium (93%).  One might suggest that a significant selenium reduction in colon tumor incidence may be obtained in future experiments by either reducing the dose of MAM injected or by reducing
the total number of MAM injections.

The total number, size, and location of tumors were recorded
for intact colons resected at the cecal and rectal junctures.  Sum-
ming the total number of tumors observed in each group of DMH-

treated animals, selenium reduced the number of colon tumors more
than three-fold.  DMH-treated rats had 39 total tumors, while DMH
plus selenium decreased the total number of colon tumors induced
by MAM to 42 tumors as compared to a total of 73 tumors in the
group of rats receiving only MAM.

TABLE 3

| Group | Total No. | No. Tumors Per Rat | Incidence (%) | Rats with Tumors Total Rats Per Group |
|-------|-----------|--------------------|----------------|----------------------------------------|
| DMH + Se | 11 | 0.7 | 40 | 6/15 |
| DMH | 39 | 2.6 | 87 | 13/15 |
| MAM + Se | 42 | 2.8 | 93 | 14/15 |
| MAM | 73 | 5.2 | 100 | 14/14 |

In Table 4, the volume of each tumor is given for different
locations of the tumors in the colon.  In the DMH-treated animals,
with and without selenium, the majority of tumors are 10 $mm^3$ or less
in volume.  Considering the limited data available, selenium im-
posed no striking influence on the size of the DMH-induced tumors.
MAM clearly induced a greater number of total tumors than DMH (DMH,
50; MAM, 115).  Although the MAM-induced tumors in the presence and
absence of selenium appeared to be of greater volume, statistically,
70% of all tumors induced by either carcinogen were 10 $mm^3$ or less.
Relative to the distance from the cecum, the tumors are referred to
as being in the proximal (0-5 cm), transverse (5-10 cm), and distal
(10-16 cm) colon.  In Table 5, the sum of the tumors in the proximal
plus distal colon is compared with the number of tumors in the
transverse colon.  Selenium supplementation tended to favor tumor
induction by DMH in the transverse colon.  Tumors induced by MAM ±
selenium were more evenly distributed by size and by location
throughout the three colonic regions described.  Approximately 50%
of all tumors induced by MAM + selenium were in the transverse region with no influence of selenium on the redistribution of induced
tumors in a specific colonic region.  Whether or not there is a
valid distinction between the distribution of DMH- and MAM-induced
tumors in the presence of selenium may not be definitely answered,
due to the limited number of induced tumors considered in this study;
it is possible, however, that the role of the bacterial flora of the
colon and the biochemical events relating selenium and carcinogen
metabolism to tumor formation cause differences in these distributions.

TABLE 4

TUMOR VOLUMES IN mm$^3$

| Location* cm | DMH + Se | DMH | MAM + Se | MAM |
|:---:|:---:|:---:|:---:|:---:|
| 0- | | 125 | 2 | 6,4,2,1,1 |
| 1- | | 1 | | 32 |
| 2- | | 9,8 | 7 | 15,9,6 |
| 3- | 30 | 15,3 | 9,3 | 56,15,12,4,2 |
| 4- | | 1,1,1 | 4 | 100,6,4,4 |
| 5- | | 2,1,1,1,1, 1,1,1 | 2 | 125,125,4,4,2 |
| 6- | 168,72,4, 4,2,2 | 6,2,1 | 2 | 98,18,9,8,2,2,2,1 |
| 7- | 4 | 1,1,1 | 6,2 | 50,16,16,8,6,4,4,2,1 |
| 8- | 9 | 90,25,8,1, 1,1 | 48,32,32,32, 9,6,4,2,2,1 | 72,30,24,24,8,4,2,2 |
| 9- | | 8,4,1 | 480,16,18, 8,6,4,2 | 8,8,4,4,4,1,1 |
| 10- | | 8,1 | 32,6,2,2, 2,1,1,1 | 100,4,1 |
| 11- | 2 | | 4 | 6,2,2,2,1 |
| 12- | | 53,8,1 | 36,32 | 288,8,4,4,1,1,1 |
| 13- | | 1 | 108,4 | 9 |
| 14- | | 18 | 30,4 | 84 |
| 15- | 4 | | 2 | 350 |
| Tumor Number | 11 | 39 | 42 | 73 |

*   From cecum to rectum.

TABLE 5

|          | Tumor Location<br>Proximal + Distal | Transverse |
|----------|:-----------------------------------:|:----------:|
| DMH + Se | 3  | 8  |
| DMH      | 16 | 23 |
| MAM + Se | 21 | 21 |
| MAM      | 36 | 37 |

B.   Mutagenesis Assays

Selenium reduction of the mutagenicity of 2-acetylaminofluorene
(AAF), N-hydroxy-2-acetylaminofluorene (N-OH-AAF) and N-hydroxyamino-
fluorene (N-OH-AF) was observeved in the *Salmonella typhimurium*
TA 1538 bacterial tester system, Jacobs et al.(*16*)  In order to
effect the reduction in mutagenicity of AAF and N-OH-AAF, selenium
was mixed with the mutagen in melted top agar (45°C) containing
bacteria, a TPNH-generating system and a rat liver homogenate fraction.  The vortexed mixture was poured on an agar plate and incubated
two days at 37°C.  The his$^+$ revertants were counted.  For microsomal
activation of AAF, the supernatant (S9) fraction from a rat liver
homogenate obtained by centrifugation at 9,000 g was added to the
above.  Centrifugation of S9 at 150,000 g yielded the microsome-
free homogenate fraction incubated with N-OH-AAF above.  Neither the
rat liver homogenate fraction nor the TPNH-generating system were
present in the incubation mixture of N-OH-AF with selenium and bacteria in the top agar since this chemical is mutagenic in its native
state (Stout, et al.(*21*)

Figure 5 illustrates decreased number of revertants per plate
and thus decreased activity of AAF, N-OH-AAF, and N-OH-AF when incubated in the presence of increased selenium concentrations.  Additions of 4 and 20 mM selenium to 4.5 mM AAF reduced the activity to
approximately 80 and 65%, respectively, of the activity of the AAF
mutagen alone.  Increasing the selenium addition to 40 mM sustained
the reduction of AAF mutagenic activity of about 65%.

Combination of the N-OH-AF metabolite of AAF with selenium
yielded a similar pattern of reduced mutagenic activity.  Addition
of 0.1 and 20 mM selenium to 0.065 mM N-OH-AF reduced the activity

to about 80% and 60%, respectively, of the control number of rever-
sions observed with mutagen alone.  Again, further increased selenium addition; e.g., 40 mM selenium, sustained the reduction to about
60% mutagenicity.

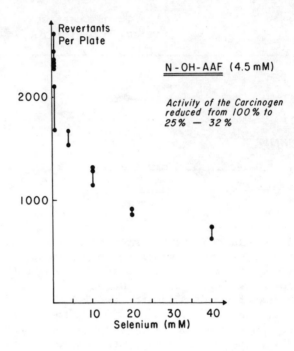

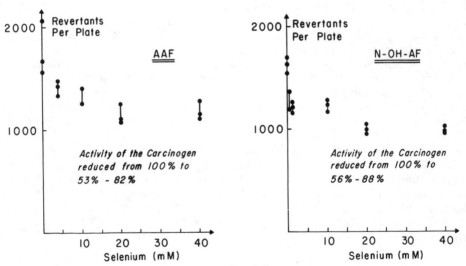

Figure 5

In contrast, a progressive inhibitory effect by increasing the selenium concentration over a 100-fold concentration range could be demonstrated with N-OH-AAF. Additions to 0.45 mM N-OH-AAF of 0.4, 4.0, 10, 20, and 40 mM selenium reduced the mutagenicity of N-OH-AAF to approximately 80, 68, 53, 37, and 28%, respectively, to that of mutagen alone.

An average background of 14 revertants per plate was noted for 0.1 to 40 mM selenium in the absence of mutagen. Selenium effects above 40 mM selenium were not tested because of the formation of a red complex of low solubility. This red complex may be elemental selenium in analogy with the finding of elemental selenium as the end product of selenite reduction by *Salmonella heidelberg* as reported by McCready et al.(22) The mutagen concentrations were selected such that each compound tested in the absence of selenium would yield approximately 2,000 his$^+$ revertants per plate. Reduction of the mutagen concentrations of AAF and N-OH-AF in order to test for selenium-inhibitory effects comparable with those observed with N-OH-AAF was not attempted because of the inherently low number of revertants that could be produced optimally per plate.

## C. Assays with Human Lymphocytes in Culture

The methodology for culturing human lymphocytes and observing sister chromatid exchanges (SCE) in chromosomes from these cell cultures has been described in detail by Latt.(23,24) The primary modification of the cited technique was that cells were grown for only one replication cycle in medium containing 5-bromodeoxyuridine (BrdU). Sister chromatid exchanges were detected in metaphase chromosomes, due to the differential affinities of each chromatid for Giemsa stain. BrdU-substituted DNA was weakly fluorescent, while brightly fluorescing DNA retained thymidine and a high affinity for the stain. Sister chromatid exchange involved breakage of sister chromatids at coincident locations with subsequent interchange and repair. Such rearrangements were detectable by differential fluorescence along each chromatid.

Table 6 shows the mean SCE/cell from an analysis of 20 metaphase spreads from each of the described culture conditions. Control cultures exhibited a mean background frequency of 6-7 SCE/cell. In toxicity studies with selenium exposure of the lymphocytes to $1.27 \times 10^{-9}$M to $1.59 \times 10^{-5}$M selenium for the last 15 hours of culture resulted in no change in SCE frequency relative to the control (6-7 SCE/cell). Addition of $10^{-4}$M methylmethane sulfonate (MMS) to the culture for 15 hours increased the SCE to 32 exchanges per metaphase; however, coexposure of the cultures to $10^{-4}$M MMS and $1.27 \times 10^{-6}$M selenium for the last 15 hours resulted in a decreased frequency of 25 SCE/cell. The significance of this reduction was statistically verified by a P value less than 0.01.

TABLE 6

EFFECT OF Se AND SELECTED CARCINOGENS ON SCE FREQUENCY

| Carcinogen (M) | Se (M) | Mean SCE/Cell |
|---|---|---|
| - | - | 6-7 |
| - | $1.59 \times 10^{-5}$ to $1.27 \times 10^{-9}$ | 6-7 |
| MMS $(10^{-4})$ | - | 32 |
| MMS $(10^{-4})$ | $1.27 \times 10^{-6}$ | 25 |
| - | - | 6.2 |
| AAF $(4 \times 10^{-5})$ | - | 6.2 |
| N-OH-AAF $(4 \times 10^{-5})$ | - | 16.3 |
| N-OH-AAF $(4 \times 10^{-6})$ | - | 7.6 |

Current toxicity studies illustrate the differential effects of AAF and N-OH-AAF on the SCE frequency. Control cultures and cultures exposed for 15 hours to $4 \times 10^{-5}$ M AAF yielded equivalent frequencies of 6.2 SCE/cell. In contrast, cultures exposed to $4 \times 10^{-5}$ M N-OH-AAF for 15 hours yielded an increased frequency to 16.3 SCE per cell. By lowering the N-OH-AAF concentration ten-fold to $4 \times 10^{-6}$ M, a decrease in the mean frequency to 7.6 SCE per cell was observed. These data are consistent with the lower mutagenicity of AAF relative to N-OH-AAF and to the more extensive requirement for activating components for AAF as opposed to N-OH-AAF in the assay for mutagenicity described earlier. Studies are currently in progress to determine the SCE frequency of lymphocyte cultures co-exposed to N-OH-AAF and selenium. Although the process by which MMS and N-OH-AAF produce sister chromatid exchanges has not been elucidated, preliminary data suggest selenium can interrupt some event essential for MMS to increase the SCE frequency.

REFERENCES

1.  Rogers, A. E., Herndon, B. I. and Newberne, P. M., Cancer Res. 33, Page 1003, 1973.

2.  Sporn, M. B., Dunlop, N. M., Newton, D. L. and Smith, J. M., Federal Proceedings 35, Page 1332, 1976.

3.  Wattenberg, L. W., J. National Cancer Institute 54, Page 1005, 1975.

4.  Shamberger, R. J. and Willis, C. E., CRC Crit. Rev. Clin. Lab. Science 2, Page 211, 1971.

5.  Shamberger, R. J., J. National Cancer Institute 44, 931, 1970.

6.  Kubota, J. and Allaway, W. H., Micronutrients in Agriculture, Soil Science of America, Inc., Madison, Wisconsin, Page 525, 1972.

7.  Mason, T. J. and McKay, F. W., Cancer Mortality by County: 1950-1969, DHEW Publishers (NIH) pp 74-615, 1974.

8.  Mason, T. J., McKay, F. W., Hoover, R., Blot, W. J. and Fraumeni, J. F., Atlas of Cancer Mortality for U. S. Counties: 1950-1969, DHEW Publishers (NIH), pp 75-780, 1975.

9.  Jannson, B., Seibert, G. B. and Speer, J. F., Cancer 36, Page 2373, 1975.

10.  McConnell, K. P., Broghamer, W. L., Jr., Blotcky, A. J. and Hurt, O. J., J. Nutrition 105, Page 1026, 1975.

11.  Broghamer, W. L., Jr., McConnell, K. P. and Blotcky, A. J., Cancer 37, Page 1384, 1976.

12.  Clayton, C. C. and Baumann, C. A., Cancer Research 9, Page 575, 1949.

13.  Harr, J. R., Exon, J. H., Weswig, J. H. and Whanger, P. H., Clin. Toxic 6, Page 287, 1973.

14.  Schrauzer, G. N. and Ishmael, D., Annals Clin. Lab. Science 2, Page 441, 1974.

15.  Jacobs, M. M., Jansson, B. and Griffin, A. C., Cancer Letters in press.

16.  Jacobs, M. M., Matney, T. S. and Griffin, A. C., Cancer Letters, in press.

17.  Jansson, B., Malahy, M. A. and Seibert, G. B., Proceedings International Symposium Detection and Prevention of Cancer, New York, 1976.

18.   Jansson, B. and Jacobs, M. M., Proceedings Selenium and
      Tellurium in the Environment, University of Notre Dame, 1976.

19.   Schrauzer, G. N., Medical Hypotheses 2, No. 2, 1976.

20.   Doll, R., Payne, P. and Waterhouse, J., Editors, Cancer
      Incidence in Five Continents, UICC, Geneva, Switzerland, 1966.

21.   Stout, D. L., Baptist, J. N., Matney, T. S. and Shaw, C. R.,
      Cancer Letters 1, Page 269, 1976.

22.   McCready, R. G. L., Campbell, J. N. and Payne, J. T., Canadian
      J. Microbiology 12, Page 703, 1966.

23.   Latt, S. A., Proceedings National Academy Science 71, 3162, 1974.

24.   Latt, S. A., Science 185, Page 74, 1974.

# Part IV

# Trace Elements and Nutrition
# in Cancer Prevention

*CHAPTER 22*


TRACE ELEMENTS, NUTRITION AND CANCER:

PERSPECTIVES OF PREVENTION


Gerhard N. Schrauzer

Department of Chemistry,
University of California at San Diego,
Revelle College, La Jolla, California 92093


## I.  INTRODUCTION

A number of inorganic compounds and elements are known to have significant effects on tumor development.  Certain metals or compounds of metals induce tumorigenesis directly and thus are genuine carcinogens.  Others promote the growth of tumors, and hence, must be regarded as inorganic cocarcinogens.  A few elements of compounds have benign or anticarcinogenic properties.  Selenium, iodine, and possibly arsenic and manganese fall into this group, not to speak of the complexes of platinum and other metals that are about to gain acceptance as cancer chemotherapeutic agents.  In the present account, the anticarcinogenic properties, particularly of selenium, or possess carcinogenic, cocarcinogenic, or anticarcinogenic propmally present in foods that may either act as selenium antagonists or possess carcinogenic, cocarcinogenic, or anticarcinogenic properties of their own.  The emphasis on selenium appears justified in view of a growing body of direct and indirect evidence that suggests that this trace element will have to be considered in future cancer prevention programs.

## II.  ANTICARCINOGENIC ACTIVITY OF SELENIUM

### A.  Historical Development

Selenium was first suggested for cancer *therapy* by Dalbert in 1912(*1*) and by Walker and Klein in 1915.(*2*)  The latter authors entitled their article "Selenium - Its Therapeutic Value - Especially

Selenium
Tumors

in Cancer" and reported on their success in the treatment of human
cancer patients.  They claimed that subcutaneous tumors underwent
"liquefactive necrosis followed by healing" and point out that deeper tumors failed to respond.  They also mention that A. von
Wasserman (1866-1925) apparently studied the effect of selenous acid
on tumor-bearing mice and rats and conclude that..."studies show
that selenium unquestionably exerts a therapeutic effect on malignant tumors."(2)   Interestingly, Walker and Klein correctly described selenium as a catalyst of hydroperoxide decomposition, thus
anticipating the existence of glutathione peroxidase, and linked
cancer development to a disturbance of cellular respiration.  However, their paper failed to attract attention.  In 1935, Todd(3)
announced that selenium exerts a beneficial effect in the treatment
of mammary metastases in conjunction with X-ray therapy, but his
paper went unnoticed as well.  From 1942 until a few years ago,
selenium gained notoriety as a hepatocarcinogen, largely through
the work of Nelson et al. and Tscherkes et al.(4,5)  Even Schroeder
considered selenium to be carcinogenic,(6) in spite of the fact that
his experiments seemed to show the opposite.  The design of these
experiments has been criticized(7,8) and the unanimous opinion has
since been reached that simple, soluble inorganic selenium compounds
are not carcinogenic.  In 1949, Clayton and Baumann(9) discovered
that dietary selenite lowers the incidence of tumors in rats exposed
to p-dimethylaminoazobenzene.  Shamberger(10)  in 1966 and Riley(11)
in 1968 demonstrated that topical selenide, as well as dietary selenite lowered the incidence of skin papillomas in mice receiving DMBA-
croton oil or benzpyrene.   Harr et al.(7) observed an inverse relationship between dietary selenium and tumors in rats exposed to
fluorenylacetamide.  Attempts(12) to repeat this work have produced
inconclusive results, presumably due to seemingly minor differences
in experimental design.

     Single doses of parenteral sodium selenite were reported to
retard the growth of transplanted Ehrlich ascites, Guerin carcinoma
and sarcomatous $M^{-1}$ neoplasms in rodents.(13)  Dietary selenite also
lowers the incidence of colon tumor induction by 1,2-dimethylhydra-
zine and methylazoxymethanol acetate.*(14)

     Aleksandrowicz(15) recently showed that selenium at low dosage
levels increases the resistance of rats to $^{60}$Co-$\gamma$-radiation.  In
view of Todd's earlier claims(3) it thus would seem to be of interest to reinvestigate the effect of selenium in breast cancer patients
receiving radiation treatment.  It also has been reported that selen-

---

*    After submission of this manuscript, A. C. Griffin and M. M.
     Jacobs demonstrated an inhibitory effect of selenium ($Na_2SeO_3$) an
     and of "high-selenium yeast" on hepatocarcinogenesis induced by
     the carcinogenic dye 3'methyl-4-dimethylaminoazobenzene (3'MeDAB)
     in male Sprague-Dawley rats (to appear in Cancer Letters).

ium prevents the growth of carcinogenic fungi and reduces cytotoxicity of aflatoxins.(16)   Several authors have demonstrated a stim-
ulatory effect of selenium on antibody production.(13,17,10)   Recently, the element has been implicated in playing a role in pros-
taglandin biosynthesis.(19)   As a protective agent in heavy metal
poisoning,(20) selenium could prevent metal-induced mutagenesis,
and has, in fact, been shown to possess antimutagenic properties
in bacterial test systems.(21)

## B.   Early Epidemiological Associations

Following the discovery of an inverse relationship between the
blood selenium levels of adult males and the total cancer mortality
in certain U. S. cities, Shamberger and Frost(22) suggested that
selenium has anticancer activity in man.   Later studies reaffirmed
these conclusions.(23-25)   Schrauzer et al.(26,27) independently
reinvestigated a simple "plasma cancer test" described(28,29) shor-
tly after World War II, and demonstrated that it actually was a
crude assay for plasma selenium.   What at the time was considered a
positive test for cancer, thus in reality indicated subnormal plasma
selenium levels.   The selenium content in forage crops has been used
as an indicator of the regional availability of selenium.   Selenium
maps of the continental United States such as shown in Figure 1
demonstrate an inverse relationship with cancer incidence and mortality.   The inverse association between the regional selenium content in forage crops and the cancer incidence is statistically significant with $r = -0.467$ (P=0.01).(27)   The cancer incidence or
mortality also correlates with other exogenous variables such as
population density or average annual precipitation, but with a lower
degree of statistical significance.   The apparent association with
rainfall could also mean that soil selenium is leached out in regions with high annual precipitation.   Using neutron activation analysis, W. L. Broghamer, Jr., et al.(30) determined the serum selenium
levels on 110 patients with carcinoma, reporting an association between the serum selenium levels and patient survival time.   They
concluded that lower selenium levels in patients with carcinoma are
"more likely to be associated with (1) distant metastasis; (2) multiple primary tumors which in many instances, appeared in different
organ systems; (3) multiple recurrences".   Higher selenium levels
were found in cases wherein the tumor (1) "is more likely to remain
confined to the region of its origin; (2) distant metastasis is
less likely to occur; and (3) multiple primary lesions and recurrences seldom appear".(30) Subnormal blood or plasma selenium levels
in cancer patients do not necessarily indicate that selenium possesses anticarcinogenic properties.   Moreover, most of the documented
evidence on the protecting effects of selenium was based on experiments with chemically induced or transplanted tumors.   Schrauzer
and coworkers accordingly investigated the effects of selenium on
the genesis of *spontaneous* mammary tumors in mice, an animal model
system believed to be related to human cancer, and subsequently ex-

tended their studies to include selenium antagonistic elements such
as arsenic and to zinc.

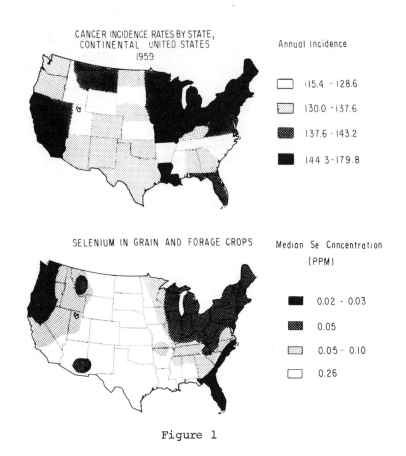

Figure 1

Top:    The cancer incidence rates for the continental
        United States, 1959.

Bottom: Median selenium concentrations (ppm) in grains
        and forage crops in the continental United
        States. Adapted from Ref. 27, loc. cit.

B.  Effects of Selenium and of Selenium Antagonistic Elements
    on the Genesis of Spontaneous Mammary Tumors in C$_3$H Mice

    1.  Inhibition of Tumorigenesis by Selenium
        Inbred virgin female C$_3$H mice exhibiting an 80% to 100%
incidence of "spontaneous" mammary adenocarcinoma were exposed to

2 ppm of selenium in the form of selenite in the water supply immediately after weaning, and were otherwise kept under normal maintenance conditions.  Only 10% of these animals developed tumors during
their full life span.  In the simultaneous control group, the total
tumor incidence was 82%.(*31*)  The protecting effect of selenium was
noticed at lower (0.1 - 1.0 ppm) and higher (5 - 15 ppm) dosage
levels.  At 0.1 ppm, the tumor incidence was not significantly different from that in the controls, but the first tumors began to
appear six months later than expected.  The tumor incidence was
< 10% in the group of animals receiving 1 ppm of Se; at the dosage
level of 5 ppm or more, the diminution of tumor incidence was still
statistically significant, even though it began to be masked by
effects of chronic Se toxicity; however, even at 15 ppm, the diminution of tumor incidence was significant at the P = 0.005 level, in
spite of a 50% mortality due to chronic selenium poisoning.(*32,33*)
The few tumors developing in Se-exposed animals grew more slowly
than those in the normally fed controls, but the growth of transplanted tumors on animals receiving selenium was not markedly different from that of the controls (Figures 2 and 3).

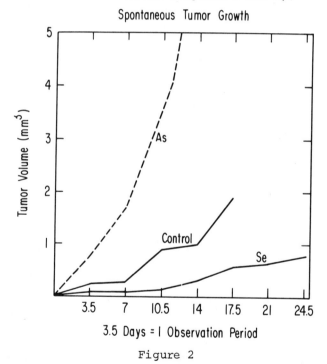

Figure 2

Growth curves of spontaneous mammary tumors in $C_3H/St$
mice receiving 2 ppm of Se and 10 ppm of As in the
water supply.  From Ref. 31, loc. cit.  Reproduced
with permission.

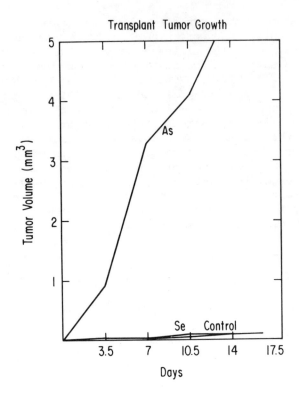

Figure 3

Growth curves of transplanted mammary tumors in C$_3$H mice.
(Mammary tumor cells from Se-exposed mice were transplanted
into Se-fed animals. Tumor cells from As-exposed animals
were similarly transplanted into As-exposed mice). Reproduced from Ref. 31, with permission.

2.    Effect of Arsenic

     Arsenic behaves as an antagonist of selenium in that it
increases the biliary excretion of selenium in the rat(34) and
thus could induce selenium deficiency. Schrauzer and Ishmael(31)
exposed female C$_3$H mice to 10 ppm of arsenic in the form of arsenite
and observed a lowering of the total tumor incidence from 82% in the
simultaneous control group to 27% in the experimental group. Animals developing mammary adenocarcinoma under these conditions had
short survival times and exhibited extremely rapid tumor growth.
The effect of arsenic cannot be due to selenium depletion alone

since tumor growth in Se-deficient animals was not markedly accelerated.(32)   A lowering of the tumor incidence was still noticeable
at toxic As levels of 80 ppm; tumor growth rates were again exceedingly high.   The tumors grew to enormous size, doubling in two weeks
as compared to five to seven weeks in the controls, or Se groups.(32)
The growth rate of transplanted tumors in arsenic-exposed animals
was ca. 50 times faster than that of transplanted control tumors
(see Figure 3).   It was concluded that selenium prevents tumorigenesis at early stages of development and that arsenic has benign
as well as adverse effects on tumor development under the chosen
conditions.

### 3.   Effect of Zinc

Although zinc is not a selenium antagonist to the degree
of arsenic, it does have a high chemical affinity for selenium and
was expected to show an effect on tumorigenesis in $C_3H$ mice.   The
joint administration of 5 ppm of Se in the form of selenite, with
200 ppm of zinc (as the chloride) via the supply water *abolished
the cancer-protecting effect of selenium* and raised the tumor incidence to 94%.   The selenium levels in tissues of these animals were
lower than in those of normally fed controls receiving no extra-
dietary selenium.   It thus appears that zinc in the supply water
prevents the uptake of inorganic selenium.

### 4.   Effects of Other Selenium Antagonists

Certain metals normally present in food have a high chemical affinity for selenium and thus may act as selenium antagonists.
Sulfate ion is a specific antagonist of selenate.(35)   Sulfur-con-
taining amino acids such as methionine are known to alleviate selenium toxicity,(36) just as linseed oil and vitamin E.(37)   It is
possible, therefore, that diets rich in sulfur containing amino acids
diminish the physiological activity or availability of selenium.
Other metals; i.e., Cu, Cd, Sn, Pb, Sb, Bi, Tl,and Te could behave
similarly to zinc or arsenic and dimish the anticarcinogenic effect
of selenium.   Some of these elements are essential for the maintenance of human or animal health; others are industrial or environmental pollutants.   Studies are needed to evaluate the effect of
these metals on selenium metabolism.

### 5.   Mechanism of Anticarcinogenic Action

Selenium is often defined as a biological "antioxidant,"
which is a fair description of some of its functions, but ignores
other important roles outlined in Scheme 1.   We believe that stimulation of immune response is the main mechanism by which selenium
prevents tumor development.

SCHEME 1

PROPERTIES AND FUNCTIONS OF SELENIUM THAT MAY BE
RELATED TO ITS ANTICARCINOGENIC ACTION

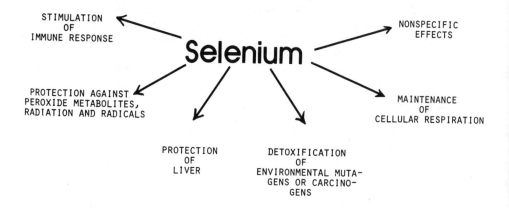

III.   RECENT EPIDEMIOLOGICAL EVIDENCE

A.   <u>Association of Cancer Mortality with Blood Selenium Levels</u>

Schrauzer, White, and Schneider(*38*) collected pooled whole human
blood from bloodbanks in 22 different countries and observed statistically significant inverse association between the blood selenium
levels and the age-corrected mortalities from cancers at major sites.
Similar results were obtained with data for 19 states of the United
States of America.  A tumor-site classification system was employed,
which places cancers of colon, rectum, prostate, breast, ovary, lung,
pancreas, skin, bladder, and leukemia into a group designated "Type
A" on the basis of mortality intercorrelation calculations and observed association of mortality with food consumption variables.(*39*,
*40*)  Type B cancers (buccal cavity and pharynx, esophagus, and larynx), those belonging to Type C (uterus and thyroid), as well as
Type D cancers (stomach and liver) as a rule did not show significant association with the blood selenium concentration (see Table 1).

The type A cancer mortality in a given population should become very low if the mean blood selenium concentration were in the
order of 0.35 micrograms/ml, based on the linear extrapolation of
the least-squares fitted line of cancer mortalities versus blood Se
concentration.(*38*)  The average selenium concentration in whole blood
from healthy male donors in the United States is in the order of
0.20 micrograms/ml; however, concentrations of 0.35 micrograms/ml

were observed in blood samples collected from donors living in
"high-selenium" areas.(41)   Blood Se concentrations from 0.41 to
0.49 micrograms/ml were seen in samples from Costa Rica,(38) and
the highest values reported to date were found in blood from normal subjects living in certain areas of Venezuela, ranging from 0.7
to 1.5 micrograms/ml, with a mean of 0.83 micrograms/ml,(42) with
no evidence for chronic selenium poisoning.  On the other hand,
selenium levels of between 0.070 to 0.133 micrograms/ml were measured in whole blood from infants in San Diego, California,(43)
which is in the same order of the selenium content of kwashiorkor
patients.(44)   Selenium intakes are particularly low in New Zealand.(45)   They may also be inadequate in certain regions of the
United States.

TABLE 1

OBSERVED CORRELATION BETWEEN THE AGE-CORRECTED MORTALITIES
FROM CANCERS AT MAJOR SITES AND THE MEAN CONCENTRATION OF
Se, Zn, Cd, Cu IN WHOLE BLOOD FROM HEALTHY DONORS FROM 19
COLLECTION SITES IN THE UNITED STATES(38,46)

| Type | Site (sex)[a] | Apparent Associations[b] | | | | | |
| | | *Direct* | | | *Inverse* | | |
| | P: | 0.001 | 0.01 | 0.05 | 0.05 | 0.01 | 0.001 |
|---|---|---|---|---|---|---|---|
| A-D | All sites (m,f) | Zn(f) | | | | | Se |
| A | Intestine(m,f) | Zn | | Cu | | | Se |
| | Rectum (m,f) | Zn | | | | | Se |
| | Breast(f) | Zn | | Cu | | | Se |
| | Ovary | | Zn | | | | Se |
| | Lung(m,f) | | Zn(f) | Cu(f) | Se | | |
| | Pancreas(m) | | | (Zn) | Se | | |
| | Leukemia(f) | | | (Zn) | | Se | |
| | Bladder(m,f) | | | Zn | | Se(f) | |
| B | Buccal cavity, pharynx(m,f) | | Zn | | | Se | |
| | Esophagus(m) | | | | | Se | |
| | Larynx(m) | | | | Se | | |
| C | Thyroid(f) | | | Cu | | | |
| | Uterus | | | | Cd | | |
| D | Stomach(f) | | | Cd | | | |

[a] Sites not included (prostate,skin,liver) show no significant correlations.
Associations observed for one sex only are indicated by (m) or (f).

[b] With state mortalities, 1959-1961.

B.    Association with Blood Zn(Cu, Cd, Pb-) Levels

Following the hypothesis that zinc may prevent dietary selenium
uptake, the mean zinc and selenium concentrations in U. S. blood
from healthy donors(41,47) were compared with each other, revealing
an inverse association with P=0.05.(46)   The mean blood zinc concentration in U. S. blood, as published by Kubota et al.(47) was
in turn found to be directly correlated with most Type A cancer
mortalities; in some cases, with very high statistical significance.
For example, the age-corrected female breast cancer mortality correlates with the mean zinc concentration, with r = 0.82 (P<0.001).
Employing the mean selenium and zinc concentrations as independent
variables, the expectation values for the age-corrected female breast
cancer mortality can be calculated from the equation of the least-
squares fitted plane,(46) the agreement between calculated and observed mortalities is satisfactory, with r = 0.87 (P<<0.001) but
could probably be improved, once more data for average blood zinc
and selenium concentrations become available for other states.   Even
the *total* age-corrected cancer mortality can be calculated from the
mean blood Zn and Se concentrations; the agreement with the observed
mortality is again quite good, with r = 0.76 (P<0.001)(Figure 4 and
Table 1).   The blood *cadmium* concentrations are low, ranging from
0.005 to 0.14 micrograms/ml, in which the mean is 0.0177 micrograms
per ml, in samples of whole human blood collected from 19 locations
in the United States.(47)   The mean blood cadmium concentration
failed to correlate with cancer mortalities except those from cancer
of the uterus and related parts, where an *inverse* association was
observed, with P<0.05.   It could be argued that this association
is spurious.   This need not be so, since it has been established
that cadmium has a destructive effect on the placenta of pregnant
animals.(50)   It would therefore be of interest to study the effect
of subtoxic levels of cadmium on developing carcinoma of the uterine
cervix.

The blood *lead* concentration from Reference 47 are essentially
uncorrelated with cancer mortality, but the corresponding *copper*
levels exhibit marginally significant direct association with most
Type A cancer mortality.   It is noteworthy that the female mortality
from cancer of the thyroid is also directly correlated with the blood
copper concentration, with r = 0.63 (P<0.05).

In concluding this chapter, it should be noted that the zinc
concentrations in U. S. blood are exceedingly variable [observed
range:   0.60 - 19.87 micrograms/ml],(47) for reasons that are not
understood.   Although the average U. S. diet provides relatively
high levels of zinc, it is difficult to interpret the wide range of
blood Zn levels to variations of the dietary zinc intakes alone.
Some water supplies may contain 1.0 - 1.2 mg/L of zinc, as evidenced
from analyses reported for samples taken from Lake Erie and the
Cuyahoga River at Cleveland, Ohio,(51) but this still does not explain the variation of the blood zinc levels.

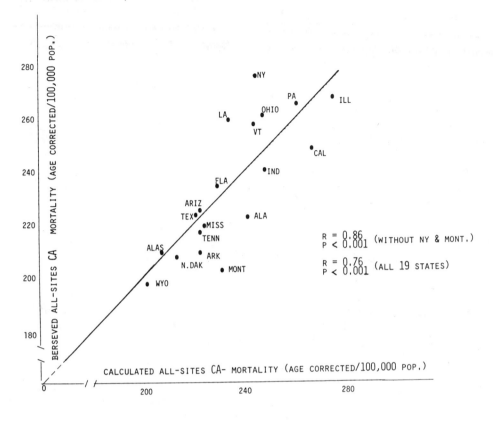

Figure 4

Comparison of calculated and observed total age-
corrected cancer mortalities in different states
from the mean blood zinc and selenium concentrations
in healthy male donors.  Values were calculated from
the least-squares fitted plane (Schrauzer and White,
unpublished).

IV.   CORRELATION OF CANCER MORTALITY WITH
        CALCULATED TRACE ELEMENT INTAKES

A.   Introductory Remarks

The observed association of blood selenium and zinc levels with
cancer mortality (see Sections III, A and B) led to a study in which

cancer mortalities were correlated with the estimated apparent dietary intakes of a number of trace elements. Using food-consumption
tables(48) a data bank of calculated trace-element intakes for 28
countries has been established.(49) The dietary intake of the elements Se, Zn, Cd, Cr, As, and Mn were calculated from known average
levels of these elements in major food items. The average per
capita intake, range, and values for the United States are given in
Table 2. The 28 countries include most European states, the United
States, Canada, Japan, Taiwan, and Australia, and other countries for
which reliable food consumption statistics are available. The calculated apparent intake for the United States is in good agreement
with estimates reported in the literature. Table 3 shows that the
age-corrected *total* cancer mortality is inversely correlated with
the apparent dietary selenium intake. Significant inverse association is also observed for all sites classified as Type A. Significant direct association was found for most Type A cancer mortality and the apparent dietary intake of Zn, Cd, Cu and Cr, even
after contributions to the linear correlation coefficients due to
intercorrelation were partialed out. The observed direct association with the zinc intake is of interest in view of the results
outlined above (see Sections III, A and B). However, the association
cannot be treated independently of those with cadmium, since the intake of zinc and cadmium is strongly intercorrelated, with r = 0.9.
The direct association of cancer mortality with copper and chromium
is of interest, and led to a study of their effect on the development of spontaneous mammary tumors in $C_3H/St$ mice, which is currently in progress. In addition to selenium, manganese and arsenic exhibit inverse association with the mortality from cancers at certain
sites.

TABLE 2

CALCULATED PER CAPITA INTAKE OF SEVEN ELEMENTS.
From Food Consumption Data, Average for 1964-1966,
Including Estimates of Intakes by Other Methods

| Apparent Intakes ( µg/day): | Se | Zn | Cd | Cu | Cr | As | Mn |
|---|---|---|---|---|---|---|---|
| Mean, 28 Count-ries | 213 | 11860 | 216 | 2180 | 47 | 405 | 2286 |
| Range | 156-296 | 6500 - 21000 | 109-397 | 1370-3290 | 32-70 | 218-753 | 1260-3233 |
| U.S.A. | 167 | 14000 | 239 | 2300 | 69 | 365 | 1786 |
| U.S.A.(Lit.)[*] | 150 | 12000 - 15000 | 200-500 | 2300 | 80 | 400 | 2400 |

[*]Most entries taken from Ref. 52.

TABLE 3

OBSERVED CORRELATION BETWEEN THE AGE-CORRECTED MORTALITY
FROM CANCER AT VARIOUS SITES AND THE APPARENT DIETARY IN-
TAKE OF TRACE ELEMENTS. Except where indicated, Data are
for 28 Countries. Doubtful Associations in Parentheses.
(Adapted from Ref. 46)

| TYPE | SITE (SEX, I.S.C.) | DIRECT 0.001 | DIRECT 0.01 | DIRECT 0.05 | INVERSE 0.05 | INVERSE 0.01 | INVERSE 0.001 [a] |
|---|---|---|---|---|---|---|---|
| A-D | All sites (m) | | | | Se | | |
| | (f) | | | Cr | | | Se |
| A | Intestine (m) (f) (152,153) | Cr,Zn,Cd | | Cu | | | Se |
| | Rectum (m,f) (154) | | | (Cr,f) | | | Se |
| | Breast (f) (170) | Cr,Zn,Cd, | | Cu | | | Se |
| | Ovary [b] (175) | | | | Mn | Se | |
| | Prostate (177) | Zn,Cd,Cr | | | | | Se |
| | Lung (m) (162,163) | | | | | Se | As |
| | Pancreas (m,f) [c] (157) | | | | Se,(Mn,f) | Mn (m) | |
| | Leukemia (m) (204) (f) | Cd Zn / Cd,Zn | Cr | Cr,Cu / Cu | | Se | Se |
| | Bladder (m,f) [b] (181) | | | | (Se) | | |
| | Skin (m) (190,191) (f) | Cd,Zn,Cu / Zn, Cd | | Cu | (Se,As) / (As) | | |
| B | B.C.&Phar. (m,f) (140-148) | | As | | | Mn(f) | |
| | Esophagus (m,f) (150) | | | | Mn(f) | | |
| | Larynx (m) (161) | | | | | Mn | |
| C | Thyroid (m,f) [c] (194) | | | | As(f) | | |
| | Uterus (171-174) | | | | Cd | | |
| D | Stomach (m,f) (151) | | | | (Cd,Cr,Zn) | | |
| | Liver (m,f) [c] (155,156) | | | | (Zn,m) | Cd | |

[a] Data from Ref. 40. (b) Data for 17 countries. (c) Data for 19 countries.

B.    Specific Associations

Table 3 reveals that the mortality of sites classified as
Type A are inversely correlated with the apparent dietary selenium
intake.  Most Type A cancers show direct association with the dietary intake.  From the apparent dietary selenium and zinc intakes,
the mortality from female breast cancer can be calculated empir-
ically with reasonably good accuracy (see Figure 5).  From the in-
tercepts of the least-squares fitted lines, it is estimated that
Type A cancer mortality should become very low if the per capita
selenium intake were raised to about 300 micrograms per day, which
is approximately twice the current U. S. intake level.  At this
selenium intake, a concentration of between 0.25 and 0.35 micrograms
per ml of selenium in whole blood should result.  We have analyzed
the blood of a normal healthy man of age 52 years who had been tak-
ing 150 micrograms of Se/day in the form of commercial supplements
(Se-yeast) during the past 15 months(15) and observed a concentration of 0.28 micrograms/ml, in good agreement with our initial
estimate.

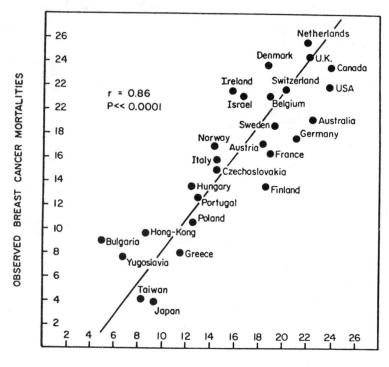

CALCULATED BREAST CANCER MORTALITIES

Figure 5

Comparison of Calculated and Observed Age-corrected Female Breast
Cancer Mortalities.  Calculated values were obtained from the
apparent dietary zinc and selenium intakes (least-squares fitted
plane).  From Reference 46, loc. cit.

Table 3 reveals a significant inverse association between the male lung cancer mortality and apparent dietary intake of *arsenic*. Since seafood is a major source of dietary arsenic, this result also expresses the empirical fact that the lung cancer mortality among males is lower in countries with a high consumption of seafood. A pertinent example of this is Japan where the per capita cigarette consumption is comparable to that in western industrialized nations and the male lung cancer mortality is disproportionately low. The idea that life-term feeding of arsenicals could be used to decrease the incidence of spontaneous lung cancer has been mentioned by Kanisawa and Schroeder[54] and even earlier, Bayard[55] recommended arsenic as a human cancer prophylactic, quoting the results of animal experiments in which arsenic displays anticarcinogenic action on joint administration with carcinogens. Although we cannot support this idea on the basis of our own work with the $C_3H$ mice, further research on arsenic is clearly desirable. It is necessary, in particular, to investigate the effects of $As^{+3}$ (arsenite) and $As^{+5}$ (arsenate) on tumor development. While arsenite seems to have stimulating effects, this may not be true for arsenate. Questions concerning arsenic are discussed in much greater detail in D. V. Frost's account in the present volume.

The mortality from cancer of the pancreas shows a weak inverse association with the dietary selenium intake that is statistically significant for females with $P=0.05$ (Table 3). The dietary *manganese* intake is also inversely correlated with the pancreas cancer mortalities; in fact, significantly for both sexes. The pancreatic gland normally contains high levels of manganese.[56] It thus would seem worthwhile to investigate if manganese deficiency predisposes to the development of cancer of the pancreas. The mortality from cancer of the ovary, buccal cavity and pharynx, esophagus, and larynx are also inversely correlated with the dietary manganese intake. Manganese could well be yet another of the cancer-protecting trace elements, but has not yet been investigated as to this effect.

Buccal cavity and pharynx cancer mortalities exhibit direct association with dietary arsenic intake that could be spurious, while the mortality from cancer of the uterus and related parts is again inversely correlated with the cadmium intake (see Section IVA).

Mortality from cancer of the stomach and liver show weak inverse correlation with apparent intake of Zn, Cd, and Cr (Table 3). These could be spurious in view of the existing inverse association between Type A and Type D cancer mortality.[40] On the other hand, the latter are not correlated with the dietary selenium intake.

## V. SELENIUM SUPPLY AND SUPPLEMENTATION

The present hypothesis challenges the common view that a well-balanced diet provides all nutritionally essential trace elements in sufficient amount.  It suggests that our knowledge of what constitutes a balanced diet is still insufficient and that imbalances occur that in part are caused by differences in regional or national dietary habits, food supply, and variations in the geographical distribution of trace elements such as selenium.  Even though acute deficiency symptoms do not appear, it is possible that the typical American diet provides an insufficient amount of selenium except in certain "high-selenium" regions.*  An increase in the consumption of seafood, organ meat (liver, kidney) and of whole grain wheat cereal products (from Se-adequate fields) could raise the dietary intake sufficiently; i.e., to about 300 micrograms per day per adult, which corresponds to about twice the amount presently supplied by the average U. S. diet.  Ultimately, selenium supplementation may become necessary.  On a national scale, supplementation of the entire U. S. population with 100 micrograms of selenium per day would require approximately two percent of the present U. S. annual selenium production.  Although a shortage need not be feared at present, it is worth remembering that the element as such is not in unlimited supply.

Questions as to how to supplement also arise.  The addition of sodium selenite to table salt comes to mind but is, in fact, difficult to recommend in view of the ease with which selenium is reduced to the elemental state or the volatile hydrogen selenide, or converted to insoluble metal derivatives (selenides or selenates). This could lead to loss of selenium during food processing or to its conversion into physiologically inactive compounds.  Although some water wells in the United States contain selenium, present regulations have prevented their use (the maximum allowable concentration is set at 10 micrograms/liter).  Conversely, the selenization of the water supply would be wasteful and potentially hazardous, and cannot be recommended, just as selenium fertilization of soil for agricultural crop production, although the latter possibility is not entirely excluded.  For individual selenium supplementation, health food stores carry products derived from selenium-containing brewer's yeast which provides an adequate source of the element in organically bound form.

_____

*    The calculated dietary selenium intake in 27 countries, as reported in Reference 38, indicates that the apparent U. S. selenium intake is the lowest next to that of the Netherlands.

## VI.   SUMMARY AND CONCLUSIONS

An increasing body of experimental and epidemiological evidence
indicates that selenium possesses anticarcinogenic properties in
animals and man.  A comparison of national per capita food consumption statistics reveals that the dietary selenium intake in different countries or population groups are variable and not necessarily
adequate.  A substantial increase of the dietary selenium intake
could be accomplished by a change of diet; i.e., increasing the
consumption of whole-wheat-grain cereal products, seafood, liver,
and kidney at the expense of sugar, fats, and excessive meat.  Theoretically, such a diet could lower, for example, the female breast
cancer mortality to 1/10th the current U. S. rate.  Diets rich in
zinc should be avoided, and since whole wheat grain bread or flour
has a high content of phytate, the recommended diet would lead to
diminished zinc uptake as compared to traditional meat-based diets.
It is possible that the typical American diet furnishes sufficient
amounts of zinc in adolescence but too much for adults or in old
age.  Elderly persons should certainly not be encouraged to take
zinc supplements; regrettably, zinc is occasionally also prescribed
to cancer patients to improve their appetite.

There is little to be said about copper and manganese and
chromium in this context; the average diet probably contains adequate amounts of these elements whose roles in tumor development
are not yet understood.  Arsenic is controversial, as it has been
for many years.  As research continues, its value in cancer prevention will be properly recognized.

As none of the trace elements with anticancer properties can
be expected to provide absolute protection against all forms of
cancer, customary methods of prevention will have to be retained
(see Scheme 1).  Efforts must continue to identify new environmental
carcinogens and to minimize all forms of carcinogenic stress.

Table 4 lists the cancer sites that are probably responsive to
selenium prophylaxis.  For other cancer sites, selenium may also be
beneficial, even though other causative factors play prominent roles.
Thus, the high incidence of Type B cancer among men is attributable
to the deleterious effects of smoking and alcoholism.  Alcoholism
may also contribute to liver cancer development, but dietary factors
are undoubtedly more important.  Although selenium is known to prevent azo dye-induced hepatocarcinogenesis, it appears that other
protective factors are lacking in populations with high liver CA
incidence, since liver cancer death rates are high in Japan where
dietary Se intake seems adequate.  If cirrhosis is accepted as a
liver cancer-predisposing condition, overall liver-protecting diets
would have preventive effects.  Of interest is the very significant
inverse correlation between liver cancer mortality and the per

SCHEME 2

CANCER CAUSES AND PREVENTION

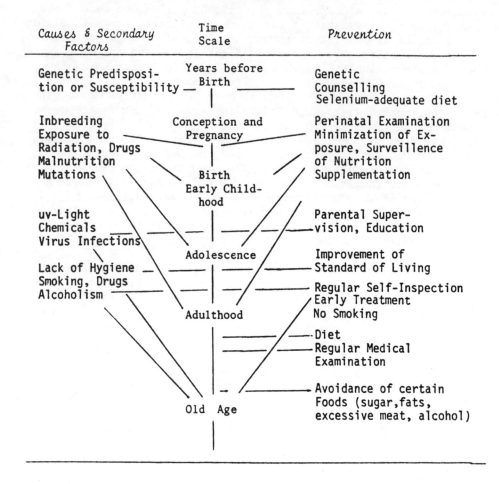

| Causes & Secondary Factors | Time Scale | Prevention |
|---|---|---|
| Genetic Predisposition or Susceptibility | Years before Birth | Genetic Counselling Selenium-adequate diet |
| Inbreeding Exposure to Radiation, Drugs Malnutrition Mutations | Conception and Pregnancy | Perinatal Examination Minimization of Exposure, Surveillence of Nutrition Supplementation |
| | Birth Early Childhood | |
| uv-Light Chemicals Virus Infections | | Parental Supervision, Education |
| | Adolescence | Improvement of Standard of Living |
| Lack of Hygiene Smoking, Drugs Alcoholism | | Regular Self-Inspection Early Treatment No Smoking |
| | Adulthood | |
| | | Diet Regular Medical Examination |
| | Old Age | Avoidance of certain Foods (sugar, fats, excessive meat, alcohol) |

capita sugar consumption [r = -0.92, for males in 18 countries].(40)
The sugar consumption is also inversely correlated with the liver
cirrhosis mortality [r = -0.75, both sexes].(40)  Stomach cancer,
finally, is another example of a neoplastic disease in which many
factors contribute to the etiology, and of these, only a few, if
any, have been rigorously identified.  The high male/female mortality ratio (ca 2.0 in the majority of countries) may be a sign of
greater male indulgence or quantity of food consumed rather than
attributable to a specific dietary component.  It is a fateful
property of the Japanese diet to protect against cancer of Type A
(listed in Table 4) while while giving rise to a stomach and liver

TABLE 4

CANCER SITES ARRANGED ACCORDING TO TYPES
ON THE BASIS OF MORTALITY AND FOOD CONSUMPTION
CORRELATION CALCULATIONS(40)

| TYPE | A | B | C | D |
|------|---|---|---|---|
| CANCER SITES | Large intestine* <br> Rectum <br> Breast* <br> Ovary <br> Lung <br> Pancreas <br> Bladder <br> Prostate <br> Leukemia <br> Skin* | Buccal cavity & <br> pharynx <br> Esophagus <br> Larynx | Uterus <br> Thyroid | Stomach <br> Liver* |
| REMARKS | Inversely correlated with consumptions of cereals and seafoods, directly correlated with consumptions of meat,eggs,milk,fat &/or sugar | Directly correlated with (wine-) alcohol consumption. Smoking believed to be contributing or primary factor | Weakly correlated with food consumption variables | Directly correlated with consumptions of cereals, seafoods; inversely correlated with consumptions of meat,milk, sugar |

*Cancer sites for which selenium prevents or retards tumorigenesis in animal experiments.

cancer mortality that nearly compensates for the diminished Type A
cancer mortality relative to that in the U. S. population.  The
adoption of a diet that would lower the breast cancer risk thus
might increase the liver or stomach cancer risk.  We can be fairly
certain that this would not be because of the increased selenium
intake, but that obviously, the factor(s) contributing to increased
susceptibility to stomach and liver cancer need identification.  For
the time being, it thus should be emphasized that the high selenium
diets will not necessarily offer increased protection against stomach or liver cancer, and that this diet in fact is not recommended
to individuals suspected of having a predisposition to cancer at
these sites.

*REFERENCES*

1.  Dalbert, P., Bulletin Assoc. Franc. Etude Cancer 5, Page 121, 1912.

2.  Walker, C. H. and Klein, F., American Medicine, Page 628, 1915.

3.  Todd, A. T., British Medical Journal, Page 172, 1935.

4.    Nelson, A. A., Fitzhugh, O. G. and Calvery, H. O., Cancer
      Research 3, Page 230, 1943.

5.    Tscherkes, L. A., Volgarev, N. M. and Aptekar, S. G., Acta Uv
      Int. Cancer 19, Page 632, 1963.

6.    Schroeder, H. A. and Balassa, J. J., J. Chronic Disease 23,
      Page 227, 1970; ibid, 25, Page 415, 1972.

7.    Harr, J. R., Exon, J. H., Whanger, P. D. and Weswig, P. H.,
      Clinical Tox. 5, Page 187, 1972; ibid 6, Page 487, 1973.

8.    Shapiro,J.R., Annals New York Academy Science 192,Page 215,1972.

9.    Clayton,C. C. and Baumann,C.A.,Cancer Research 9,Page 575, 1949.

10.   Shamberger,R.J.and Rudolph,G., Experientia 22, Page 116, 1966.

11.   Riley, J. F., ibid Ref. 10, 24, Page 1237, 1968.

12.   Whanger, P. D., personal communication.

13.   Abdullaev, G. B., Gasanov, G. G., Ragimov, R. N., Teplyakova,
      G. V., Mekhitiev, M. A. and Dzhafarov, A. I., Dokl. Akad.
      Nauk Azerb. SSR 29, Page 18, 1973.

14.   Jacobs, M. M., Jansson, B. and Griffin, A. Clark, Cancer Let-
      ters, in press, 1976.

15.   Aleksandrowicz, J. and Wazewska-Czyzewska, M., in press, per-
      sonal communication.

16.   Aleksandrowicz, J., Kuliczycki, A. and Smyk, B., Polish Med.
      Science Hist. Bulletin, Page 453, 1975.

17.   Martin, J. L. and Spallholz, J. E., Abstract, Symposium on
      Selenium and Tellurium in the Environment, University of
      Notre Dame, May 11-13, 1976, Page 16.

18.   Aleksandrowicz, J., Rev. Espan. de Oncologia 22, 335, 1975.

19.   Vincent, J. E., Prostaglandins 8, Page 339, 1974.

20.   Jansson, B., Proceedings Conference Inorganic and Nutritional
      Aspects of Cancer.

21.   Frost, D. V., Annual Review Pharmacology 15, Page 259, 1975.

22.   Shamberger, R. J. and Frost, D. V., Canadian Medical Assn J.
      100, Page 682, 1969.

23.    Shamberger, R. J., Critical Reviews in Clin. Lab. Science 2, Page 211, 1971.

24.    Shamberger, R. J., S. Tytko, Price, J. W. and Willis, C. E., Clinical Chem. 17, Page 643, 1971.

25.    Shamberger, R. J., Rukovena, E. F. and Willis, C. E., Proc. American Association Cancer Research 13, Page 41, 1973.

26.    Schrauzer, G. N. and Rhead, W. J., Experientia 27, Page 1069, 1971.

27.    Schrauzer, G. N., Rhead, W. J. and Evans, G. A., Bioinorganic Chemistry 2, Page 329, 1973.

28.    Savionac, R. J., Gant, J. C. and Sizer, I. W., American Assoc. Adv. Science Conference Cancer, Page 241, 1945.

29.    Black, M. M., Cancer Research 7, Page 321, 1947.

30.    Broghamer, W. L., Jr., McConnell, K. P. and Blotcky, A. L., Cancer 37, Page 1384, 1976.

31.    Schrauzer, G. N. and Ishmael, D., Annual Clin. and Lab. Science 4, Page 441, 1974.

32.    Schrauzer, G. N., White, D. A. and Schneider, C. J., Bioinorg. Chemistry 6, Page 265, 1976.

33.    Schrauzer, G. N., White, D. A. and Schneider, C. J., Publication in preparation.

34.    Levander, O. A. and Baumann, C. A., Toxicol. Applied Pharmacology 9, Page 106, 1966.

35.    Ganther, H. E. and Baumann, C. A., J. Nutrition 77, pp. 208 and 408, 1962.

36.    Lewis, H. B., Schultz, J. and Gortner, R. H., J. Pharmac. Exp. Therapy 68, Page 292, 1940.

37.    National Academy Science, Washington, D. C., Selenium, pp. 115, 116, 1976; references cited therein.

38.    Schrauzer, G. N., White, D. A. and Schneider, C. J., Bioinorg. Chemistry 7, Page 23, 1977.

39.    Schrauzer, G. N., Medical Hypotheses 2, Page 31, 1976.

40.    Schrauzer, G. N., ibid, Page 39.

41.  Allaway, W. H., Kubota, J., Losee, F. and Roth, M., Arch.
     Environmental Health 16, Page 342, 1968.

42.  Jaffe, W. G., ibid Reference 17, Page 14.

43.  Rhead, W. J., Cary, E. E., Allaway, W. H., Saltzstein, S. L.
     and Schrauzer, G. N., Bioinorganic Chemistry 1, Page 289, 1972.

44.  Burk, R. F., Pearson, W. H., Wood, R. P. and Viteri, F.,
     American Journal Clinical Nutrition 20, Page 723, 1967.

45.  Watkinson, J. H., New Zealand Medical Journal, Page 202, 1974.

46.  Schrauzer, G. N., White, D. A. and Schneider, C. J., Bioinorg.
     Chemistry 7, Page 36, 1977.

47.  Kubota, J., Lazar, V. A. and Losee, F., Arch. Environmental
     Health 16, Page 788, 1968.

48.  Food and Agriculture Organization of the United Nations,
     Food Balance Sheets, Average for 1964-1966, Rome, 1971.

49.  Schrauzer, G. N. and White, D. A., unpublished.

50.  Parizek, J., J. Reprod. Fert. 9, Page 111, 1965.

51.  Kopp, J. F. and Kroner, R. C., Trace Metals in Waters of the
     United States, 1962-1967, U. S. Department of the Interior,
     Federal Water Pollution Control Administration, Cincinnati,
     Ohio, 1967.

52.  Underwood, E. J., Trace Elements in Human and Animal Nutrition,
     Third Edition, Academic Press, New York, London.

53.  Schrauzer, G. N., et al., to be published.

54.  Kanisawa, M. and Schroeder, H. A., Cancer Research 27,
     Page 1192, 1967.

55.  Bayard, O., Oncologia (Basel) 2, Page 193, 1949.

56.  Tipton, I. H. and Cook, M. J., Health Phys. 9, Page 103, 1963.

# CONTRIBUTOR INDEX

THE LIBF